Combining Visual Intelligence and Federated Learning in Smart Healthcare

Manisha Guduri
Lawrence Technological University, USA

Chinmay Chakraborty
Kalinga Institute of Industrial Technology, India

Martin Margala
University of Louisiana at Lafayette, USA

IGI Global
Scientific Publishing
Publishing Tomorrow's Research Today

Vice President of Editorial Melissa Wagner
Director of Acquisitions Mikaela Felty
Director of Book Development Jocelynn Hessler
Production Manager Mike Brehm
Cover Design Jose Rosado

Published in the United States of America by
IGI Global Scientific Publishing
701 East Chocolate Avenue
Hershey, PA, 17033, USA
Tel: 717-533-8845
Fax: 717-533-7115
Website: https://www.igi-global.com E-mail: cust@igi-global.com

Library of Congress Cataloging-in-Publication Data

Names: Guduri, Manisha, 1988- editor http://id.loc.gov/rwo/agents/n2024060769 | Chakraborty, Chinmay, 1984- editor http://id.loc.gov/authorities/names/n2018186309 | Margala, Martin editor http://id.loc.gov/authorities/names/nb2017004100
Title: Combining visual intelligence and federated learning in smart healthcare / edited by Manisha Guduri, Chinmay Chakraborty, Martin Margala.
Description: Hershey, PA : IGI Global Scientific Publishing, [2026] | Includes bibliographical references and index. | Summary: "The objective of this book aims to implement emerging technology to transforms images from the original grayscale and reveals hidden patterns, into new well-defined structured patterns empowering research community, and computer analytics to remove indicative uncertainty"-- Provided by publisher.
Identifiers: LCCN 2024056682 (print) | LCCN 2024056683 (ebook) | ISBN 9798369360941 h/c | ISBN 9798369360958 s/c | ISBN 9798369360965 eISBN
Subjects: LCSH: Computer vision in medicine http://id.loc.gov/authorities/subjects/sh95001351 | Federated learning (Machine learning) http://id.loc.gov/authorities/subjects/sh2024001385
Classification: LCC R859.7.C67 C658 2025 (print) | LCC R859.7.C67 (ebook) | DDC 610.285--dc23/eng/20250321
LC record available at https://lccn.loc.gov/2024056682
LC ebook record available at https://lccn.loc.gov/2024056683

British Cataloguing in Publication Data
A Cataloguing in Publication record for this book is available from the British Library.

Table of Contents

Detailed Table of Contents

approach significantly outperforms traditional methods, achieving higher accuracy in identifying cardiac conditions such as arrhythmias. The results underscore the potential of real-time monitoring capabilities in telemedicine, facilitating timely interventions and improved patient outcomes. The study concludes that addressing the limitations of existing ECG classification systems is crucial for their effective integration into clinical practice, ultimately contributing to the advancement of remote healthcare solutions.

K. Priyadharshini, Department of Computing Technologies, SRM Institute of Science and Technology, Chennai, India
R. Purushothaman, Department of Computer Science and Engineering (Artificial Intelligence and Data Analytics), Sri Ramachandra Institute of Higher Education and Research, Chennai, India
Bobby N. D., Department of Biomedical Engineering, St. Peter's Institute of Higher Education and Research, Chennai, India
Syed Musthafa A., Department of Information Technology, M. Kumarasamy College of Engineering, Karur, India
V Jaiganesh, Department of Mechanical Engineering, Bharath Institute of Higher Education and Research, Chennai, India
M. Sudhakar, Sri Sai Ram Engineering College, Chennai, India

Visual intelligence, building on the thrust of AI through machine learning (ML), revolutionizes the smart health devices, aiding in more accurate diagnostics, real-time monitoring, and better care of patients by integrating computer vision algorithms that allow the analysis of medical images and monitoring of physiological parameters in developing early signs of diseases such as diabetic retinopathy, cardiovascular conditions, and skin cancers. By combining these with edge computing, systems provide real-time insights while preserving data privacy. Key innovations that underlie new visual intelligence applications in this chapter include deep learning models, CNNs, and reinforcement techniques all properly customized for healthcare environments. Challenges would include data scarcity, model interpretability, and more regulatory compliance, as well as opportunities for the future in personalized medicine and remote care. The integration of visual intelligence with ML into healthcare devices promises a paradigm shift in providing accessible and effective healthcare solutions.

Preface

The rapid advancements in artificial intelligence, federated learning, and visual intelligence are transforming the landscape of modern healthcare. The integration of these technologies is not merely an evolution but a revolution in how medical diagnostics, monitoring, and patient care are conducted. As editors, we have curated this book, *Combining Visual Intelligence and Federated Learning in Smart Healthcare*, to provide a comprehensive exploration of these groundbreaking developments. Our goal is to offer an in-depth understanding of how these emerging technologies contribute to more efficient, accurate, and patient-centered healthcare solutions. This volume brings together cutting-edge research and innovative applications from experts across the globe, shedding light on the transformative impact of visual intelligence, federated learning, and smart healthcare systems.

This book is structured to provide a balanced perspective, beginning with foundational discussions on software testing and AI-driven mental health solutions, followed by in-depth analyses of robotics, IoT, and deep learning applications in healthcare. Topics such as smart healthcare robotics, real-time monitoring, and federated learning highlight the potential of these technologies in enhancing patient outcomes while maintaining privacy and data security. The inclusion of research on wearable sensors, telemedicine, and IoT-enhanced additive manufacturing further expands the discourse on how digital health innovations are paving the way for more effective and accessible healthcare services. Each chapter has been carefully selected to present a holistic view of the latest developments, challenges, and opportunities in this rapidly evolving field.

Chapter 1: 5W+1H Automated Testing in Healthcare – A Case Study

This chapter presents a systematic approach to improving software usability and deployment in healthcare testing environments. It introduces the 5W+1H framework as a structured methodology for categorizing, classifying, and extracting conceptual models to enhance software testing processes. By addressing critical research questions in healthcare application development, the study provides a roadmap for mitigating software bugs and risks while ensuring high-quality deployment. The findings contribute to the broader field of healthcare technology by offering a well-defined research approach to enhance software reliability and efficiency.

Chapter 2: AI, IoT, and Cognitive Computing for Mental Health Enhancement and Object Detection

This chapter explores how artificial intelligence (AI), the Internet of Things (IoT), and cognitive computing can be leveraged to improve mental health care and object detection technologies. AI-driven cognitive models can analyze behavioral patterns and provide early warnings for mental health conditions, enabling proactive intervention. Additionally, object detection capabilities powered by cognitive computing help identify environmental factors that impact mental well-being. The integration of these technologies is paving the way for a shift from reactive mental health services to a preventive and data-driven approach, ultimately enhancing patient outcomes.

Chapter 3: An Innovative Obstacle Detection Smart System for Robot Navigation in Healthcare Industry

Robotic systems are increasingly being integrated into healthcare environments, necessitating reliable navigation mechanisms. This chapter introduces an innovative obstacle detection system that ensures seamless and safe robot navigation in complex healthcare settings. By utilizing a vision-based, low-cost detection technique, the system enhances efficiency and reliability while operating even with low-resolution images. The chapter highlights extensive testing conducted in both structured and unstructured environments, demonstrating the effectiveness of this approach in real-world applications.

Chapter 4: Enhancing Telemedicine with Deep Learning-Based Classification of ECG Heartbeats Using Continuous Wavelet Transform

This chapter presents an advanced approach to ECG classification for telemedicine applications, utilizing deep learning techniques in conjunction with Continuous Wavelet Transform (CWT) for feature extraction. A convolutional neural network (CNN) is employed to enhance the accuracy and reliability of ECG signal classification, enabling more precise detection of cardiac conditions such as arrhythmias. The findings highlight the potential for real-time monitoring solutions in telemedicine, facilitating timely interventions and improving patient care outcomes.

Chapter 5: Integrating Machine Learning for Accurate Diagnostics and Real-Time Monitoring with Visual Intelligence

The integration of machine learning (ML) with visual intelligence is revolutionizing healthcare by enabling more accurate diagnostics and real-time patient monitoring. This chapter explores how AI-powered computer vision models can analyze medical images and physiological data to detect early signs of diseases such as diabetic retinopathy and cardiovascular conditions. By incorporating edge computing, these systems provide real-time insights while ensuring data privacy. The discussion also covers key challenges, including data scarcity, model interpretability, and regulatory compliance, as well as opportunities for personalized medicine and remote healthcare solutions.

Chapter 6: Integrating Visual Intelligence with Federated Learning and IoT in Healthcare

This chapter examines the role of visual intelligence in healthcare and its integration with federated learning and IoT technologies. By leveraging decentralized AI models, federated learning allows collaborative data training across various sources without compromising patient privacy. The chapter discusses multiple applications, including remote patient monitoring and diagnostic imaging, highlighting how these technologies contribute to improved patient outcomes, personalized treatments, and optimized healthcare workflows. The integration of these cutting-edge approaches presents new opportunities to address contemporary challenges in healthcare data management.

Chapter 7: IoT-Enhanced Additive Manufacturing and Federated Learning for Smart Healthcare Systems

The convergence of IoT-driven additive manufacturing and federated learning is transforming healthcare by enabling the production of customized medical devices while maintaining stringent data privacy standards. This chapter explores the privacy-utility trade-offs associated with these technologies and examines strategies such as differential privacy, homomorphic encryption, and secure multi-party computation. Through case studies and comparative analyses, the chapter provides a framework for developing secure and scalable IoT-augmented healthcare systems, ensuring both regulatory compliance and technological efficiency.

Chapter 8: Challenges and Future Prospects of Glomerulus-on-a-Chip: A Pathway for Future Kidney-on-Chip Technology

This chapter presents an in-depth review of glomerulus-on-a-chip (GoC) technology, a groundbreaking advancement in microfluidic organ-on-a-chip research. The technology replicates the filtration barrier of the glomerulus and is instrumental in studying kidney diseases, testing drug nephrotoxicity, and eliminating the need for animal testing. The chapter highlights current challenges in verifying selective permeability and outlines potential future innovations required for advancing kidney-on-a-chip technology.

Chapter 9: Synergistic Integration of Federated Learning and Visual Intelligence for Disease Diagnosis and Prediction

This chapter explores how the integration of federated learning and visual intelligence is redefining healthcare diagnostics. AI-enabled diagnostic systems enhance disease detection through the analysis of medical images from various modalities, such as X-rays and MRI scans. Federated learning further strengthens these capabilities by facilitating collaborative model training across multiple healthcare institutions while ensuring data privacy. The discussion encompasses real-time applications, benefits, challenges, and use cases demonstrating the impact of this synergistic approach on next-generation healthcare solutions.

Chapter 10: Unleashing Sensors and Wearable Technologies in Digital Health and Human Augmentation

The growing adoption of wearable sensors is revolutionizing digital healthcare by enabling real-time patient monitoring and personalized treatments. This chapter discusses how AI-powered sensors enhance data analysis, facilitating remote diagnostics, early interventions, and proactive health management. With the expansion of wearable technology, healthcare accessibility is significantly improving, particularly in underserved regions. The chapter explores emerging trends in human augmentation, emphasizing the potential for connected and data-driven healthcare ecosystems to enhance the quality of life.

Chapter 11: Wearable Sensors, Real-Time Monitoring, and Data Assimilation in Healthcare

This chapter highlights the role of wearable sensors in modern healthcare, focusing on their ability to collect and analyze real-time physiological data. Continuous monitoring empowers healthcare professionals to track patient vitals, detect anomalies, and adjust treatment plans dynamically. The chapter examines various wearable sensor applications and their impact on improving patient outcomes. By integrating advanced data assimilation techniques, healthcare providers can leverage real-time insights to enhance disease control and treatment adherence.

We believe this book will serve as a valuable resource for researchers, practitioners, and students interested in the intersection of artificial intelligence, federated learning, and smart healthcare. By examining real-world case studies, theoretical frameworks, and emerging technologies, this volume offers insights that will inspire further exploration and innovation. We extend our sincere gratitude to all contributing authors for their dedication and expertise in shaping this work. Their efforts have made it possible to present a diverse collection of research that highlights the ongoing advancements in smart healthcare. We also thank our readers for their interest in this critical domain, and we hope that this book will serve as both an informative and inspirational guide to the future of intelligent healthcare systems.

The advancements discussed in this book are not just theoretical; they have the potential to redefine the future of healthcare by making it more data-driven, personalized, and efficient. The challenges associated with implementing these technologies, such as data privacy, regulatory compliance, and ethical considerations, are also addressed, ensuring that this volume provides a realistic perspective on both the opportunities and limitations. We encourage readers to critically engage with the content, explore interdisciplinary collaborations, and contribute to the ongoing evolution of smart healthcare. The synergy between visual intelligence and federated learning presents immense possibilities, and we are confident that this book will serve as a catalyst for future research and innovation in the field.

Chapter 1
5W+1H Automated Testing in Healthcare: A Case Study

Mehboob Zahedi
https://orcid.org/0000-0002-3421-9786
Indian Institute of Engineering Science and Technology, Shibpur (IIEST), Howrah, India

Abhishek Das
https://orcid.org/0000-0002-5546-6188
Aliah University, Kolkata, India

ABSTRACT

This paper contains the solution to enhance software usability and deployment during testing, addressing industry needs for effective software testing research to identify applications and technologies. Those help clients from avoiding software bugs and risks may be mitigated. In this study, a systematic mapping guide categorizing, classifying, and extracting conceptual models about the 5W+1H process has been developed. The mapping process begins with the Health care research where the study is being conducted and initially asks specific questions about that field. In this stage, the investigator formulates a list of research questions that can provide an overarching framework for research into a particular research topic. Investigators must decide the minimum number of key questions they need to answer in order to generate a unique research question. The minimum number of key questions needed for better software testing development in the healthcare domain has been provided.

DOI: 10.4018/979-8-3693-6094-1.ch001

INTRODUCTION

There is a standard software testing model "ISO/IEC/IEEE 29119" that was published in 2013 (Wegener, Baresel, & Sthamer, 2001). Because software testing has become increasingly important due to its critical role in verifying that the software is reliable, an ongoing series of software testing standards has been created. This series of standards software testing should be regarded as an important component for software testing practice. The International Conference on Software Engineering was held it's first "Future of Soft-ware Engineering" in 2000. Software testing standards was announced software testing standards: methodology and international standards in 2001 and included both biological specification and a product-oriented version. In 1992, the genetic algorithm is suggested to use for the structural test (Díaz, Tuya, Blanco, & Dolado, 2008). But this is frequently used from the 1995 for the automatic generation test (Watkins, 1995).

In 2013, the NISTS was established by ISO and IEC. The ISO/IEC/IEEE 29119 introduced as a standard series novel which includes systems and software testing. Firstly, it makes a set of standards and which are agreed internationally. Secondly, those standards should be accepted in different perspective scenarios that bind with running technological advancement in software development (Wegener, Baresel, & Sthamer, 2001). The essential part of research in software testing is Experiment (Andrews, Briand, & Labiche, 2005). The various level of testing processes can be visualized in the New International standard comprehensively. It includes documentation, design test technique, testing vocabulary and concepts. In this paper, we have proposed 5W+1H pattern in automated testing in the Heath Care domain (Jia, Cai, Yu, & Tse, 2016). The essential part of research in software testing is Experiment (Andrews, Briand, & Labiche, 2005). The various level of testing processes can be visualized in the New Inter-national standard comprehensively. It includes documentation, design test technique, testing vocabulary and concepts. In this paper, we have proposed 5W+1H pattern in automated testing in the Heath Care domain (Jia, Cai, Yu, & Tse, 2016). The following have been proposed in this paper:

- To ease the difficulty of conducting literature surveys using 5W+1H pattern.
- Help to formulate initial questioning and structural reports (Jia, Cai, Yu, & Tse, 2016).
- To know the acceptancy level of any software.

Software testing is a special kind of method to inspect the given software working correctly or giving the desired output or not. It contains some processes to execute or examine. It also includes the functional and non-functional requirements (Hooda & Chhillar, 2015).

It's main objective to identify the errors, gaps or missing actual contrasts requirements.

- We evaluate the software according to the desired requirements at the different stages.
- When a unit is developed, it is tested and it is also tested when we integrate with another one.
- We test the whole system when all the units are integrated.
- We have to test the software multiple times before available it to the customer.
- In some testing types, we directly deal with code known as White Box testing.
- When we don't look the code of any software and it have to be tested, is called as Black box testing.
- Mixture of these two known as Grey Box testing.
- The testing is a complete separate world contains slots of experts.

5W+1H Method

This part includes the different types of testing which are used during the SDLC in software testing (Lawanna, 2012) (Jamil, Arif, Abubakar, & Ahmad, 2016).

- **Manual Testing**. The process, by which we can test any software manually i.e. without using any automated tool, is called Manual Testing (Fraser & Arcuri, 2012). Here, the tester can identify any kind of improper behavior of software which leads the role of the end user (Abbas, Sultan, & Bhatti, 2017) (Lawanna, 2012). The stages of manual testing are Unit testing, Integration testing, and System Testing and User Acceptance testing.

Here, there are some steps to find out the Manual Testing:

i. Understanding the requirements (BRS,SRS,FRS, Mock-Ups)
ii. Test Plan
iii. Test Scenarios
iv. Test cases
v. Test Execution Expected Result Arrived Result
vi. Defect reporting & Re-testing
vii. Test Closer

- **Automation Testing**. This is the process where we can test the software using some automation tools and the third-party tools (Lawanna, 2012) (Jamil, Arif, Abubakar, & Ahmad, 2016). This leads the process easy and comfortable. It is quite fast than manual testing (Jamil, Arif, Abubakar, & Ahmad, 2016).

Here, there are few steps to test in automated mode:

i. Understanding the requirements (BRS,SRS,FRS, Mock-Ups)
ii. Test plan
iii. Test Scenarios
iv. Test cases
v. Using Testing Tools

DISCUSSION

It includes various different steps of process and methods of the software testing methodology. In various companies, there are different teams to evaluate or test the software according to the requirements. In some cases, the developers also evaluate the software that is called Unite testing. But mostly, there are some professionals hired for testing a software with some desired capability. These are Software Tester, Software Developer, Project Lead/Manager and End User.

Sometime before the SDLC, the testing activities start (Unterkalmsteiner et al., 2011). There is an urgent need to complete all the tasks during the last two months of the SDLC (Jamil, Arif, Abubakar, & Ahmad, 2016). The testing needs to be performed on a large number of employees during the SDLC in order to achieve its complete success. During the SDLC, the testing is performed on individual employees by a team of testers. The testers need to find all the defects that could be found at that time (Unterkalmsteiner et al., 2011).

Start Testing. Functional testing and Acceptance testing are the two prominent types of testing. It is also broadly categorized as compliance testing and risk-based testing (Unterkalmsteiner et al., 2011). This testing indicates how a software/hardware solution meets the requirements of an end-user, as specified by the business people. The development process consists of coding, documentation and code testing. The tools for this type of testing are, Automated testing tools use automation software such as automated unit testing suites and graphical user interface testers to check that a software or application fully meets the required specifications (Anand et al., 2013).

Stop Testing. The software will never be 100% ready – software never gets ready. Every day some small issue would be uncovered in the testing and that would need to be addressed. So, stopping the testing can be done only when a reasonable amount of time has been wasted in producing a system which would not be useful or efficient.

- Deadlines of Testing
- Test case execution of Testing (Keane & Topol, 2018)
- Completion of code coverage and functional to a certain point.
- If the bug rate drops below a given threshold and no high-priority bugs are found.
- Decision Management

5W+1H Method

As it relates to the theme and the arguments in favor of your position, give your viewpoint on the disputes, problems, issues, etc. In relation to the particular topic of the chapter and the book's overall theme, compare and contrast what has been done or is being done now. It is a method of asking some questions to the software such that we can identify the real objective that testing. It follows a pattern that we call 5H+1H pattern. The "5W+1H" word contains of 6 words i.e. Who, Why, What, Where, When and How (Jia, Cai, Yu, & Tse, 2016). This method includes the major needy things to know about the given software. It arises the Questions:

- Who do this activity in the software?
- Why do this happen?
- What are the activities and what will happen as an output?
- Where does the activity take place?
- When does the activity happen?
- How do the activities inter-connected to each other?

The tool or thing which is used to test any given software whereas it is working correctly or giving the correct and desired output (Lawanna, 2012) (Mustafa, Al-Qutaish, & Muhairat, 2009). Basically, in the market we can get these tools in 2 types:

i. **Open Source**. We can get these tools in the market with free of cost i.e. it is available in open source. Just open any browser with internet and download it. It contains fewer features. There are some tools named as:

    - Selenium
    - Sahi
    - Auto-IT
    - Sikoli
    - UserTesting

- PractiTest
- LambdaTest
- Sauce Labs
- Panaya Change Intelligence
- Rainforest QA
- Provar
- Zephyr-E
- TestRail

In Open-source testing tool, Selenium is the most useful tool in the market. **Selenium**. It is one of the market's free (Open Source) automated testing tools. Web applications are validated using it on various platforms and browsers. It is composed of multiple software tools which are available in the market i.e. Selenium IDE, Selenium RC (selenium 1.0), and Selenium webdriver (Gojare, Joshi, & Gaigaware, 2015). It supports multiple languages that means it supports 6 languages i.e. Java, C#, Python, php, Perl, Ruby. It runs in both Operating system Windows and Linux as well.

It was first introduced in 2004 as JSFT (Java Script Functional Tool). While working with the Selenium, we need to know about the basic programming like the core JAVA knowledge. In a single shot, all the features of Selenium are not come in the market. As per the requirement of the testers, it comes one by one.

There are some components in Selenium available in the market:

I. **SelIDE:** It was the first Component of Selenium. There is no need of programming. It works on Record and Play. It means we just record the steps and play. It is so easy for working. But we do not able to do complex programming i.e. API, Loop etc. For the current market, it is totally outdated.
II. **SelRC:** To overcome above problem of programming, there was introduced SelRC. It was also known as Sel1.0 . There is no concept of SelRC in the current market.
III. **SelWebDriver:** This is the advanced version of SelRC, also known as Sel2.0, Sel3.0, Sel4.0 etc. The whole market is running with the SelWebDriver.
IV. **SelGrid:** It is used to execute automation script in multiple browsers or multiple system.

Selenium is an API with having a group of components. We do not need to install (.exe) file, we need to work with individual component. Based on the project requirement, we need to use individual component. We can integrate the third-party tools with the component as per our requirement.

There are few third-parties available here:

a) **Testng or Junit:** In that, we can know how many test cases pass or fail. This kind of report could be known by this (Keane & Topol, 2018).
b) **Auto-IT or Sikuli:** The drawback of Selenium is that it is not support on the window based application. So, while working with the web based application related with the windows, Selenium is not capable to handle. For that purpose, we can use Auto-IT or Sikuli.
c) **Automation Framework:** There are many automation frameworks available in the market e.g. Hybrid framework, Modular framework, Testng framework, POM framework etc. But we need to work with these for the scratch level.
d) **Another tool:** While working with the automation framework, we need to get the knowledge about some tools like: Maven, CuCumber, Jenkings, Log4j, Github. Besides we need to know about the Web-Service testing and API testing.

Commercial tools. We cannot get these tools with free of cost. We need to take licensed to that respected company to use any particular tool • (Gurcan & Cagiltay, 2019). These tools are owned or exclusively licensed to Supplier or company. It contains more features. There are some tools named as:

- QTP/UFT
- RFT
- Test Complete

Methodology

Testing is necessary in every aspect in software analysis like industry and other personal standards. Firstly we have to develop a test environment to measure all the data flow and control flow of the software (Wegener, Baresel, & Sthamer, 2001). According to the required test purpose and control flow graph, the structural testing is divided into four categories. These are:

i. **Node-oriented methods**: It needs the knowledge of the particular nodes to get the control flow graph. The main objective of this is to get the test dataset that performs the control flow graph of every desired nodes. The "test" word represents all the nodes to be imagined and the "condition" word represents the branching nodes. We have to check the branching conditions carefully to predict True and False. To calculate the approximation level, the nodes need to be grouped together. The following characteristics belong to each node group: Only one entry node, Nodes that belong to one path from entry to target node, Node group is made according to the rules and don't violate the other characteristics.

ii. **Path-oriented methods**: It needs certain paths for execution the control flow graph. To complete the path coverage, the variations of all the path tests are got from the reduced path test belong to this category. So, the paths which are needed to satisfy the structural test criteria and identify as partial aim.
iii. **Node-path oriented methods**: It needs the knowledge of a specific node and from that node the execution of a particular path through the control flow graph. LCSAJ (Linear code sequence and jump) and the branch test belong to this category.
iv. **Node-node oriented methods**: At last, it performs the program to the path which covers the node combinations according to the determined sequence to get the control flow graph between nodes. There are many data flow oriented methods belong to this category (Wegener, Baresel, & Sthamer, 2001).

Process. In the Software Testing Process, 11 steps could be followed for getting the solution. Those could be explained as follows:

- **Step-1: Assess Development Plan and Status**. Intended to evaluate every aspect of implemented software solution, all testing is now to be completed with above functionality (Jamil, Arif, Abubakar, & Ahmad, 2016). This step has to do with ensuring functionality and presentation of data associated with the software solution. There are varied testing activities in implementation stage for efficient execution of the project plan. The activities are outlined under seven Project Development Activities. They include 8 basic tasks – system testing, operating system testing, application testing, data analysis, functional testing, cross-functional testing, user acceptance testing, and overall system testing.
- **Step-2: Test Plan Development**. Taking a plan for testing will be going to follow a particular pattern for process to software testing. The format of planning should be followed as mentioned in the pattern we have taken, but content of unit modules may vary at the developer easiness and risks of the software (Jamil, Arif, Abubakar, & Ahmad, 2016).
- **Step-3: Testing the Software Requirements**. The cause of any software failures could be as incomplete, inaccurate or inconsistent. The impotence of getting the requirements at the collecting requirement phase time, could be increased the cost of implement significance. In the verification, testers must identify those requirements accurately, completely and whether they conflict to each other.
- **Step-4: Testing Software Design**. External design work consists of verifying hardware and software and confirming that mechanical interface supports desired features. These hardware design issues are best tackled through simu-

lation analysis. Internal design work provides a sense of cohesive design and helps implement the associated hardware features. Information required for internal de-sign.

- **Step-5: Build Phase Testing**. Characteristics of automation testers, the position of the automation tester are a dynamic one, with no strict physical conditions. Automation tester takes the best solution to get the right functionality from both the developer and the business (Jamil, Arif, Abubakar, & Ahmad, 2016). When making software, he doesn't need to adhere to particular methodology, as he can use the solution with relative ease. He takes an active part in the development process.
- **Step-6: Executing and Record Result**. While dynamic state occurs, it includes testing of code. That executable code actually would not be validated the approach, methods and tools which are laid out in test plan meeting stated software requirements, and designing the structural specifications.
- **Step-7: Acceptance Test**. Applicability and usefulness of software are enabled the acceptance testing of users in the performance day by day. Those tests include what the user thinks about the software to be performed against what the outputs are desired from the documented requirements of the software.
- **Step-8: Report Testing Results**. In software testing, test reporting is continuous process. It could be both oral and written. The AMU program requires a certain number of annual quality indicators for each project, to provide an independent review of the quality of the AMU efforts.
- **Step-9: Installation of the Software**. When test team has confirmed that soft-ware is prepared for production use, power to execute, then software during production environment should be tested (Jamil, Arif, Abubakar, & Ahmad, 2016). When any software is prepared for production which is confirmed by the Team and power to execute that software during production environment should be tested.
- **Step-10: Test Software Changes**. Test plan formulation is similar to other phases in software development. When goals are developed and given directions to development teams, the team must deliver this information to development management and obtain approval. This approval creates the infrastructure within which they can implement the system and make necessary changes to the system as they go along.
- **Step-11: Evaluate Test Effectiveness**. Top of a software testing assignment should be related to success or failure of the feature development effort (Galin, 2004). A test tester should be empowered to take ownership of tests in a delivery team in order to make it a true objective assessment. Further,

the evaluation should be factored with the rate at which the software is developed, software quality and impact on business.

Testing Phases

After the software implementation is finished, there is a separate testing phase that is carried out by numerous test teams. The test team's viewpoint is taken into consideration when choosing the testing methodology. We can use various techniques to check robustness, modularization and cost-estimation of any software like: Hill Climbing (easy to implement (Wegener, Baresel, & Sthamer, 2001)). In this paper, there are three steps in the testing phase as mentioned below:

- **Verification**: Technical reviews, software inspections, walkthroughs, and attempts to verify the design elements, software requirements, conduct requirements, acceptance testing, and audit are all included (Richardson, Iezzi, Khan, & Maxwell, 2014). The software's purpose, according to the user, is to determine what is right. This includes testing the application of the correct procedure, such as figuring out whether the software was created correctly.
- **Validation**: It determines whether the created software complies with the needs of the user (Richardson, Iezzi, Khan, & Maxwell, 2014) (Christodorescu & Jha, 2004) (Fraser & Arcuri, 2012). It makes sure that we evaluate the specific software by user (Jan, Shah, Johar, Shah, & Khan, 2016).
- **Testing**: It is a helpful technique for both validation and verification (Rana, Goswami, & Maheshwari, 2019). Of course, walkthroughs, inspections, reviews, and static analysis are additional methods that are helpful for verification. There are other various useful techniques for verification i.e. static analysis, inspection, reviews and walkthroughs etc. Rest of another techniques i.e. prototyping and early release are used for validation.

Need of Testing

Software testing is so important; there are some reasons as follows:

- Helps in saving money
- Satisfaction of the customer
- Easy while adding new features
- Enhancing the development process
- Quality of the product
- Determining the performance of the software.
- Security

Health Care Testing Domain

The process by which we can test the healthcare applications or software in a standard, safety and compliance manner such that we can ensure about the quality, reliability, performance, safety and efficiency of that particular application.

In 21st century, there are many smart types of software with AI used in the Healthcare field (Panch, Mattie, & Celi, 2019). We can predict the Heart disease with the advent of the digital era and technological advancement. The Healthcare field stores a large amount of distributed data but the separation is very difficult to get the valuable data from it. For that, we are using much software to detect and predict the disease such that we can take precaution. From the report, we know that the special physicians can diagnose with 79.97% of accuracy, but using software we could do the same thing with 91.1% of accuracy (Arumugam et al., 2021). We can evaluate our models by different evaluating methods to determine the accuracy of the software. We have to look about the true and false cases as well for improving the software model.

The 5W+1H method—Who, What, Where, When, Why, and How—is a systematic approach to explore and analyze various aspects of a topic. Applying this method to automated testing in healthcare can help outline key considerations and components:

i. Who:
   – Stakeholders: This includes a wide range of people like doctors, nurses, patients, lab technicians, IT teams, regulatory agencies, and even insurance companies.
   – Beneficiaries: Primarily, patients benefit from quicker and more accurate diagnoses. Healthcare providers also gain from more reliable data, and healthcare facilities can operate more efficiently.

ii. What:
   – Automated Testing: It involves using technology to perform medical tests, diagnostics, or quality checks without needing direct human intervention.
   – Examples: This could include things like automated blood tests, analyzing medical images, genetic testing, or even monitoring patient vital signs through smart devices.

iii. Where:
   – Healthcare Settings: These technologies are used in hospitals, clinics, and labs, but also extend to remote or at-home settings with devices that monitor patients' health.

– Remote Monitoring: Patients can use wearables and smart devices at home to keep track of their health, which is especially helpful for chronic conditions.

iv. When:

– Timing: Automated testing can be done continuously or on a scheduled basis, depending on the medical requirements or system checks.
– Adoption: The speed at which these technologies are adopted varies, influenced by factors like technology integration, regulatory approvals, and costs.

v. Why:

– Accuracy: One of the biggest advantages is reducing human error, which leads to more accurate results.
– Efficiency: These systems can handle a large number of tests quickly, speeding up the diagnostic process.
– Cost Savings: Automated testing can cut down on labor costs and minimize errors, which can be expensive.
– Patient Safety: With accurate and timely diagnoses, patients can receive the right treatment sooner, improving their overall care.

vi. How:

– Technology: This includes AI, machine learning, robotics, and advanced data analytics, all working together to automate the testing process.
– Integration: These systems are integrated with existing healthcare IT infrastructures, like Electronic Health Records (EHRs), to streamline data flow and improve accuracy.
– Regulation: Ensuring that these systems comply with healthcare regulations is crucial for safety and reliability.
– Quality Control: Regular updates and maintenance are necessary to keep the automated systems functioning correctly and to meet performance standards.

It also allows us to maximize the time and effort spent in creating more robust products to serve more customers. For instance, all the testing that happens in a digital manufacturing application can happen in a safety test environment before the application is released in the market. It also gives us more control over the time-to-market. We can develop products before they are released in the market for better development of the software. From the Fig.1, we can understand the testing domain needed in the healthcare. Moreover, it plays a vital role for figure it out the better performance as well as better accuracy without having high risk.

Figure 1. Healthcare-Testing Domain

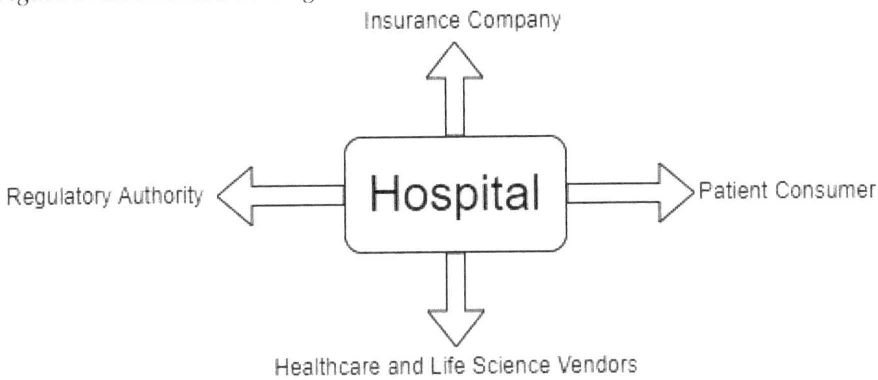

Consequently, testing becomes a very crucial part of digital transformation because not only does it help to create better products or services but also it helps us to secure our customer's data and protect our consumers [9]. Various enterprises are being engaged in discussions to better understand their needs. Future testing offerings are planned to be rolled out, integrating past capabilities and expertise in functional safety, digital transformation, and add-on testing for diverse applications such as IoT, artificial intelligence, and digital materials. This will enable the transition from testing only safety-critical applications to also encompassing safety-critical and other types of applications.

These days, software is used extensively in this industry. It has already been observed in a number of fields, including computer networks, intelligent control, speech recognition, computer vision, computer graphics, and natural language processing (NLP). By automating some routine tasks, machine learning (ML) with IoT helps to improve the quality of human lives. Through the use of applications and body-attached sensors, it is able to monitor human parts. Additionally, we are able to collect data from wearable technology, social media, the internet, medical records, genomic data, mobile phone data, and environmental data, among other sources. It could compile all the data necessary to use big data or historical data to predict the disease.

Business Process of Health-Care. The organizational Health-Care software must be worked in a smooth manner such that we can know all the information in a single shot for each entity deadline [9]. To create the whole interconnecting system, it is huge task to make so it could be decided into modules such that it could fewer complexes.

Figure 2. Business Process of HealthCare

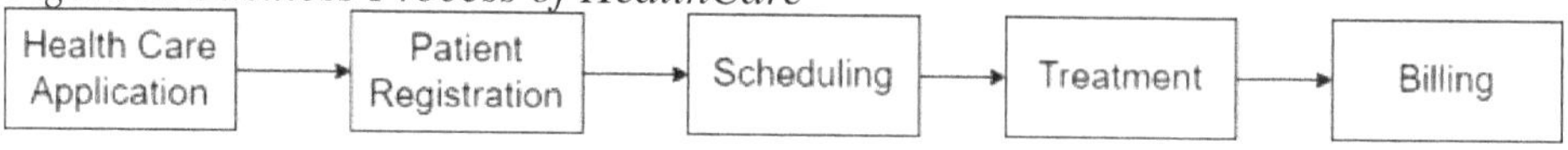

Applications. In this domain, Software application is increasing day by day. There are several software introduced to produce powerful models that can diagnose automatically (Keane & Topol, 2018). There are also various applications such as:

i. Prognosis: It is the process of predicting the expected development of dis-ease (Jordan & Mitchell, 2015).
ii. Identifying the medicine
iii. Medical Image Diagnosis
iv. Colleting the medical data in a smart way
v. Medical trial and research
vi. Good Radiotherapy
vii. Disease prediction and diagnosis.

By using this technique, we are facing some challenges like: Big data analysis, interoperability, Resource scarcity, Security & Privacy, Energy management, safety etc.

Mathematical Model

It involves using software tools and frameworks to test healthcare systems, devices, or applications with minimal human intervention. This process is crucial to ensure that systems function correctly, securely, and in compliance with regulatory standards (Balch et al., 2023) (Magrabi, Lyell, & Coiera, 2023). The methodology can be detailed using the 5W+1H framework and a more mathematical approach, including statistical analysis and computational models.

i. System Modeling and Risk Assessment

- System Model:

    – State Space Representation: This is a mathematical model representing all possible states (conditions or configurations) of a healthcare system, including normal operation, failure states, and transitions between these states.

    – States (S): These are distinct conditions or outputs of the system. For example, a state could represent a system functioning correctly, while another state could represent a system failure.

$S=\{S_1,S_2,\ldots,S_n\}$

– Transitions (T): These represent the probability of moving from one state to another due to various factors, such as system inputs or environmental conditions.

$T=\{T_{ij}:S_i\rightarrow S_j, P(T_{ij})\}$

- Risk Assesment

Failure Modes and Effects Analysis (FMEA): This is a structured approach to identifying and prioritizing potential failure modes within a system (Ahamad, Al-Shehri, & Keshta, 2022). A failure mode is a way in which a system could fail.

– Risk Priority Number (RPN): This is a numerical score used to prioritize risks based on their severity, occurrence, and detection likelihood (Khinvasara, Shankar, & Wong, 2024).
– Severity: The impact of a failure mode if it occurs, ranging from minor inconveniences to catastrophic events affecting patient safety.
– Occurrence: The likelihood of a failure mode happening.
– Detection: The probability that the failure mode will be detected before it reaches the patient or user.

RPN = Severity* Occurrence * Detection

ii. Test Design and Coverage Analysis

- Test case Generation:

  – Functional Requirements (FR): These are specific capabilities or functions that the system must perform, as defined by regulatory standards or user needs.
  – Test Cases (TC): Detailed, systematic instructions to test whether the system meets its functional requirements.

$TC=\{TC_1,TC_2,\ldots,TC_k\}$

- Coverage Metrics:

– Measures the extent to which the source code is tested by the test cases (Nawaz, Khan, & Ahmad, 2024). It helps ensure that all parts of the system are tested.

$$\text{Code Coverage} = \frac{\textit{Number of Requirement Tested}}{\textit{Total Number of Requirements}} * 100\%$$

iii. Test Execution and Monitoring

- Automated Test Execution:
  – Execution Environment: The physical or virtual setup where testing occurs, which should mimic real-world conditions to provide accurate results.
  – Automated Testing Tools: Software tools used to automate the testing process, such as Selenium or QTP.
- Monitoring and Data Collection:
  – Event Logs: Records of all actions and responses during test execution, used for analysis and debugging.
  – Performance Metrics: Key indicators such as system response time, throughput, and error rates.

iv. Statistical Analysis and Validation

- Hypothesis Testing
  – Null Hypothesis (H_0): Assumes that the system performs as expected without defects.
  – Alternative Hypothesis (H_1): Suggests that there are deviations or defects in the system's performance.

Statistical tests (e.g., Chi-square test, t-test) are used to validate these hypotheses by comparing observed test results with expected outcomes.

H_0: Observed Results = Expected Results
H_1: Observed Results $\neq$ Expected Results

- Confidence Intervals (CI):
  – These provide a range within which the true performance metrics of the system are expected to fall, with a certain level of confidence (usually 95%).

$$\text{CI} = \hat{\theta} \pm z\frac{\sigma}{\sqrt{n}}$$

where:
$\hat{\theta}$ is the sample mean.
z is the z-score corresponding to the desired confidence level.
σ is the standard deviation.
n is the sample size.

v. Error and Reliability Analysis

- Error Rate Calculation:
  – False Positive Rate (FPR): The proportion of non-defective cases that were incorrectly identified as defective.
  – False Negative Rate (FNR): The proportion of defective cases that were incorrectly identified as non-defective.

$$FPR = \frac{False\ Positives}{False\ Positive + True\ Negatives}$$

$$FPR = \frac{False\ Negatives}{False\ Negatives + True\ Positives}$$

- Reliability Metrics:
  – Mean Time Between Failures (MTBF): A measure of system reliability, representing the average time between failures.

$$MTBF = \frac{Total\ Operational\ Time}{Number\ of\ Failures}$$

  – Mean Time to Repair (MTTR): The average time taken to repair a system after a failure.

$$MTTR = \frac{Total\ Repair\ Time}{Number\ of\ Repairs}$$

vi. Reporting and Continuous Improvement

- Test Results Reporting:
  – Defect Density (DD): The number of defects found in the system relative to its size (e.g., lines of code).

$$Defect\ Density = \frac{Total\ Defects}{Size\ of\ the\ System\ (Lines\ of\ Code)}$$

- Continuous Improvement:

– Root Cause Analysis (RCA): A process used to identify the underlying causes of defects and failures to prevent future occurrences (Abd Rahman, Ibrahim, Hasikin, & Abd Razak, 2023).

– Process Improvement: Implementing changes in the testing process based on RCA findings to improve overall system quality.

- Mathematical Models in Healthcare Testing

  – Bayesian Networks for Risk Assessment: Bayesian networks are probabilistic graphical models that represent the dependencies between different components and their failure probabilities. They are particularly useful in healthcare for assessing risks and understanding how various factors influence system behavior.

$$P\left(Fi \middle| Ci\right) = \frac{P(\mathrm{CiFi})P(\mathrm{Fi})}{P(Ci)}$$

Where:

$P(F_i|C_i)$ is the probability of a failure occurring given a specific cause.

$P(Ci|\, F_i)$is the likelihood of the cause occurring given the failure.

$P(F_i)$ is the prior probability of the failure occurring.

$P(C_i)$ is the probability of the cause occurring.

This comprehensive methodology, integrating both qualitative and quantitative analyses, ensures that automated testing in healthcare is thorough, reliable, and capable of identifying and mitigating risks. It emphasizes the importance of patient safety, data integrity, and compliance with healthcare standards.

Practical Implementation and Execution of Automated Testing in Healthcare

Following the development of mathematical models for automated testing, the next step involves applying these models in practical, real-world healthcare settings. This process includes detailed strategies for test execution, monitoring and data collection, validation and verification, error analysis and correction, and continuous improvement (Jiwani, Gupta, & Whig, 2023). Each step is crucial to ensuring the reliability, safety, and compliance of healthcare systems.

i. Test Execution Strategies

- Preparation and Setup:

  – Test Environment: A controlled setup that mirrors the real-world conditions where the healthcare system will operate. This includes hardware, software, network configurations, and simulated clinical scenarios.

– Test Data Preparation: Creating datasets that include typical, boundary, and exceptional cases to thoroughly evaluate system performance under various conditions.

- Execution Process:

  – Automated Test Scripts: Utilizing automation tools to execute predefined test cases. These scripts cover different testing dimensions, such as functionality, performance, security, and compliance.

  – Functional Testing: Ensures that each function of the system operates in conformance with the requirement specifications.

  – Performance Testing: Assesses the system's response time, throughput, and resource utilization under various conditions.

  – Security Testing: Identifies vulnerabilities and ensures data protection mechanisms are effective.

  – Compliance Testing: Verifies that the system meets regulatory and standards requirements.

  – Real-time Monitoring: Implement real-time monitoring tools to track system behavior throughout the testing process.

ii. Monitoring and Data Collection

- Key Metrics Collection:

  – Performance Metrics: Key indicators of how the system handles workloads, including:

    - Load Times: The time taken to load various system components or data.
    - Throughput: The amount of data processed over a specific period.
    - Scalability Metrics: How well the system can handle increasing workloads.

  – Error Logs: Comprehensive logging of all system errors, including:

    - Error Type: Categorizing errors by type (e.g., data errors, system crashes).
    - Occurrence: Frequency and conditions under which the errors occur.
    - Severity: The impact of each error on system operation and patient safety.

  – User Interaction Data: In usability testing, this involves:

    - Tracking User Actions: Understanding how users interact with the system.

- Identifying Usability Issues: Finding points where users encounter difficulties or errors.

- Data Analysis:
  – Statistical Analysis: Applying statistical techniques to interpret the data, identify trends, and compare system performance against expected benchmarks.
    - Descriptive Statistics: Summarize the basic features of the data, providing simple summaries about the sample and the measures.
    - Hypothesis Testing: Test assumptions about the data, such as system performance under different conditions.
  – Anomaly Detection: Using machine learning models to detect anomalies in the data, which may indicate potential system malfunctions or inefficiencies.
    - Outliers: Data points significantly different from the rest, which could indicate potential issues.
    - Pattern Recognition: Identifying patterns that may suggest underlying problems.

iii. Validation and Verification

- Validation:
  – Requirement Validation: Ensuring that the system fulfills all specified requirements, both functional (e.g., accuracy of diagnostics) and non-functional (e.g., system speed).
  – Clinical Validation: Particularly in healthcare, validating that the system accurately processes clinical data and provides correct outputs, such as diagnoses or treatment recommendations.
- Verification:
  – Regulatory Compliance: Verifying adherence to healthcare regulations and standards.
  – Security Verification: Ensuring the system is secure from potential threats.

iv. Error Analysis and Correlation

- Root Cause Analysis (RCA):
  – Identifying Root Causes: Systematically identifying the underlying causes of system errors and failures:
    - Data Analysis: Reviewing error logs and system data to pinpoint the source of issues.

- System Component Analysis: Examining specific components (software modules, hardware components) that might be responsible for failures.

– Prioritizing Issues: Using metrics like the Risk Priority Number (RPN) to prioritize which issues to address first:

- Severity (S): Impact of the issue on patient safety and system functionality.
- Occurrence (O): Likelihood of the issue occurring.
- Detection (D): Likelihood of detecting the issue before it affects users.

$$RPN = Severit * Occurance * Detection$$

- Correlation and Retesting:

  – Implementation of Fixes: Addressing the identified issues and implementing necessary changes:

  - Bug Fixes: Correcting software errors.
  - System Updates: Applying patches or updates to improve system stability and security (Tang, Li, & Fantus, 2023).

  – Retesting: Conducting regression testing to ensure that:

  - No New Issues: The fixes do not introduce new problems.
  - System Integrity: All system components work together seamlessly post-correction.

v. Continuous Improvement and Iteration

- Feedback Integration:

  – User Feedback: Gathering input from healthcare professionals and patients to:

  - Identify Improvement Areas: Understanding practical challenges and user needs.
  - Enhance Usability: Making the system more user-friendly based on feedback (Jha, Sahu, Bisoy, & Sain, 2022).

  – Post-Deployment Monitoring: Continuously monitoring the system in the field to:

  - Detect New Issues: Identifying any issues that arise in real-world use.
  - Adapt to Changes: Quickly adapting to new requirements or changing regulations.

- Process Optimization:

– Continuous Learning: Incorporating insights from each testing cycle into the next:
  - Refining Test Cases: Updating and improving test cases based on previous results.
  - Optimizing Testing Tools: Enhancing the efficiency and coverage of automated testing tools.
– Automation Enhancements: Continuously improving the automation of testing processes:
  - Script Optimization: Reducing redundancy and improving the accuracy of automated scripts.
  - Integration of New Technologies: Incorporating new tools and technologies to improve testing outcomes.

- Documentation and Reporting:
  – Comprehensive Reporting: Detailed documentation of all testing activities, including:
    - Test Results: Outcomes of each test case, including any deviations from expected results.
    - Defects and Resolutions: Detailed descriptions of identified defects and the steps taken to resolve them.
  – Traceability and Auditing: Maintaining records that link tests to requirements and changes:
    - Traceability Matrix: A document that maps test cases to specific requirements, ensuring comprehensive testing.
    - Audit Trails: Detailed records that support regulatory compliance and facilitate audits.

Ethical Considerations in Automated Testing

Ethical considerations are crucial in healthcare, where patient safety and data confidentiality are paramount. The automated testing process must be guided by these principles:

- Informed Consent: Patients should be informed about how their data will be used in testing and consent to its use. This includes understanding the scope of data collection and the purposes for which it will be used (Tang, Li, & Fantus, 2023).
- Data Privacy and Security: Ensuring that all patient data is handled in compliance with privacy regulations and protected against unauthorized access

(Al Naam et al., 2022). This involves implementing strong encryption, access controls, and regular security audits.

By following this comprehensive, detailed approach, healthcare systems can achieve high levels of reliability, safety, and compliance. This not only ensures the smooth operation of healthcare technologies but also enhances patient trust and outcomes.

Post-Implementation Review and Continuous Monitoring

In the lifecycle of healthcare systems, the post-implementation phase is critical for ensuring that the systems continue to operate effectively, securely, and in compliance with regulatory standards (Davis, Walsh, & Matheny, 2023). This phase involves a comprehensive review of the system's performance, ongoing monitoring, and continuous improvement based on real-world usage and feedback.

i. Post Implementation Review

- Performance Evaluation:

  – System Performance Analysis: After deployment, the system's actual performance needs to be rigorously evaluated against the expected benchmarks. Key performance indicators (KPIs) such as response times, system uptime, throughput, and resource utilization are measured and analyzed. This ensures that the system performs optimally under real-world conditions, maintaining efficiency and reliability. For instance, we can use metrics like Mean Time Between Failures (MTBF) and Mean Time to Repair (MTTR) to assess system reliability and maintainability:

$$MTBF = \frac{Total\ Operation\ Time}{Number\ of\ Failures}$$

$$MTTR = \frac{Total\ Repair\ Time}{Number\ of\ Repairs}$$

These metrics help in understanding the system's robustness and identifying areas that require improvement.

  – User Feedback Collection: Engaging with healthcare professionals and patients is crucial for gathering insights into the system's usability and effectiveness. This feedback helps identify practical challenges and areas where the system may need enhancements

(Davis & Shepheard, 2024). Techniques such as surveys, interviews, and direct observation can be employed to collect qualitative data, which can then be analyzed to pinpoint common issues and areas for improvement.

- Compliance and Regulatory Review:
  – Regulatory Compliance Check: Continuous compliance with healthcare regulations such as HIPAA (Health Insurance Portability and Accountability Act) and FDA guidelines is essential. This involves regularly reviewing data protection protocols, access controls, and other security measures to ensure patient data confidentiality and integrity. The system must be audited to verify that all legal and regulatory requirements are being met. For example, compliance can be quantified using a compliance score, calculated by evaluating the extent to which the system adheres to various regulatory criteria.
  – Audit and Documentation Review: Maintaining detailed records and documentation of all system activities, including data processing, user interactions, and system changes, is crucial for accountability and traceability. This documentation supports audits and helps demonstrate compliance with regulatory standards. A traceability matrix can be used to map test cases and requirements to specific regulatory standards, ensuring comprehensive coverage and easy verification.

ii. Continuous Monitoring

- Ongoing System Monitoring:
  – Real-Time Monitoring Tools: Implementing real-time monitoring solutions is critical for continuously tracking the system's performance. These tools should monitor metrics such as CPU and memory usage, network latency, and transaction volumes. Anomaly detection algorithms can be employed to identify deviations from normal behavior, which may indicate potential issues such as security breaches or system failures (Nawaz & Ahmed, 2022).
  – Security Monitoring: Security is a top priority in healthcare systems. Continuous monitoring for unauthorized access attempts, unusual data transfers, and other security threats is necessary to protect sensitive patient information. Security Information and Event Management (SIEM) systems can be used to aggregate and analyze logs from various sources, helping to detect and respond to security incidents promptly.

- Data Quality and Integrity Checks:
  – Data Validation: Ensuring the accuracy, completeness, and consistency of data is vital for the system's integrity. Regular data validation checks help identify and correct errors, such as duplicate records or incorrect data entries. Data integrity can be maintained using checksums or hash functions to verify that data has not been altered unexpectedly [46].
  – Error and Anomaly Detection: Machine learning models and statistical methods can be employed to identify anomalies in the data. For example, a healthcare system might use a control chart to monitor lab results over time, identifying outliers that could indicate equipment malfunctions or data entry errors.

iii. Continuous Improvement and Iteration

- Feedback Integration and System Updates:
  – User Feedback Analysis: Continuous analysis of feedback from users helps prioritize system updates and improvements. Techniques like sentiment analysis and natural language processing can be used to analyze qualitative feedback from surveys and interviews, providing insights into user satisfaction and identifying areas for enhancement.
  – Regular System Updates: Implementing updates based on the feedback and monitoring results is crucial for maintaining system performance and security (Jain & Rakesh, 2024). These updates might include software patches, new features, or process optimizations. An effective update strategy involves scheduling regular updates and communicating with users about upcoming changes to minimize disruptions.
- Proactive Issue Resolution:
  – Proactive Monitoring: Predictive analytics can be used to anticipate potential issues before they impact the system. For example, trend analysis might reveal increasing system load, prompting preventive measures such as server scaling or optimization of resource usage (Yari et al., 2023).
  – Incident Response Planning: Having a well-defined incident response plan is essential for addressing system failures or security breaches. This plan should outline the steps to take in response to different types of incidents, including roles and responsibilities, communication protocols, and recovery procedures. Regular drills and reviews of the incident response plan help ensure preparedness.

The post-implementation review and continuous monitoring phase is integral to the long-term success of healthcare systems. By rigorously evaluating performance, ensuring compliance, monitoring security, and integrating continuous improvements, healthcare organizations can maintain the reliability, safety, and effectiveness of their systems. This proactive approach not only protects patient data and privacy but also enhances user satisfaction and trust in the technology.

Change Management and Future Enhancements

Following the post-implementation review and continuous monitoring, it is crucial to manage changes effectively and plan for future enhancements. This ensures that the healthcare system remains adaptable and aligned with evolving technological advancements and user needs. The change management process and planning for future enhancements focus on incorporating feedback, addressing emerging requirements, and maintaining system relevance and efficiency.

i. Change Management

- Change Planning and Impact Analysis:

  – Change Requests: Collecting and evaluating requests for modifications or enhancements from stakeholders (Larsson & Thesing, 2024). Each request is assessed for potential impacts on system performance, security, and compliance. This includes:

  - Impact Analysis: Assessing how proposed changes will affect the system. This involves:

$$Impact\ Score = Severity\ of\ Change * Probability\ of\ Issues$$

where:

  - Severity of Change is a qualitative measure of the potential impact on the system.
  - Probability of Issues is a qualitative measure of the likelihood that the change will cause problems.

  – Approval Process: Establishing a structured process for approving changes, including review by relevant stakeholders and decision-makers (Popescu, El-Chaarani, El-Abiad, & Gigauri, 2022). This ensures that all proposed changes are thoroughly vetted before implementation.

- Change Implementation and Testing:

– Executing approved changes in a controlled environment to minimize disruptions. This includes:
– Development and Configuration: Making the necessary updates or modifications to the system.
– Testing: Conducting comprehensive testing to ensure that changes do not introduce new issues. This involves:

$$\textit{Testing Coverage} = \frac{\textit{Number of Test Cases Passes}}{\textit{Total Number of Test cases}}$$

– Deployment: Rolling out changes to the live system. This involves:
- Deployment Strategies: Using strategies such as phased rollouts or blue-green deployments to mitigate risks and ensure smooth transitions.

- Change Monitoring and Review:
  – Post-Change Monitoring: Monitoring the system after changes are implemented to detect and address any issues that arise. This includes:
  – Performance Monitoring: Continuously tracking performance metrics to ensure that the system operates as expected.
  – User Feedback: Gathering feedback from users to identify any issues or areas for improvement related to the recent changes (Haux, 2006).
  – Review and Documentation: Reviewing the change process and documenting outcomes. This includes:

ii. Future Enhancements

- Identifying and Prioritizing Enhancements:
  – Needs Assessment: Continuously assessing user needs and technological advancements to identify potential enhancements (Okolo et al., 2024). Enhancement Roadmap: Developing a roadmap for future enhancements. This includes:
- Research and Development:
  – Innovative Solutions: Exploring and integrating innovative solutions to address emerging challenges and opportunities. This includes:
  - Research: Conducting research on new technologies and methodologies that can enhance system capabilities.
  - Prototyping and Testing: Developing prototypes and conducting tests to evaluate the feasibility and benefits of new solutions.

- Continuous Learning and Adaptation:
  - Training and Development: Providing ongoing training and development for staff to ensure they are up-to-date with the latest technologies and practices (Olaboye, 2024).
  - Adaptation and Flexibility: Maintaining flexibility to adapt to changes in the healthcare environment and technology landscape. This includes:

Effective change management and planning for future enhancements are essential for maintaining the relevance and effectiveness of healthcare systems. By systematically managing changes, identifying and prioritizing enhancements, and fostering a culture of continuous learning and adaptation, healthcare organizations can ensure that their systems remain robust, efficient, and aligned with evolving needs and technologies.

Importance of Testing

Software testing helps to eliminate time waste and money waste. There is no better a way to achieve this. There are several cost benefits of software testing. If the software test is done right, then the software product is expected to be error free. The measurement of any software quality is done based on defects of the final product (Turhan & Bener, 2007).

Table 1. Comparison between 5W+1H and other methods

5W+1H method	Other methods
i. It has the various important problem solving methodologies that could be applied in various personal as well as business field.	It has less problem solving methodologies.
ii. It can detect the bugs or errors easily at the time of software testing easily.	It takes some complicacies.
iii. It gives better accurate result.	It gives less accurate result.
iv. It is very much testing friendly.	Less testing friendly.
v. Testing questions are more organized so that we can develop a software with good accuracy.	Testing questions are placed in a scattered way so it is very difficult to check and understand the errors.
vi. Verification, validation and testing can be performed within less time and an efficient way.	It takes more time and is not so much efficient.
vii. It is used for the precious output.	It is used in general way.
viii. In Healthcare, it saves millions of lives for correct software testing.	Not quite efficient.

Result

There are different types of software and also various number of techniques for software testing. Some of these easier and some of them are difficult to test. Software testability is a thing in which a software is how much supportive in a given context. If the degree of software testability is high, then it is easier to find bugs in the software otherwise it would be difficult. We should increase the testability of a software such that the cost can be decreased and we can increase the quality of the software. There are six factors in a software testability. These are the following described as Software requirements, Implementation characteristics, Test capability while Built-in, Test cases, Test environment, Software process for testing.

A large number of techniques and frameworks should be proposed to improve the software testability. At last, we have seen that there is no clear guideline for software testing as well as handling the errors, it just varies on the aspect of software.

Table 2. Usage rates of testing using testing tools

<table>
<tr><th rowspan="3">Test Evaluation</th><th colspan="2">Activities</th><th>Evaluating test effort</th><th>Evaluating cost involved</th><th>Did Not Use</th></tr>
<tr><td rowspan="2">Usage Rates</td><td>Methods</td><td>59%</td><td>40%</td><td>19%</td></tr>
<tr><td>Tools</td><td>20%</td><td>24%</td><td>52%</td></tr>
<tr><th rowspan="3">Test Planning</th><th colspan="2">Activities</th><th>Deciding Test items</th><th>Finding testing risks</th><th>Did Not Use</th></tr>
<tr><td rowspan="2">Usage Rates</td><td>Methods</td><td>59%</td><td>35%</td><td>19%</td></tr>
<tr><td>Tools</td><td>22%</td><td>0%</td><td>55%</td></tr>
</table>

- **Test Evaluation**. It is a technique to calculate the resources, approximate time and cost needed to execute testing in a particular environment. From Table 2, we discover that about 19% of querists don't use the software testing methods. Evaluating test effort is an important part of it.

$$\text{Number of Test Cases} = (\text{Number of function Points}) \times 1.2 \qquad (1)$$

When we get the number of test cases, we can know the productivity of data from the unorganized data. According to the Table 2, the usage of tools and price estimation are quite low. There are various accurate techniques of Test Evaluation i.e. UCP method, WBS, PERT, Percentile distribution, Based on Experience, Function point technique. It needs various experience in different software life cycle to calculate the participation of tools and methods for testing. From the Table 2, there are 52% of querists using the software tools. It is the half of the querists. There are various accurate techniques of Test Evaluation. These are,

- UCP method
- WBS
- PERT
- Percentile distribution
- Based on Experience
- Function point technique
- **Test Planning**. It is a documentation in which test objectives, targets, schedules deadline, required resources etc. are described in detailed manner. It is also knows as a blue print of software testing. From Table 2, we know that approx. 55% of querists don't use the test planning tools. And about 19% of users don't use the testing methods which is quite low.

Table 3. Test report using test levels

Test Design		**Activities**		**Identifying test design**	**Identifying test cases**	**Did Not Use**
Test Levels	Unit Test	**Usage Rates**	Methods	35%	40%	25%
			Tools	12%	25%	51%
	Integration Test		Methods	51%	68%	15%
			Tools	22%	31%	39%
	System Test		Methods	51%	67%	12%
			Tools	29%	31%	24%
	Acceptance Test		Methods	30%	41%	35%
			Tools	12%	15%	53%
Test Execution		**Activities**		**Performing Tests**	**Recording test logs**	**Did Not Use**
Test Levels	Unit Test	**Usage Rates**	Methods	42%	32%	41%
			Tools	35%	29%	31%
	Integration Test		Methods	51%	48%	10%
			Tools	59%	64%	21%
	System Test		Methods	61%	61%	15%
			Tools	45%	29%	24%
	Acceptance Test		Methods	48%	37%	37%
			Tools	40%	35%	41%

Test Report	Activities		Writing test report	Documenting report	Did Not Use
	Usage Rates	Methods	61%	64%	19%
		Tools	55%	41%	21%

- **Test Design**. It is an action of obtaining and enumerating the test cases according to the test conditions for software testing. From the Table 3, we get to know that an average of 38% of users use the method of unit test which is quite low. We also discovered that an average of 19% of users use the testing tools.
- **Test Execution**. It is a process of performing the action code and expecting the desired result for software testing. We need to assign the test cases for test execution in any testing (Lee, Kang, & Lee, 2012). From the Table 3, the rate of test execution is comparatively high from the Test design. We can see that testing methods in test execution is widely used by the user for the Integration testing and system testing.
- **Test Report**. It is a documented summary of software testing activities, objectives and desired results. It can help the analysists, testing team, developers and product manager for understanding the quality of the software. It assures the acceptable level to our software application (Lee, Kang, & Lee, 2012). Form Table 3, an average of 63% of users use the testing method and an average of 76% of users use the testing tool for test reporting.

CONCLUSION

5W+1H testing is a guider for testing a software with the help of developers and can find the bugs as well as report the bugs to the software developer. It contains some questions to be asked to the software so that we can get the performance status of any software. With the help of this, we can develop the software according to our requirements. It is imperative to take into account the crucial issues related to testing, such as the organization of source codes and the overall system. With the help of 5W+1H, we can control our software cost with the help of the reports it will generate. We can test our software manually as well as automated as per our case. In this paper, we have de-scribe the open source and commercial tools that are available in the market for testing any software. With the help of these tools, we can apply the described methods that are mentioned in the paper. These methods include some node-path steps such that we can understand the data flow and testing flow of any software. Besides there are eleven steps for processing the testing easily with their requirements and output report that could be given. After that, we can also evaluate and validate the software comparing our needs from the software. The software needs i.e. security, price, speed etc. are very much essential for our software performance. Anyone can loss a life for single software bug. With this method, we decrease the software risks in the healthcare domain. This method is much better than the other normal comparing methods or any random method that is applied for software testing as shown in our results. As it can find the bugs very easily with the help of the questioning and can give better performance.

REFERENCES

Abbas, R., Sultan, Z. and Bhatti, S.N. (2017, April). Comparative analysis of automated load testing tools: Apache jmeter, microsoft visual studio (tfs), loadrunner, siege. In 2017 interna-tional conference on communication technologies (comtech) (pp. 39-44). IEEE.

Abd Rahman, N. H., Ibrahim, A. K., Hasikin, K., & Abd Razak, N. A. (2023). Critical device reliability assessment in healthcare services. *Journal of Healthcare Engineering, 2023*(1), 3136511. DOI: 10.1155/2023/3136511 PMID: 36860328

Ahamad, S. S., Al-Shehri, M., & Keshta, I. (2022). A secure and resilient scheme for telecare medical information systems with threat modeling and formal verification. *IEEE Access : Practical Innovations, Open Solutions, 10*, 120227–120244. DOI: 10.1109/ACCESS.2022.3217230

Al Naam, Y. A., Elsafi, S., Al Jahdali, M. H., Al Shaman, R. S., Al-Qurouni, B. H., & Al Zahrani, E. M. (2022). The impact of total automaton on the clinical laboratory workforce: A case study. *Journal of Healthcare Leadership, 14*, 55–62. DOI: 10.2147/JHL.S362614 PMID: 35586661

Anand, S., Burke, E. K., Chen, T. Y., Clark, J., Cohen, M. B., Grieskamp, W., Harman, M., Harrold, M. J., McMinn, P., Bertolino, A., Jenny Li, J., & Zhu, H. (2013). An orchestrated survey of methodologies for automated software test case genera-tion. *Journal of Systems and Software, 86*(8), 1978–2001. DOI: 10.1016/j.jss.2013.02.061

Andrews, J. H., Briand, L. C., & Labiche, Y. (2005, May). Is mutation an appropriate tool for testing experiments? In *Proceedings of the 27th international conference on Software engineering* (pp. 402-411).

Arcuri, A., & Yao, X. (2008). Search based software testing of object-oriented containers. *Information Sciences, 178*(15), 3075–3095. DOI: 10.1016/j.ins.2007.11.024

Arumugam, K., Naved, M., Shinde, P. P., Leiva-Chauca, O., Huaman-Osorio, A., & Gon-zales-Yanac, T. (2021). Multiple disease prediction using Machine learning algo-rithms. *Materials Today: Proceedings.*

Balch, J. A., Ruppert, M. M., Loftus, T. J., Guan, Z., Ren, Y., Upchurch, G. R., Ozrazgat-Baslanti, T., Rashidi, P., & Bihorac, A. (2023). Machine learning–enabled clinical information systems using fast healthcare interoperability resources data standards: Scoping review. *JMIR Medical Informatics, 11*, e48297. DOI: 10.2196/48297 PMID: 37646309

Budnik, C., Fraser, G., Lonetti, F., & Zhu, H. (2018). Special issue on automation of software testing: Improving practical applicability. *Software Quality Journal, 26*(4), 1415–1419. DOI: 10.1007/s11219-018-9410-1

Christodorescu, M., & Jha, S. (2004). Testing malware detectors. *Software Engineering Notes, 29*(4), 34–44. DOI: 10.1145/1013886.1007518

Davis, J., & Shepheard, J. (2024). Clinical documentation integrity: Its role in health data integrity, patient safety and quality outcomes and its impact on clinical coding and health information management. *The HIM Journal, 53*(2), 53–60. DOI: 10.1177/18333583231218029 PMID: 38073462

Davis, S. E., Walsh, C. G., & Matheny, M. E. (2023). This article was submitted to Health Informatics, a section of the journal Frontiers in Digital Health RECEIVED 31 May 2022 ACCEPTED 11 August 2022. Surfacing best practices for AI software development and integration in healthcare, 62.

Díaz, E., Tuya, J., Blanco, R., & Dolado, J. J. (2008). A tabu search algorithm for structural software testing. *Computers & Operations Research, 35*(10), 3052–3072. DOI: 10.1016/j.cor.2007.01.009

Fraser, G., & Arcuri, A. (2012, Jun). Sound empirical evidence in software testing. In 2012 34th International Conference on Software Engineering (ICSE) (pp. 178-188). IEEE. DOI: 10.1109/ICSE.2012.6227195

Galin, D. (2004). *Software quality assurance: from theory to implementation.* Pearson Education.

Gojare, S., Joshi, R., & Gaigaware, D. (2015). Analysis and design of selenium webdriver automation testing framework. *Procedia Computer Science, 50*, 341–346. DOI: 10.1016/j.procs.2015.04.038

Gurcan, F., & Cagiltay, N. E. (2019). Big data software engineering: Analysis of knowledge domains and skill sets using LDA-based topic modeling. *IEEE Access : Practical Innovations, Open Solutions, 7*, 82541–82552. DOI: 10.1109/ACCESS.2019.2924075

Haux, R. (2006). Health information systems–past, present, future. *International Journal of Medical Informatics, 75*(3-4), 268–281. DOI: 10.1016/j.ijmedinf.2005.08.002 PMID: 16169771

Hooda, I., & Chhillar, R. S. (2015). Software test process, testing types and techniques. *International Journal of Computer Applications, 111*(13), 10–14. DOI: 10.5120/19597-1433

Jain, A., & Rakesh, S. K. (2024, July). IoT-driven predictive healthcare system for proactive treatment and improved patient management. In AIP Conference Proceedings (Vol. 3111, No. 1). AIP Publishing. DOI: 10.1063/5.0221495

Jamil, M. A., Arif, M., Abubakar, N. S. A., & Ahmad, A. (2016, November). Software test-ing techniques: A literature review. In 2016 6th international conference on information and communication technology for the Muslim world (ICT4M) (pp. 177-182). IEEE.

Jan, S.R., Shah, S.T.U., Johar, Z.U., Shah, Y. and Khan, F. (2016). An innovative approach to investigate various software testing techniques and strategies. International Journal of Sci-entific Research in Science, Engineering and Technology (IJSRSET), Print ISSN, 23951990.

Jha, P., Sahu, M., Bisoy, S. K., & Sain, M. (2022). Application of Model-Based Software Testing in the Health Care Domain. *Electronics (Basel)*, *11*(13), 2062. DOI: 10.3390/electronics11132062

Jia, C., Cai, Y., Yu, Y. T., & Tse, T. H. (2016). 5W+ 1H pattern: A perspective of systematic mapping studies and a case study on cloud software testing. *Journal of Systems and Software*, *116*, 206–219. DOI: 10.1016/j.jss.2015.01.058

Jiwani, N., Gupta, K., & Whig, P. (2023). Machine Learning Approaches for Analysis in Smart Healthcare Informatics. In Machine Learning and Artificial Intelligence in Healthcare Systems (pp. 129-154). CRC Press.

Jordan, M. I., & Mitchell, T. M. (2015). Machine learning: Trends, perspectives, and pro-spects. *Science*, *349*(6245), 255–260. DOI: 10.1126/science.aaa8415 PMID: 26185243

Keane, P. A., & Topol, E. J. (2018). With an eye to AI and autonomous diagnosis. *NPJ Digital Medicine*, *1*(1), 1–3. DOI: 10.1038/s41746-018-0048-y PMID: 31304321

Khinvasara, T., Shankar, A., & Wong, C. (2024). Robustness and Reliability Testing in Healthcare Using Artificial Intelligence. *Asian Journal of Research in Computer Science*, *17*(7), 103–118. DOI: 10.9734/ajrcos/2024/v17i7482

Larsson, E., & Thesing, M. (2024). Change Management Strategies for Seamless Adoption of Digital Healthcare Solutions in the Healthcare Industry.

Lawanna, A. (2012). The theory of software testing. *AU Journal of Technology*, *16*(1).

Lee, J., Kang, S., & Lee, D. (2012). Survey on software testing practices. *IET Software*, *6*(3), 275–282. DOI: 10.1049/iet-sen.2011.0066

Li, W., Chai, Y., Khan, F., Jan, S. R. U., Verma, S., Menon, V. G., & Li, X. (2021). A com-prehensive survey on machine learning-based big data analytics for IoT-enabled smart healthcare system. *Mobile Networks and Applications*, *26*(1), 234–252. DOI: 10.1007/s11036-020-01700-6 PMID: 40477400

Magrabi, F., Lyell, D., & Coiera, E. (2023). Automation in contemporary clinical information systems: A survey of AI in healthcare settings. *Yearbook of Medical Informatics*, *32*(01), 115–126. DOI: 10.1055/s-0043-1768733 PMID: 38147855

Mustafa, K. M., Al-Qutaish, R. E., & Muhairat, M. I. (2009, December). Classification of software testing tools based on the software testing methods. In *2009 Second International Conference on Computer and Electrical Engineering* (Vol. 1, pp. 229-233). IEEE. DOI: 10.1109/ICCEE.2009.9

Nawaz, A., Khan, S. S., & Ahmad, A. (2024). Ensemble of Autoencoders for Anomaly Detection in Biomedical Data: A Narrative Review. *IEEE Access : Practical Innovations, Open Solutions*, *12*, 17273–17289. DOI: 10.1109/ACCESS.2024.3360691

Nawaz, M., & Ahmed, J. (2022). Cloud-based healthcare framework for real-time anomaly detection and classification of 1-D ECG signals. *PLoS One*, *17*(12), e0279305. DOI: 10.1371/journal.pone.0279305 PMID: 36574391

Okolo, C. A., Ijeh, S., Arowoogun, J. O., Adeniyi, A. O., & Omotayo, O. (2024). Reviewing the impact of health information technology on healthcare management efficiency. *International Medical Science Research Journal*, *4*(4), 420–440. DOI: 10.51594/imsrj.v4i4.1000

Olaboye, J. A.Queen-Mary Akudo EbugosiJanet Aderonke Olaboye. (2024). Optimizing healthcare resource allocation through data-driven demographic and psychographic analysis. *Computer Science & IT Research Journal*, *5*(6), 1488–1504. DOI: 10.51594/csitrj.v5i6.1249

Orso, A., & Rothermel, G. (2014). Software testing: a research travelogue (2000–2014). In Future of Software Engineering Proceedings (pp. 117-132).

Panch, T., Mattie, H., & Celi, L. A. (2019). The “inconvenient truth” about AI in healthcare. *NPJ Digital Medicine*, *2*(1), 1–3. DOI: 10.1038/s41746-019-0155-4 PMID: 31453372

Popescu, C., El-Chaarani, H., El-Abiad, Z., & Gigauri, I. (2022). Implementation of health information systems to improve patient identification. *International Journal of Environmental Research and Public Health*, *19*(22), 15236. DOI: 10.3390/ijerph192215236 PMID: 36429954

Qayyum, A., Qadir, J., Bilal, M., & Al-Fuqaha, A. (2020). Secure and robust machine learning for healthcare: A survey. *IEEE Reviews in Biomedical Engineering*, *14*, 156–180. DOI: 10.1109/RBME.2020.3013489 PMID: 32746371

Rafi, D. M., Moses, K. R. K., Petersen, K., & Mäntylä, M. V. (2012, June). Benefits and limitations of automated software testing: Systematic literature review and practitioner survey. In 2012 7th International Workshop on Automation of Software Test (AST) (pp. 36-42). IEEE.

Rana, I., Goswami, P., & Maheshwari, H. (2019). A review of tools and techniques used in software testing. *Int. J. Emerg. Technol. Innovative Res*, *6*(4), 262–266.

Richardson, J., Iezzi, A., Khan, M. A., & Maxwell, A. (2014). Validity and reliability of the Assessment of Quality of Life (AQoL)-8D multi-attribute utility instrument. *Patient*, *7*(1), 85–96. DOI: 10.1007/s40271-013-0036-x PMID: 24271592

Tang, L., Li, J., & Fantus, S. (2023). Medical artificial intelligence ethics: A systematic review of empirical studies. *Digital Health*, *9*, 20552076231186064. DOI: 10.1177/20552076231186064 PMID: 37434728

Turhan, B., & Bener, A. B. (2007, Jul). Software Defect Prediction: Heuristics for Weighted Naïve Bayes. In ICSOFT (SE) (pp. 244-249).

Unterkalmsteiner, M., Gorschek, T., Islam, A. M., Cheng, C. K., Permadi, R. B., & Feldt, R. (2011). Evaluation and measurement of software process improvement—A systematic litera-ture review. *IEEE Transactions on Software Engineering*, *38*(2), 398–424. DOI: 10.1109/TSE.2011.26

Watkins, A. L. (1995). "The automatic generation of test data using genetic algorithms." In *Proceedings of the 4th software quality conference*, vol. 2, pp. 300-309. 1995.

Wegener, J., Baresel, A., & Sthamer, H. (2001). Evolutionary test environment for automatic structural testing. *Information and Software Technology*, *43*(14), 841–854. DOI: 10.1016/S0950-5849(01)00190-2

Yari, A., Yousefi Khoshsabegheh, H., Zarezadeh, Y., Amraei, M., Soufi Boubakran, M., & Motlagh, M. E. (2023). Iranian primary healthcare system's response to the COVID-19 pandemic using the healthcare incident command system. *PLoS One*, *18*(8), e0290273. DOI: 10.1371/journal.pone.0290273 PMID: 37607162

Chapter 2
AI, IoT, and Cognitive Computing for Mental Health Enhancement and Object Detection

K. K. Baseer
https://orcid.org/0000-0002-4524-2922
Department of Computer Science & Engineering, GITAM School of Technology, GITAM University, Bengaluru, India

Nalavala Ramanjaneya Reddy
https://orcid.org/0000-0002-7915-711X
Department of Computer Science & Engineering, RGM College of Engineering and Technology (Autonomous), Nandyal, India

T. Satyendra Kumar
Department of CS and IOT, Malla Reddy University, Hyderabad, India

Harishchander Anandaram
https://orcid.org/0000-0003-2993-5304
Department of Artificial Intelligence, Amrita Vishwa Vidyapeetham, Coimbatore, India

Alavikunhu Panthakkan
https://orcid.org/0000-0002-2065-6539
University of Dubai, Dubai, UAE

DOI: 10.4018/979-8-3693-6094-1.ch002

ABSTRACT

This chapter explores the potential of AI, IoT, and cognitive computing in improving mental health care and object detection technologies. AI-driven cognitive computing and IoT-enabled devices could enhance personalized, efficient, and real-time mental health solutions. Cognitive computing models will be able to analyze the huge streams of data coming from wearables, for instance, and enable early warnings of mental health issues. Monitoring behavioral patterns will be provided through cognitive computing models, with proactive interventions delivered based on early warning signs. Object detection powered by cognitive computing will offer the capability to identify with precision various environmental factors that may exert effects on one's mental well-being, including crowding, noise, or temperature changes. The integration of these technologies will transform mental health care from a reactive service to a preventive and data-driven approach, thereby enhancing patient outcomes.

INTRODUCTION

A deep intersection of AI, IoT, and cognitive computing is transforming mental health care and object detection from its very roots, thus opening up fresh avenues for innovation. Transiently increasing mental health concerns worldwide have led to the need for preventive, accessible, and personalized solution interventions in mental health care. Conventional approaches to mental health fundamentally rely on time-consuming and subjective in-person assessments through self-report measures, which are limited in scope and not entirely timely. Instead, integration of AI and IoT heralds a new era in mental health care-that will use real-time data on the detection of mental health concerns, assess related environmental influences, and provide targeted interventions(Gál et al., 2021). This chapter addresses how cognitive computing AI, along with the capabilities of IoT, may revolutionize mental health care and improve detection techniques of objects, showing how these two technologies complement each other toward advancement in better patient outcomes while also opening pathways to increased accessibility of services and changing the face of mental health services towards the preventive care model.

Mental health issues have already seen the light of how advantageous AI can become, through predictive analytics, pattern recognition, and superior data processing. For example, these machine learning algorithms will enable detection of behavioral patterns, voice tone, and facial expressions so that you can notice initial signs of depression or anxiety or some other disorder. Connected with IoT devices-wearables, for instance-AI will also be able to monitor your vital signs, sleep patterns, and levels of physical activity-all critical indicators of mental health(Salami et al.,

2019). These data points are continuously being collected from IoT devices, which send such information to cognitive computing platforms; AI algorithms then work to process and interpret them in an effort to deliver actionable insights. This will mean that cognitive computing and IoT devices are synergistically collaborating in the collection, analysis, and interpretation of complex datasets to allow health professionals to monitor their patients' mental health better and intervene at an earlier stage. This integration allows to heighten the personalization of care by creating real-time, evolving individual health profiles, based on the user's ongoing behavior, physiological metrics, and even their surroundings(Ströhle, 2019).

Object detection is one of the most widely known and critical capabilities at the intersection of cognitive computing and IoT, such as identifying elements within the physical environment that could impact a person's mental state. Object detection enables cognitive computing systems to identify various environmental stressors such as loud noises, dim lighting, or crowded spaces that can contribute or add on mental health conditions(Smith & Merwin, 2021). For instance, a person diagnosed with anxiety may be abnormally discombobulated by crowded public places or loud environments. The cameras or sensors can detect these factors and alert the cognitive computing systems, thus soliciting precautionary actions. These metrics can be referred to a person's real-time behavioral metrics for a 360° perspective of stimulation factors that affect mental health. These impacts are understood and addressed through cognitive computing and IoT technology(Foy et al., 2019).

Wearable devices will form the heart of IoT, especially health applications, to add a layer of non-intrusive but efficient real-time monitoring. Devices like smartwatches, fitness bands, and even specific wearables monitoring mental health take persistent reading on heart rate variability, quality of sleep, activity levels-all signals pointing to the mental and emotional status of a person. All of these data streams are then transmitted to powerful platforms empowered with AI capabilities, where data sets are subjected to crossing cognitive models to detect anomalies. For example, it can identify the onset of depression or even anxiety by significant change in activity or sleep quality(Hrabok et al., 2020). These devices can alert health practitioners to step in and provide an intervention at early times, or send notifications to relax or even alert the family members or providers for the judgment of a serious mental health problem. Therefore, while IoT integration in the mental health field allows continued tracking of health, it also offers quick and context-specific responses that empower patients and caregivers alike.

Cognitive computing benefits in mental health are greatly valued due to their ability to process and interpret high volumes of data within a sensitive understanding. It is the type of model that mimics human thought processes through a computerized model; therefore, it learns from vast datasets, identifies patterns, and even simulates the emotional response to a degree. In the mental health case, cognitive computing may analyze diverse sources of information—to enumerate: text from therapy session transcripts, speech patterns, and social media posts—leading to the detection of slight cues for mental illness(Almeida et al., 2020). For example, linguistic analytics may uncover depression through change in vocabulary and tone, while social media monitoring may also help in discovering the withdrawal behaviors of people at risk. Coupled with IoT data, cognitive computing provides a multi-dimensional view of an individual's mental wellness, thus enabling predictive modeling and personalized recommendations for care.

Preventive mental health care is one of the promising aspects in putting together AI, IoT, and cognitive computing. Traditional approaches to mental health care largely focus on dealing with issues after they get full manifestations. This is less effective and resource-intensive. It becomes possible with real-time monitoring and data analytics. Early detection of the patterns there are before such episodes of mental health-episodes like stagnated behavior, irregular sleep, or increased social withdrawal creates opportunities for action by health providers that may prevent a full mental health crisis from unfolding. What's more, the algorithms that run cognitive computing learn over time and gradually introduce improvements to their models based on new information, further making preventive care more precise and pertinent to each person's unique situation(Hickey et al., 2021).

Despite these developments, there is still a myriad of ethical and practical issues that need to be addressed to unlock fully the potential of AI, IoT, and cognitive computing in mental health care. Data privacy and security are the most pressing concerns in this regard; people are constantly handing over sensitive personal information that is regularly transmitted and analyzed. This is a base upon which user trust is built-that the data are handled securely and responsibly. Advances in digital mental health solutions have further raised questions regarding consent and ownership of data. Evidently, patients require knowledge of what is done with their data and who accesses it(Hickey et al., 2021). There is also the risk of over-reliance on technology-based mental health solutions. AI and IoT augment the processes of mental health care but cannot replace human empathy and clinician expertise. Technology should enhance rather than substitute the traditional therapeutic relationship, thereby allowing the human element to be at the core of mental health care.

The issue of equity and access to these technologies must also be considered. While AI and IoT-enabled health solutions are more readily available in urban cities and economically developed regions, they are probably scarce in rural and low-income regions due to prohibitive cost, limited access to internet, or low infrastructure. If these technologies are to become options in handling global mental health challenges, then surely there is the need for them to be non-discriminatory and non-disparaging(Hickey et al., 2021). There is still emerging research on the long-term effects and effectiveness of AI and IoT in mental health care. To adequately assess long-term impacts on mental health outcomes, longer longitudinal studies are needed to guide future innovations and policy.

The convergence of AI, IoT, and cognitive computing is revolutionizing mental health care-from making it more data-driven, preventive, and responsive. These technologies can be harnessed by mental health professionals, and with their support, they would gain a much better understanding of the psychology behind the minds of their patients and could respond even more effectively. However, attaining such full potential requires extreme care about the ethical, practical, and societal challenges involved(Hua et al., 2024). These factors will ensure AI and IoT maintain the foreground of mental health care as highly effective enhancers of patient outcome while still respecting rights and making accessibility to all segments of populations. As AI, IoT, and cognitive computing advance, this will very likely redefine the face of mental health care: mentally healthy people whose mental health is continuously monitored, understood, and supported in ways that some of us thought unthinkable just a few years ago.

Objectives

This chapter tries to explore how the integration of Artificial Intelligence (AI), Internet of Things (IoT), and cognitive computing can be used in the enhancement of mental health care and object detection. I will therefore outline how AI and IoT can be utilized in tracking and analyzing the real-time mental health indicators, how cognitive computing promotes object detection and usage in identification of degrading or supporting environmental factors toward mental wellbeing. Then, I will continue with the point on the practical applicability of such technologies toward preventive mental healthcare before raising ethical and privacy concerns around data utilization in health monitoring. This chapter offers quite broad insight into emerging technologies that have been used toward the enactment of modern mental health practices.

THE ROLE OF AI IN MENTAL HEALTH CARE

The first application of AI to the field of mental health-a space that is sure to be highly influential-offers new ways of diagnosing, monitoring, and even treating mental health disorders with a precision and scalability impossible before. Indeed, AI technologies can fetch data from a range of sources, analyze it, identify patterns, and detect risk factors associated with mental health disorders, thus enabling clinicians to take best decisions at the right times(Dong et al., 2020). AI can be involved in every stage of mental health care-from early detection of disorders, through real-time monitoring and intervention-altering the very landscape of mental health care as a more proactive, individually tailored discipline. The pliability of machine learning and predictive analytics marries greater accuracy and efficiency, offering facilities that the mental health arena has never before seen. Applications of AI in Mental Health Disorders with the Role of Machine Learning and Predictive Analytics This chapter explains the role of machine learning and predictive analytics with benefits and limitations in the usage of AI in mental health.

Figure 1. The role of AI In Mental Health Care

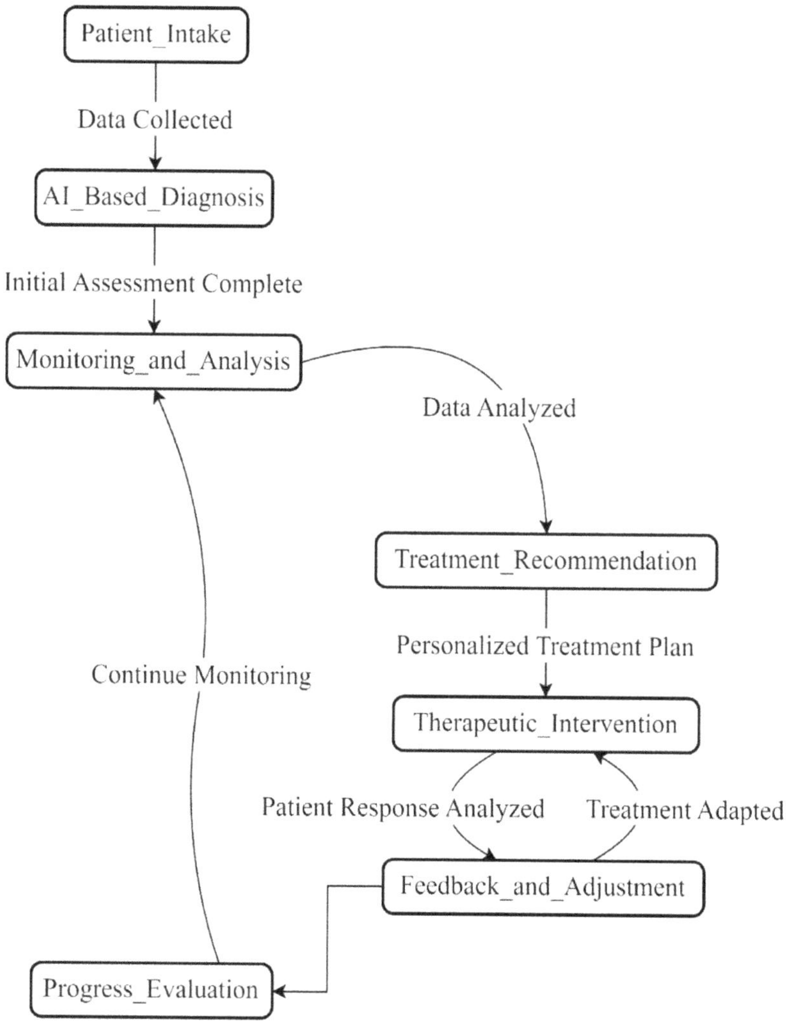

The use of AI in the stages of interaction, from diagnosis to monitoring and potential treatment, is enhancing precision and adaptability as shown in Figure 1.

Applications of AI in Detecting Mental Health Disorders

AI is transforming the ways mental health conditions are detected, by establishing patterns in speech, text, facial expressions, and even biological indicators. Mental conditions often classified as depression, anxiety, or bipolar are subjective in nature. Moreover, it is self-reporting, and the patients may hide from this mode of detection when they fail to report it in a subtle frame. Thus, AI-based systems may overcome this limitation by making use of machine learning algorithms to find pattern flows that may indicate mental health issues(Suryadevara, 2022).

One of the largest applications of AI in mental health diagnostics comes through the application of Natural Language Processing, by which algorithms can analyze the use of language both verbally and in writing. Already, research has demonstrated the possibility of proving that those individuals diagnosed with depression "use more negative words when speaking or writing, are egocentric, or exhibit another set of linguistic characteristics, such as repetition and obsessive focus on other topics.". The AI models can analyze social media posts, text messages, or spoken conversations, thereby helping clinicians to identify such patterns that may otherwise be overlooked. Indeed, it has become a valuable tool in the detection of mental conditions. This is the case since social media mostly provides a baseline view that may take place outside the clinical settings and unfiltered.

Finally, analysis of facial expressions and speech patterns can be monitored. This means that the AI-driven computer vision algorithms can analyze facial micro-expressions, the tone of voice, and speech rhythm to distinguish signs of emotional distress or instability. For example, slow and monotonous speech indicates the depressive states, and speedy, animated speech could be a marker of manic episodes. Perhaps more importantly, wearable devices like fitness trackers and smartwatches have become increasingly accessible for the measurement of physiological data, including heart rate variability and sleep patterns, which are sensitive markers of mental health. AI can spot anomalies in those biological signals that may indicate potential problems in mental health if those signals are well correlated with behavioral data. It is through this multi-modal approach that data from text, audio, and physiological monitoring converge to paint a clearer picture of an individual's mental health.

Machine Learning and Predictive Analytics in Mental Health

Machine learning and predictive analytics are two of the fundamental ingredients of AI and its role in the field of mental health. It enables the system to learn from historic data; hence the capability to recognize and make better predictions about the patterns of events over time. This is very helpful in the context of mental health, where early signs can be caught and treated before symptoms escalate. Predictive analytics is a type of machine learning that uses statistical techniques to predict future outcomes based on information drawn from both historic and real-time data(D'Alfonso, 2020).

One of the most widely applied uses of predictive analytics in the mental health domain is the prediction of suicide. With respect to past cases, and with historical data used to train predictive models, one can determine who is more likely to commit suicide based on such factors as past mental history, behavioral indicators, and environmental stressors. A few AI systems use predictive analytics to monitor the streams of information regarding patients from health records, wearable devices, and social media to predict when an individual might be likely to suffer from their mental health crisis. For example, an AI model can analyze changes in sleep patterns, social withdrawal, and negative sentiment in communication to send alerts to the caregiver or healthcare professionals.

Machine learning also produces customized treatment plans. On the other hand, responses to therapies could be greatly diverse among patients; therefore, the search for the best therapy would take a long time. AI models can help by analyzing data from various patients to identify their treatment patterns, enabling clinicians to recommend personalized interventions. For instance, machine learning may analyze the number of successes and failures through various therapies for profiles of similar patients and thus optimize treatment plans and minimize the time before relief of symptoms is obtained. In this regard, AI should inform which interventions are likely to be successful so that personalization and effectiveness in mental health care would be strengthened.

Benefits and Challenges of Applying AI in Mental Health

There are several advantages of AI integration in mental care. Most importantly, AI increases the diagnostic intensity through determinations that human diagnosis may miss. Since complexities or comorbidities can be true to diagnosis when depressive anxiety forms, and such instances call for specific therapeutic programs, an AI system equips the clinician with increased detective prowess at this level. Most importantly, the use of AI allows early intervention of mental health issues before they advance to critical stages of development. Data feedback through AI and wearable devices continues to monitor in real time, unlike traditional settings where the treatment is periodic, thus providing a dynamic impression of the patient's mental status(Swayamsiddha & Mohanty, 2020).

Accessibility is maximized by AI through the following. Digital tools, including a chatbot and mobile apps, can provide support anytime, even reaching people in remote or under-served areas lacking access to other mental health services. For instance, AI chatbots who have undergone training in CBT can help the victims of such mild and moderate mental problems. Psychological treatments are supplemented by these resources because they fill the gap toward seeking mental health services between this people group and other individuals who may not pass through regular therapy.

However, its integration into mental health care also brings with it numerous challenges. The foremost one is related to data privacy and security. Mental health-related data are highly sensitive in nature and need to be protected rigorously. It is thus crucial that the AI system must adhere to stringent standards of data protection so as to achieve the confidence of the patient. Ethical considerations involving potential misuse of personal data necessitate the presence of strong data governance policies to prevent breaches and unauthorized access.

Another issue is algorithmic bias. AI works only as well as the data that it was trained on. When diversity is lacking in the training data, so may be skewed the diagnostic and predictive capabilities of the AI model. For instance, if the principal learning of an AI system is done on a data set that applies merely to one demographic group, it will not be as effective at an exact assessment of people from different backgrounds, and there could be misdiagnoses or other less than ideal treatment recommendations. Thus, training AI systems on diverse datasets is vital to avoid those biases and move towards equal health care for all.

Such AI for mental health lacks regulations, which thereby makes it difficult to standardize and validate the technologies. Pharmaceutical clinical trials are much tougher than those developed using AI for mental health, which have no uniform regulation; therefore, their effectiveness and reliability may vary. Clear guidelines in the development and deployment of AI in mental health will be crucial to its successful integration into healthcare.

AI has the potential to radically transform mental health care, from enhancing the accuracy of diagnoses to the provision of treatment options. Applications like NLP, facial recognition, wearable monitoring, and predictive analytics can all be used by AI to understand mental health and present early interventions. However, realizing this potential requires dealing with some challenges related to data privacy, algorithmic bias, and regulatory oversight. Human care should be supplemented by AI to enhance the work of mental health professionals instead of replacing them. A balanced approach to these challenges will see AI become invaluable to improving mental health outcomes and accessibility.

Figure 2. Integration of IoT (Internet of Things) in Mental Health Monitoring

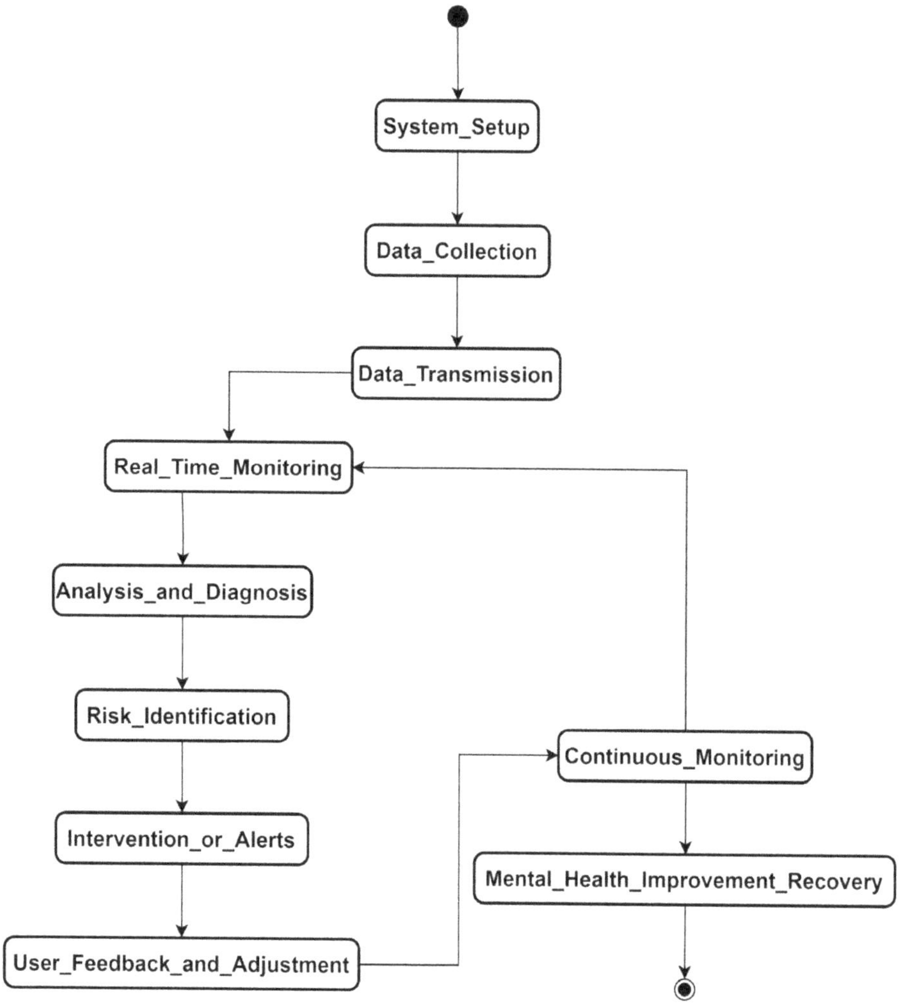

IOT IN MENTAL HEALTH MONITORING

The Internet of Things is widely revolutionizing the health sector as patients can now have data collected in real time, be continuously monitored, and improvements in patient outcomes through IoT in many areas of medicine, such as the psychological. IoT refers to a network of connected devices, which collects, transmits, and analyses data, where remote insights are derived into a patient's physical and psychological well-being. Undoubtedly, IoT has revolutionized the face of mental health care by giving opportunities for regular monitoring-which is especially important for conditions where continuous observation would be necessary(Mody & Mody, 2019). The paper breaks it down to cover the overview of the use of IoT devices in healthcare, the involvement of wearable technology in monitoring mental health, and the opportunities that the real-time collection and analysis of data present toward more personalized and responsive mental health care.'

The use of IoT in Mental Health Monitoring has been shown to improve patient outcomes, as illustrated in Figure 2. The system enables real-time data collection, continuous monitoring, and proactive intervention through wearables and environmental sensors.

IoT Devices in Healthcare

Indeed, the IoT is very dominant in health technology innovation as it provides a multiplicity of solutions either aimed at supporting a person's physical or mental well-being. Going as simple as fitness trackers to more advanced diagnostic tools even in smart home systems that assist in the gathering of information regarding one's current health status in real-time. Applications of IoE devices in healthcare include monitoring critical physiological metrics such as heart rate, blood pressure, respiratory rate, sleep patterns, and activity levels. These are important not only for physical but also mental health since physiological characteristics are highly correlated with a person's psychological states(Mody & Mody, 2019; Osifeko et al., 2020).

This is unprecedented opportunity for remote monitoring, especially for those patients who cannot frequently visit healthcare facilities. Capturing continuous data, IoT devices allow healthcare professionals to track mood changes, behavioral patterns, and even potential mental health triggers without relying heavily on patient self-reporting, which is usually plagued by memory bias and personal interpretation. Some other IoT devices could also catch the attention of a caregiver or family member if unusual patterns are observed, such as long periods of inactivity or interruptions in sleep, which might indicate some kind of mental health crisis.

One of the biggest benefits of IoT in healthcare is its ability to create a holistic image of the patient's health: there are various data points that integrate over time, and this is particularly helpful in the area of mental health because symptoms and triggers often fluctuate. Advanced data analytics allows mental health professionals to tap into the trends and patterns that are not possible to be looked into in traditional episodic assessments. Thus, IoT devices fill the bridge created between clinical visits through seamless continuity in care required for cffective management of mental health.

Wearable Technology for Mental Health

Wearable technology has become popular in the realm of mental health monitoring due to its portability, affordability, and its capacity to naturally acquire data from users. The types of wearables that can take on such physiological measurements as are associated with mental well-being include a smartwatch, fitness trackers, and health monitors, such as EDA, skin temperature, and heart rate variability, which have been well established to be connected to states of stress or emotional arousal(Hickey et al., 2021; Hua et al., 2024).

Devices can only capture record, and monitor stress, anxiety or depressive states indirectly through electrocardiogram signals such as high heart rate or increased skin conductance, for example. However low heart variability could be associated with the depressive state. Capturing these signals in wearable devices can help track the daily fluctuations of mental health as well as possible insights into symptom development. Advanced sensors and algorithms in devices such as Fitbit, Apple Watch, and Whoop make them useful not only for activity tracking and monitoring sleep patterns but also mental health insights. Most of these wearables offer some form of features that encourage relaxation, from guided breathing exercises to benefit those with anxiety or stress-related disorders.

The Muse headband and the Spire Stone are wearables dedicated totally to mental health, taking this to the level of metrics specifically relevant to mental health. For example, the Muse headband has EEG sensors tracking brain waves during meditation and monitors the ways in which the mind is relaxed and focused throughout. The Spire Stone, meanwhile monitors the breathing pattern giving instantaneous feedback and alerts in case of irregular breathing patterns that prove to be a common precursor to stress. Such machines are capable of helping the users get a better understanding of their mental health as they feed them real-time information regarding their physiological states thus enhancing self-awareness as well as proactive coping mechanisms.

The conveniences and accessibilities of wearables make them an attractive option for people unlikely to seek traditional support for mental health. Wearables blend mental health monitoring into everyday devices, making it easier for users to monitor their mental health discreetly, without the stigmas often associated with mental health assessments.

Real-Time Data Monitoring

Perhaps the greatest strength in using IoT for mental health monitoring is real-time data collection. Contrary to traditional mental health monitoring, which is check-in at scheduled intervals, IoT devices are set up to provide constant streams of data such that a more responsive approach to management can be taken. Real-time monitoring of mental health means that any particular pattern or sudden shift in a person's mental health can be detected at the point it occurs, in time for appropriate action(Lee et al., 2021; Mody & Mody, 2019).

For example, if there is an acute elevation of heart rate along with various broken sleep patterns and lesser physical exertion, IoT devices would alarmingly point to the changes in association with anxiety or depression. This data may then be passed on to mental health professionals or indicated to their care providers so interventions involving direct communication might be over telehealth sessions or automated indications to engage with care activities. Such proactive measures help prevent situations from reaching the level of mental health crisis and have a better outcome for the patient by dealing with them at an early stage.

Apart from this direct patient care, real-time data from IoT devices can be used with predictive analytics to manage mental health. The machine learning algorithm would, based on longitudinal data, identify patterns and predict the future mental status of the patient. For instance, this possibility implies that AI-driven models can predict episodes of depression or anxiety with real-time data from wearables to enable preventive care strategies and limit the severity and duration of episodes. Such predictability is also particularly useful for patients who are chronic mental health care takers and require continuous adjustment in their treatment plan.

Real-time monitoring also makes self-management easy because users can view their data and, in turn, see how changes in lifestyles impact mental health. Therefore, patients begin to track their changes and find specific triggers and modify their behavior for enhanced mental well-being. For example, if the user finds that his or her stress level increases when they sleep for less time, then he or she will be likely to regard sleep more as a worthwhile asset. This will promote self-awareness as real-time data collection empowers the individual to take control and conduct things better with themselves.

IoT is transforming the landscape of mental health monitoring by establishing a continuous data acquisition, real-time monitoring, and proactive intervention through long-serving devices that track physiological signals. Advanced analytics interpret patterns, more personalized, and responsive care for mental health professionals. In monitoring mental health, there is much that is exciting about IoT for the patient and clinician: a holistic approach towards assessment that goes beyond face-to-face practice. It carries along with it challenges such as issues of privacy and data security, but these also make a case for the benefits of IoT in mental care-thereby making it one of the most promising tools for better mental health outcome in larger scale numbers.

COGNITIVE COMPUTING IN OBJECT DETECTION FOR MENTAL HEALTH

From integrating cognitive computing with object detection, new avenues open for understanding the impact that environmental factors can make upon mental well-being. Cognitive computing is a blend of artificial intelligence, machine learning, and natural language processing put into simulating human thought processes so as to enable systems to make profoundly complex decisions based on data(Gál et al., 2021; Salami et al., 2019). The object detection technique enhances the ability to identify and interpret environmental stressors and possible mental health triggers through cognitive computing. The fundamental principles of cognitive computing and object detection are being covered in this chapter as well as the ways in which environmental factors influence mental health problems, including some practical applications of where object detection can assist in realizing influences on mental health. The figure 3 illustrates how the environment can impact individuals' mental states, providing valuable insights for implementing preventive mental health measures.

Figure 3. Cognitive Computing in Object Detection for Mental Health

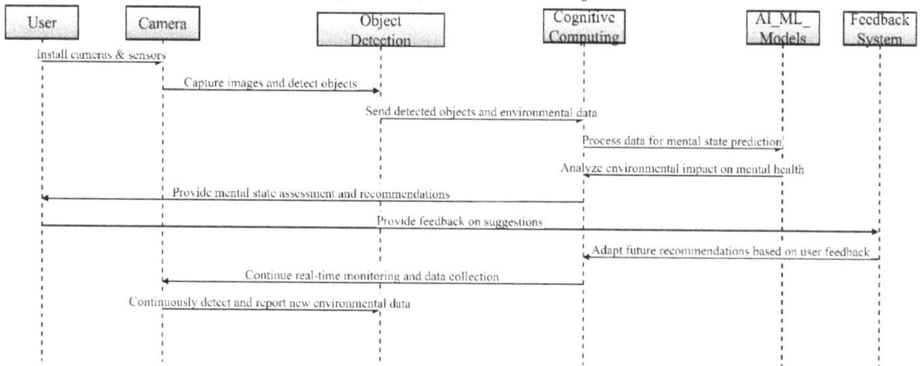

Cognitive Computing and Object Detection: Understanding Environmental Triggers for Mental Health Illnesses

Cognitive computing processes a human cognitive process and simulates the manner in which the human brain operates. Therefore, computers can scan unstructured data, learn from it, and make decisions that are reasoned upon this information. Such ability holds a lot of value particularly in areas like mental health, where conditions can be influenced by the interplay of complex psychological as well as environmental factors. Cognitive systems are engineered to handle very large volumes of information, including sensory data, text, images, or even voice recordings, and then extract insights from all this data. These data can be interpreted to imply patterns regarding mental health in terms of the emotional state and behavior change, as well as response to external stimuli, if processed by sophisticated algorithms in cognitive computing systems(Suryadevara, 2022; Zhao et al., 2022).

Object detection is computer vision, a part wherein objects present in the images or videos are identified and classified. Object detection systems could, with the help of some machine learning algorithms, analyze visual data and recognize and evaluate some specific objects and their association within their surroundings. In mental health, object detection could give insight into the visual cue of his or her surroundings, habits, and environmental stressors it may cause. For example, the determination that his environment is cluttered or chaotic might be associated with higher levels of stress, and some objects, such as bottles of alcohol or drug paraphernalia, are indicators for triggers of substance abuse.

Combining cognitive computing with object detection enables real-time capturing of a mental health monitor as to how the surrounding factors might impact one's mental state. Through chronic analysis of external influences, such technological advancements bridge this gap between influences and their consequences on mental health, thus moving towards a more holistic approach for better mental well-being.

Environmental Stressors

Mental health is not purely an internal psychological matter; significant influences often arise from external environmental stressors. Cognitive computing in alliance with object detection technology can identify and quantify the influence of such stressors to estimate how much a person could be influenced in terms of his mental state. Typical environmental stressors that can affect mental health range from noise, crowding, pollution, lighting, or visible disorder or clutter within living or working spaces. By identifying these factors and analyzing them, cognitive systems are able to infer the existence of stress-inducing conditions that might spur the affects of anxiety, depression, and stress-related disorders, among others(Smith & Merwin, 2021).

For instance, high noise levels have been known to increase stress and anxiety levels as a direct result of the massive and increased level of noise experienced within urban regions. An audio-sensitive object detection system could continuously monitor levels of noise and alert those individuals or caregivers if the noises are set too high against thresholds recognized to be distressing. The same is true for continuous exposure to low lighting or dark environments, which a person may feel could have an effect on one's mood and cause lethargy. Under such circumstances, ambient light levels can be surveilled by object detection systems and suggest changes if the perception is that the lighting environment is impacting their mental health negatively.

Clutter or disorganization of the living space can also serve as a precursor to potential depressive states. Clutter has been linked with stress, low productivity, and mental health issues, such as depression. Cognitive systems employing object detection can detect excessive messiness and offer nudges or suggestions to clean up, which may help improve the individual's mental well-being. Cognitive computing systems offer a proactive means to identify these stressors so that people can manage and reduce their exposure to environmental factors that affect their mental health.

Identifying Influences in Mental Health through Object Detection

Monitoring of Living Conditions for Depression or Anxiety Symptoms: Cognitive computing system implementing object detection will monitor an individual's living condition for signs that indicate the onset of a mental health episode. An example is a living space that becomes messy and cluttered, a sign of a depressive episode or lost motivation. Patterns of clutter will be noted by algorithms in object detection software and trigger an alert to the individual or caregiver to intervene accordingly.

Technology to monitor objects can further be utilized to monitor social interactions and activity in shared spaces. For example, when a cognitive system observes the drastic decline in activities of social interaction or continued absence of interaction in social places, the possibility is social withdrawal; a very common feature of depression and anxiety disorders as well. In such instances, the system will notify the caregivers, which results in timely visits and interventions. Object detection can enable cognitive computing to identify objects like alcohol cans or drug parading items around the person. The same can serve as an early warning for those undergoing mental health treatment or have a risk of substance abuse. Upon the detection of such objects by the system, it may alert health care providers or request mental health resources, thus allowing for timely intervention.

Environmental Trigger Analysis for PTSD Patients: Most people with PTSD have identifiable environmental triggers that cause episodes of stress or anxiety. Object detection, combined with the aid of cognitive computing, enables the environment to be analyzed such that some triggers may be detected and categorized, such as loud noises or particular objects reminding patients of traumatic experiences. For instance, if an individual is sensitized to particular visual or audio triggers, which characterize the specific traumatic experiences he had, the network can send him alerts warning him to avoid certain places or equip him with techniques to cope up with his response.

Emotions can be introduced in smart homes by incorporating object detection systems and cognitive computing to integrate with smart homes. This can change the lighting, play soothing music, or give out calming scents every time there are detected signs of stress. Therefore, individuals will be able to keep their emotions in check, and preventive measures will be undertaken to handle the situation as much as possible. It might be especially helpful in the case of anxiety disorders, with changes in environment prompting relaxation and decreased stress levels.

Combining cognitive computing with object detection would open the door for a dramatic improvement in mental care through the detection of environmental influences in relation to mental well-being. Cognitive systems using object detection technology can assess myriad stressors in the environment, ranging from disorganized living space and dim lighting to social isolation and potential substance use triggers. Reveal these forces, and cognitive computing provides insights that are ordinary mental health diagnostics stepping further toward more personalized and preventive care. The applications of cognitive computing in object detection for mental health are likely to continue expanding with the progression of technology, providing ever more sophisticated tools to understand and apply a way to manage the impact of the environment on mental health. Through continuous surveillance and analysis of external input, cognitive computing and object detection bring mental health care closer to an all-rounded, context-sensitive support provided for any human being. Ultimately, holistic well-being to mental faculties through this approach supports a more proactive and resilient conduct toward one's psychological well-being.

INTEGRATING AI, IOT, AND COGNITIVE COMPUTING FOR PREVENTIVE MENTAL HEALTH

The rapid revolution in artificial intelligence, the Internet of Things, and cognitive computing transforms the landscape of mental health care to make a transformation possible from a reactive towards a preventive model of care. This comes with a paradigm shift as the condition, management, and treatment of mental health issues are being identified based on new considerations and systematic early identification. Traditionally, the area of mental health care has been reactive, established mainly on diagnosing and treating conditions after they emerge. With advancements in AI, IoT, and cognitive computing, it is now possible to predict, monitor, and intervene early on when talking about some mental health conditions before they become full-blown and result in better overall outcomes in the long run. This chapter will be about how these technologies blend in line with the offer of proactive, data-driven approaches to mental health care, specifically early intervention, predictive modeling, and prevention. Figure 4 typically emphasizes the stages of monitoring, analysis, and intervention to ensure comprehensive and proactive mental health management(Boopathi & Khang, 2023; Malathi et al., 2024; Satav et al., 2023).

Figure 4. AI, IoT, and Cognitive Computing for Preventive Mental Health

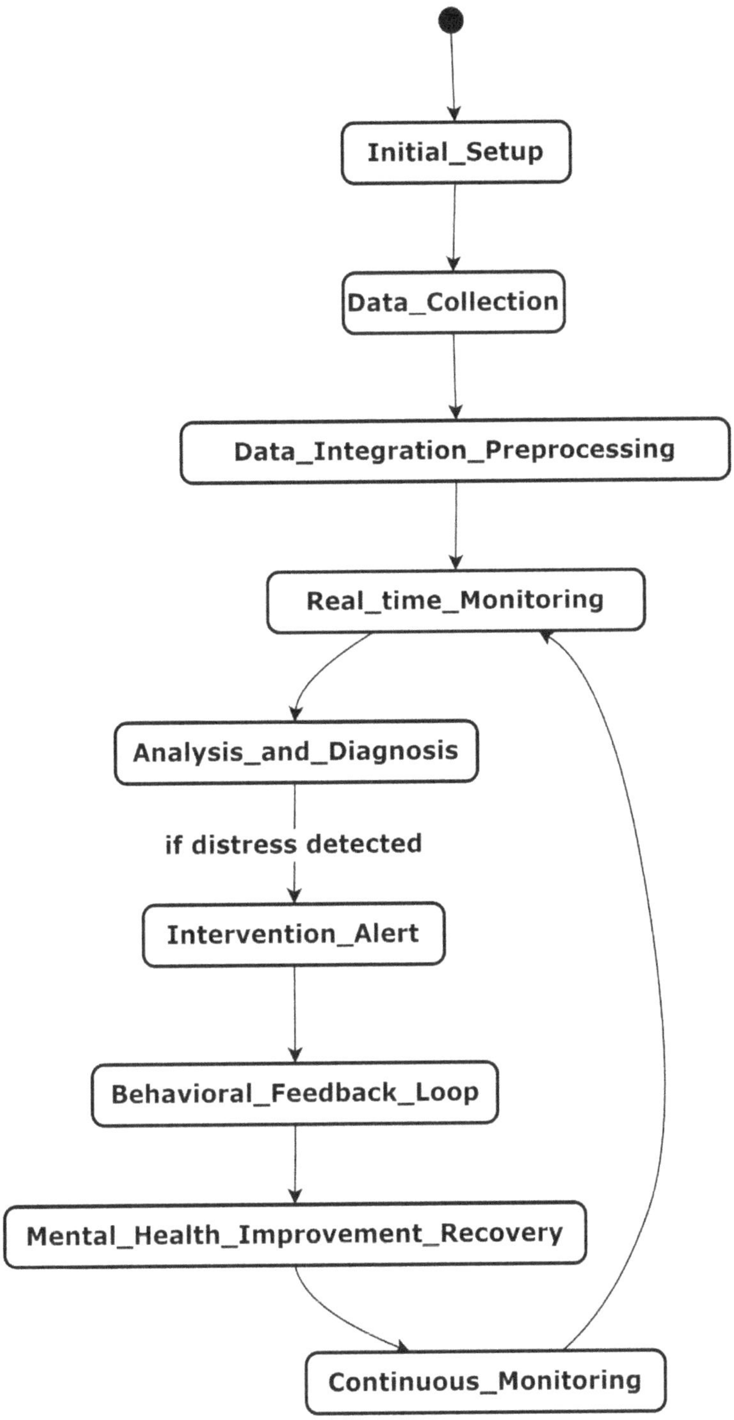

The Transition from Reactive to Preventive Mental Health Care

Generally, the mental health care has been characterized as reactive, focusing on symptoms after they had fully developed. People usually request treatment when symptoms of mental illness, such as anxiety, depression, or stress, become overwhelming and disrupt normal life. However, this usually results in delayed intervention and more intensive treatments that are costly and less effective. It's a preventive step about mental health care, changing from reactive mental health care and addressing the issues of mental health before they go full-blown and thus helping in being ahead of the risk curve and being well(Kushwah et al., 2024; Mohanraj et al., 2024).

This change will be brought about by AI, IoT, and cognitive computing capabilities that can look forward to the early detection of possible mental health issues, helping to track real-time monitoring and identify deviations from baseline states of mental well-being. All these technologies could be integrated into one platform, empowering people to continuously and personally assess their mental health so as to become more capable of taking preventive measures before problems mature into worse forms. Preventive care can also help alleviate the burden on the healthcare systems, develop quality of life, and ensure that people have better access to mental health care early enough and in time.

For instance, wearable devices enabled by IoT can continuously monitor heart rates, sleeping patterns, and activity levels-things that are critical indicators of mental health. Cognitive computing can then analyze these streams of data, using machine learning algorithms to find patterns that could indicate the early symptoms of depression or anxiety. That is, when abnormal behaviors are manifested, AI systems can send alerts to the person and their care providers to intervene early and avoid a catastrophic mental health disorder.

Early Interventions and Predictive Modeling

The early principle of preventive mental health care becomes achievable through AI and predictive modeling. Predictive modeling intends to identify, based on historical data and the use of machine learning algorithms, the patterns that can predict future issues with mental health. Models for prediction can be built from any sort of source of data: an IoT-enabled device, EHRs of electronic health records, social media activity, or NLP analysis of text or speech(Ramudu et al., 2023; Satav et al., 2023).

For instance, AI-based predictive models detect subtle symptoms of illnesses such as depression by tracing changes in sleep, physical activity, social communication —like staying away from social gatherings or less interaction. And from such models, individuals may be predicted to be at risk for a mental health crisis, which could then prompt clinicians and caregivers to intervene before things become worse. In this manner, early intervention stops the degeneration of mental disorders and provides more cost-efficient and effective care.

Use AI algorithms to assist in making real-time data-based constant updates to care plans for personalized and relevant care. For example, AI would track how an individual responded to certain types of interventions and would make corresponding adjustments to predictions or treatment recommendations. This adaptive, dynamic approach ensures that not only is the preventive approach to mental health but also adjusts and optimizes care over time.

This predictive modeling for early intervention in mental health monitoring even goes to the level of identifying the environmental triggers. Using the IoT sensors, for instance, on the environmental level, can identify particular stressors such as noise, the increase in temperature or the decrease in temperature, and social cues, which are connected with the worsening mental health outcomes. Cognitive computing can process such data, detecting environmental patterns that predict shifts in mental health outcomes. One can then use the predictive models to gain data-driven insights for action that prevents or reduces the impacts of potential negative triggers before they affect one's mental well-being.

The Role of Data-Driven Insights in Preventive Care

Data-driven insight motivates preventive mental care. Preventive mental care is a more objective measurable representation of an individual's mental health status as compared to conventional observation and assessment. Real-time data from several streams can be gathered and processed through AI, IoT, and cognitive computing technologies. The data-driven insights can then influence the preventive care strategy, providing greater decision capacity regarding the management of mental health to the customer and clinician.

There are wearable fitness trackers and sleep monitors that are examples of IoT devices, which provide data about the physical health of an individual who is directly related to mental health. For instance, poor quality sleep has been often linked with depression and anxiety. This is the kind of information that is made available to an algorithm running an AI when collecting real-time data from a sleep pattern; its analysis could look out for anomalies in trends related to the sleep cycle that could serve as an indicator of an emerging occurrence of a mental health condition. Cognitive computing may further amplify this process by crossing references of data from related sources like heart rate, physical activity, and social engagement in order to frame a more complete picture of an individual's well-being.

However, outside of wearable devices, AI can analyze other streams of data-for example, records of digital health or patterns of behavior online-to give more depth. For example, models of AI can analyze communications patterns on emails or social media posts by identifying changes in language to indicate a growing risk to mental health issues. Sentiment analysis and emotion recognition technology can also prove useful in identifying negative emotional states, which may be a haro

lder of the development of mental health disorders

The data-driven approach also allows for a better personalization of mental health care services. Continual monitoring of an individual's behavior by AI systems enables interventions that are personalized to each unique case of need, preferences, and conditions. Data-driven individualized care thus has a huge potential for bettering outcomes as well as improving long-term well-being.

For instance, an at-risk person can receive personalized advice or guidance based on their behavioral patterns, such as getting out socially and interacting with people who foster good feelings of well-being, while a person develops better sleep hygiene, maybe changing his exercise behavior, or building more positive sleep habits. Cognitive computing can provide a virtual coach or mental health assistant that helps facilitate the self-tracking of mood, stresses experienced, and therapeutic mental health exercises with real-time data insight.

Also, evidence-based information promotes teamwork among the patient and mental health professionals. Although health care providers monitor individuals in real time, data analysis automatically brings to their attention the occurring of the problem. During this situation, health care providers are in an excellent position to stop the worsening of the mental health conditions by taking prompt steps and providing appropriate therapeutic recommendations.

The integration of AI, IoT, and cognitive computing marked a shift of momentous proportions in how we care for mental health issues because the application allowed us to shift from reactive services to preventive ones. Harnessing real-time data collection through predictive modeling and cognitive computing allows mental health care providers to signal early warning signs of emerging conditions, intervene before conditions worsen, and provide individualized care to improve long-term outcomes. It thus enhances the well-being of the individual but, on the other hand, also reduces pressure on the medical system and healthcare facilities whilst enhancing efficiency and effectiveness. The data-driven insights provided by these technologies open pathways to a proactive, personalized, and sustainable approach to mental health care that ensures the right support reaches an individual at the right time. Because these technologies continue to evolve, further progress in preventive mental health care remains enormous and holds much promise for improvement in psychosocial well-being among diverse populations.

CHALLENGES IN ADOPTING AI AND IOT IN MENTAL HEALTH

Adopting AI and IoT in mental healthcare faces some of the challenges that need to be overcome to integrate it and ensure sustained impact(Kushwah et al., 2024; Mohanraj et al., 2024; Viraj Dravid et al., 2024). The adoption of AI and IoT in mental health faces several challenges as shown in Figure 5.

Figure 5. Challenges in adopting AI and IOT In Mental Health

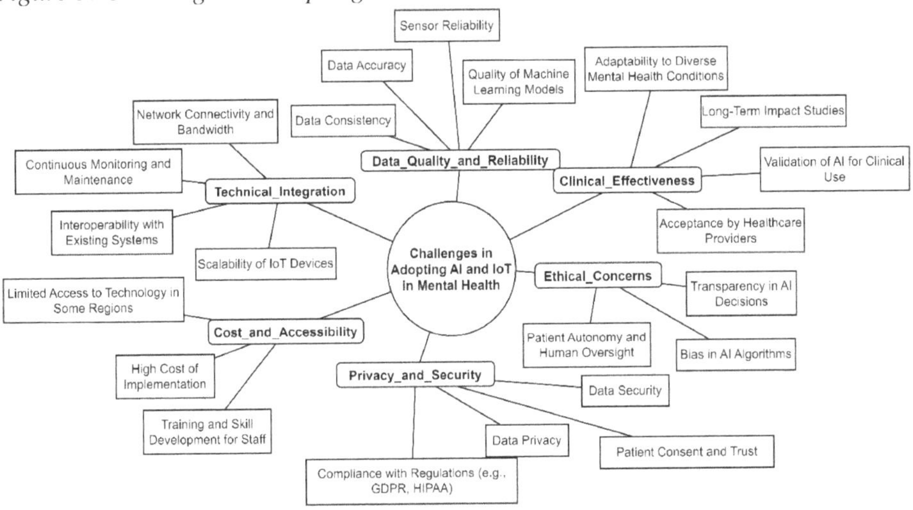

Technical and Infrastructure Barriers

The very first challenge that AI and IoT use in mental health also face is that using AI and IoT requires a solid foundation of technical infrastructure. There's a further need to equip the mental health professionals and health systems with the relevant hardware, software, and data storage solutions to ensure that advanced technologies are appropriately supported. Embedding AI models and IoT devices requires immense technology investment- ranging from high-quality sensors to secure data storage and real-time analytics platforms. Another extremely critical issue is the problem of data interoperability between different health systems, which may create an obstacle in the smooth information sharing across platforms and providers.

Access and Equity in the Utilization of Technology

In reality, AI and IoT have a lot of promise. On aspects of accessibility and equity, they face a huge challenge. Most people do not have access to the right devices or internet to properly use these technologies. Populations in rural areas or lower-income communities might face a challenge getting wearable devices, internet connectivity, or even the kind of digital literacy needed to operate these systems. This could create a digital divide and, therefore, exacerbate the existing health inequities and limit the benefits that can accrue from these technologies to certain groups.

Long-Term Impact and Effectiveness

There is a dearth of long-term efficacy data regarding AI and IoT-based interventions in the realm of mental health. Even though early outcome results are promising, issues persist about sustained impact on an individual's mental well-being over time. Data fatigue over periods, decreasing user engagement, or arising needs of mental health may dissolve such solutions. Secondly, scaling up these AI-based interventions to larger global populations will leave such scalability uncertain.

FUTURE DIRECTIONS

Emerging Trends in AI, IoT, and Cognitive Computing for Mental Health

The future of care concerning mental health will be further integrated with the use of AI, IoT, and cognitive computing to make solutions even more personalized, proactive, and accessible. Some of the emerging trends within this area include the development of advanced AI algorithms capable of detecting subtle changes in mental states through NLP and emotion recognition from voice and text. The future of IoT-enabled devices is to make them more sophisticated by offering continuous, non-intrusive monitoring of mental health indicators such as heart variability and sleep patterns. These technologies are enhanced by cognitive computing systems as they interpret complex data from multiple sources, provide actionable insights, and real-time recommendations for the maintenance of mental health(Boopathi, 2023; Ramudu et al., 2023).

Research Needs and Potential Innovations

Further research would be needed to improve the algorithms for AI and IoT towards having more sensitive and reliable detection of such issues in mental health. There would also be a need for innovation in how both technologies come together in developing virtual mental health services, such as AI-led therapy chatbots or CBT apps that use data coming from various IoT devices at real time for tailored interventions. Above all, long-term impacts of these technologies on mental well-being need to be understood and their efficacy in preventing mental health crises.

Policy Implications and Recommendations

For the widespread adoption of these technologies, policy frameworks must talk about issues of data privacy, security, and ethical concerns. Such sensitive data on the mental well-being of individuals deserve absolute confidentiality, and regulatory provisions such as GDPR or CCPA need improvement for scope to include AI and IoT in mental health applications. Policies should also create equal access to these technologies by the underprivileged to avoid discriminatory treatment in care. The governments and health organizations must make regulations that can facilitate the inclusion of AI and IoT into mental health systems in a less distorted and biased manner while applying it ethically

CONCUSION

Their inclusion in AI, IoT, and cognitive computing is the future possibility that can revolutionize mental health care, given the new paradigm, which shifts from being reactive to being preventive. With real-time data sourced from IoT-enabled devices, AI algorithms can identify early warnings for mental health concerns much before they emerge, and this can be addressed by timely intervention and support. Enrichment of the approach is further drawn by the role of cognitive computing in object detection in physical and environmental triggers that might target them, such as crowded areas or high levels of noise. These technologies not only improve the outcomes for the patient by offering personalized care, but also contribute to the widening of access for mental health care resources, and that too in remote or underserved areas. However, these advantages come with an equally vital challenge in the realm of ethics from the implementation of AI and IoT in mental health towards data privacy and consent. Thus, secure data handling must be rendered transparent, keeping such digital mental health solutions trustworthy. In conclusion, AI, IoT, and cognitive computing all promise much for the future of mental health care and therefore an approach that balances these in innovation, ethical considerations, and user trust. Future development waves should refine them into effectiveness with responsibility in improving patient care and respect toward privileges and autonomy.

REFERENCES

Almeida, M., Shrestha, A. D., Stojanac, D., & Miller, L. J. (2020). The impact of the COVID-19 pandemic on women's mental health. *Archives of Women's Mental Health, 23*(6), 741–748. DOI: 10.1007/s00737-020-01092-2 PMID: 33263142

Boopathi, S. (2023). Securing Healthcare Systems Integrated With IoT: Fundamentals, Applications, and Future Trends. In *Dynamics of Swarm Intelligence Health Analysis for the Next Generation* (pp. 186–209). IGI Global.

Boopathi, S., & Khang, A. (2023). AI-Integrated Technology for a Secure and Ethical Healthcare Ecosystem. In *AI and IoT-Based Technologies for Precision Medicine* (pp. 36–59). IGI Global. DOI: 10.4018/979-8-3693-0876-9.ch003

D'Alfonso, S. (2020). AI in mental health. *Current Opinion in Psychology, 36*, 112–117. DOI: 10.1016/j.copsyc.2020.04.005 PMID: 32604065

Dong, Y., Hou, J., Zhang, N., & Zhang, M. (2020). Research on how human intelligence, consciousness, and cognitive computing affect the development of artificial intelligence. *Complexity, 2020*(1), 1680845. DOI: 10.1155/2020/1680845

Foy, J. M., Green, C. M., Earls, M. F., Lavin, A., Askew, G. L., Baum, R., Berger-Jenkins, E., Gambon, T. B., Nasir, A. A., Wissow, L. S., & Joffe, A. (2019). Mental health competencies for pediatric practice. *Pediatrics, 144*(5), e20192757. DOI: 10.1542/peds.2019-2757 PMID: 31636143

Gál, É., tefan, S., & Cristea, I. A. (2021). The efficacy of mindfulness meditation apps in enhancing users' well-being and mental health related outcomes: A meta-analysis of randomized controlled trials. *Journal of Affective Disorders, 279*, 131–142. DOI: 10.1016/j.jad.2020.09.134 PMID: 33049431

Hickey, B. A., Chalmers, T., Newton, P., Lin, C.-T., Sibbritt, D., McLachlan, C. S., Clifton-Bligh, R., Morley, J., & Lal, S. (2021). Smart devices and wearable technologies to detect and monitor mental health conditions and stress: A systematic review. *Sensors (Basel), 21*(10), 3461. DOI: 10.3390/s21103461 PMID: 34065620

Hrabok, M., Delorme, A., & Agyapong, V. I. (2020). Threats to mental health and well-being associated with climate change. *Journal of Anxiety Disorders, 76*, 102295. DOI: 10.1016/j.janxdis.2020.102295 PMID: 32896782

Hua, Y., Liu, F., Yang, K., Li, Z., Na, H., Sheu, Y., Zhou, P., Moran, L. V., Ananiadou, S., Beam, A., & Associates. (2024). Large language models in mental health care: A scoping review. *arXiv Preprint arXiv:2401.02984*.

Kushwah, J. S., Gupta, M., Shrivastava, S., Saxena, N., Saini, R., & Boopathi, S. (2024). Psychological Impacts, Prevention Strategies, and Intervention Approaches Across Age Groups: Unmasking Cyberbullying. In *Change Dynamics in Healthcare, Technological Innovations, and Complex Scenarios* (pp. 89–109). IGI Global.

Lee, E. E., Torous, J., De Choudhury, M., Depp, C. A., Graham, S. A., Kim, H.-C., Paulus, M. P., Krystal, J. H., & Jeste, D. V. (2021). Artificial intelligence for mental health care: Clinical applications, barriers, facilitators, and artificial wisdom. *Biological Psychiatry: Cognitive Neuroscience and Neuroimaging*, *6*(9), 856–864. DOI: 10.1016/j.bpsc.2021.02.001 PMID: 33571718

Malathi, J., Kusha, K., Isaac, S., Ramesh, A., Rajendiran, M., & Boopathi, S. (2024). IoT-Enabled Remote Patient Monitoring for Chronic Disease Management and Cost Savings: Transforming Healthcare. In *Advances in Explainable AI Applications for Smart Cities* (pp. 371–388). IGI Global.

Mody, V., & Mody, V. (2019). Mental health monitoring system using artificial intelligence: A review. *2019 IEEE 5th International Conference for Convergence in Technology (I2CT)*, 1–6.

Mohanraj, G., Krishna, K. S., Lakshmi, B. S., Vijayalakshmi, A., Pramila, P. V., & Boopathi, S. (2024). Optimizing Trust and Security in Healthcare 4.0: Human Factors in Lightweight Secured IoMT Ecosystems. In *Lightweight Digital Trust Architectures in the Internet of Medical Things (IoMT)* (pp. 52–72). IGI Global. DOI: 10.4018/979-8-3693-2109-6.ch004

Osifeko, M. O., Hancke, G. P., & Abu-Mahfouz, A. M. (2020). Artificial intelligence techniques for cognitive sensing in future IoT: State-of-the-Art, potentials, and challenges. *Journal of Sensor and Actuator Networks*, *9*(2), 21. DOI: 10.3390/jsan9020021

Ramudu, K., Mohan, V. M., Jyothirmai, D., Prasad, D., Agrawal, R., & Boopathi, S. (2023). Machine Learning and Artificial Intelligence in Disease Prediction: Applications, Challenges, Limitations, Case Studies, and Future Directions. In *Contemporary Applications of Data Fusion for Advanced Healthcare Informatics* (pp. 297–318). IGI Global.

Salami, B., Salma, J., & Hegadoren, K. (2019). Access and utilization of mental health services for immigrants and refugees: Perspectives of immigrant service providers. *International Journal of Mental Health Nursing*, *28*(1), 152–161. DOI: 10.1111/inm.12512 PMID: 29984880

Satav, S. D., Hasan, D. S., Pitchai, R., Mohanaprakash, T., Sultanuddin, S., & Boopathi, S. (2023). Next generation of internet of things (ngiot) in healthcare systems. In *Sustainable Science and Intelligent Technologies for Societal Development* (pp. 307–330). IGI Global.

Smith, P. J., & Merwin, R. M. (2021). The role of exercise in management of mental health disorders: An integrative review. *Annual Review of Medicine*, *72*(1), 45–62. DOI: 10.1146/annurev-med-060619-022943 PMID: 33256493

Ströhle, A. (2019). Sports psychiatry: Mental health and mental disorders in athletes and exercise treatment of mental disorders. *European Archives of Psychiatry and Clinical Neuroscience*, *269*(5), 485–498. DOI: 10.1007/s00406-018-0891-5 PMID: 29564546

Suryadevara, S. (2022). Enhancing Brain-Computer Interface Applications through IoT Optimization. *Revista de Inteligencia Artificial En Medicina*, *13*(1), 52–76.

Swayamsiddha, S., & Mohanty, C. (2020). Application of cognitive Internet of Medical Things for COVID-19 pandemic. *Diabetes & Metabolic Syndrome*, *14*(5), 911–915. DOI: 10.1016/j.dsx.2020.06.014 PMID: 32570016

Viraj Dravid, S., Gopi, B., & Kumaresan, T. K., Nehru., Hari, B. S., & Boopathi, S. (2024). Monitoring Structural Health Using Friction Stir Techniques for Hybrid Composite Joints. In *Advances in Chemical and Materials Engineering* (pp. 221–255). IGI Global. DOI: 10.4018/979-8-3693-3993-0.ch012

Zhao, G., Li, Y., & Xu, Q. (2022). From emotion AI to cognitive AI. *International Journal of Network Dynamics and Intelligence*, 65–72.

KEY TERMS AND DEFINITIONS

AI: Machines that can perform tasks that were previously considered to be suited only to human intelligence, such as learning, reasoning, and problem-solving.

CBT: A psychotherapeutic approach predicated on the assumption that mental malfunction arises from abnormally rigid and irrational patterns of thought that can be changed through practice and insight.

NLP: It is one branch of AI that enables computers to understand, interpret, and generate human language.

EDA: Exploratory Data Analysis-Some general methods to analyze datasets through the use of visual summaries of key characteristics about the data.

EEG: The electrical activity test in the brain, often used in diagnosing mental health disorders.

PTSD: A mental health condition that results from direct exposure to or indirect eyewitness observation of traumatic events.

EHR: Electronic version of a patient's medical history and treatment kept in electronic form.

GDPR: EU regulation that has to do with data privacy and protection.

CCPA: A state regulation or rather law that gives residents of California even more rights with regard to the increased level of privacy concerning personal data.

Chapter 3
An Innovative Obstacle Detection Smart System for Robot Navigation in Healthcare Industry

Abhishek Das
http://orcid.org/0000-0002-5546-6188
Aliah University, India

Saiyed Umer
Department of Computer Science and Engineering, Aliah University, West Bengal, India

ABSTRACT

The integration of robotics in the healthcare industry is transforming how tasks are performed, enhancing efficiency, safety, and patient care. One critical aspect of robotic systems in healthcare is reliable navigation within complex and dynamic environments. The development of an innovative obstacle detection smart system is essential to ensure seamless and safe robot navigation in healthcare facilities. This chapter introduces a novel technique for Smart Robot Navigation, focusing on Obstacle Avoidance and Detection in Healthcare Industry. The proposed method is based as in reasonable and readily available electronic devices. Our Vision-based low-cost Obstacle Detection Technique for Robot Navigation demonstrates impressive speed and effectiveness, even when using low-resolution images. Extensive testing in both structured and unstructured office environments confirms the reliability of the robot platform's obstacle avoidance behavior.

DOI: 10.4018/979-8-3693-6094-1.ch003

1. Introduction

The global scientific community has displayed significant interest in the autonomous navigation of mobile platforms, driven by a wide range of contexts and applications. Mobile robots find utility in diverse areas such as mining, cleaning, maintenance, supervision, search and rescue operations in challenging environments like collapsed or radiation-prone areas, space, and deep underwater exploration. Additionally, in industrial settings, mobile-operated platforms have been developed for goods transportation, and artificial intelligence (A.I.) driver helper systems have been implemented on open roads and highways to enhance security. Moreover, military operations extensively use automated guided vehicles (AVG) (Bertozzi, Broggi, & Fascicoli, 2000) (Kastrinaki, Zervakis, & Kalaitzakis, 2003) (Roy, Bhanja, & Das, 2023)and autonomous mobile robots (AMR) (DeSouza & Kak, 2002). The field of autonomous navigation for mobile platforms is vast and spans multiple disciplines, including robotics, informatics, artificial intelligence, computer architecture, telecommunications, control theory, and mobile automation. It draws from both ancient techniques and cutting-edge space science and engineering. Regardless of the specific application, a crucial aspect of autonomous navigation is perceiving the environment in which the mobile platform operates.

Computer vision, a highly researched field within computer science, finds diverse applications in robotics, ranging from face recognition to autonomous navigation. This work focuses on exploring the computer vision's critical contributions to mobile robot navigation – obstacle detection. The approach relies on basic principles like epipolar geometry, planar homography, and image segmentation. Various obstacle detection methods are analyzed and compared based on their performance in different scenes using multi-view relations.

To gather data, a video is recorded, and image pairs are extracted from the video using a digital camera that moves between frames. The first method involves estimating the heights of corners in a scene using planar homography, accurately identifying objects by employing image segmentation. The second technique employs planar homography to generate a distinct warped image based on the initial frame. This warped image is subsequently compared with the final image for obstacle detection. Finally, the third approach employs epipolar geometry and edge detection to identify corresponding points on edges in images. Subsequently, planar homography is applied to calculate heights along the contours, facilitating obstacle detection.

1.1 AUTONOMOUS NAVIGATION SYSTEMS

In 1997, the semi-autonomous robot Sojourner Rover (Jet Propulsion Laboratory, n.d.) achieved a significant milestone by traversing the Martian surface as part of the Pathfinder mission (also known as the Mars Environmental Survey, or MESUR, Pathfinder). Sojourner Rover was a six-wheeled vehicle controlled by an Earth-based operator system. Due to the communication time delay of 6 to 41 minutes between Earth and Mars, some level of autonomous control was necessary.

Numerous robots equipped with various types of sensors have been developed to gather information about their external environments (Mondal & Das, 2023). For instance, Robocup (Veloso, Pagello, & Kitano, 2000) is an International Competition where robots play football matches. These robots are equipped with multiple sensors to comprehend the environment and the positions of other robots, along with cooperative artificial mechanisms to play the game. Another example is HELPMATE (Helpmate, 2023), a mobile robot used in hospitals for tasks such as transportation and autonomous navigation in corridors. Its primary localization sensor is a ceiling-facing camera that detects lamps on the ceiling, acting as reference landmarks.

In the industrial sector, Automated Guided Vehicles (AGV) like the one developed by VOLVO (Danaher Motion, 2023), represent the latest generation of mobile platforms used for transporting motor blocks between assembly stations. These AGVs are guided by an electrical wire installed in the floor but also possess the ability to deviate from the wire to avoid obstacles. Another notable example of Automated Guided Vehicles is the DARPA Challenge (DARPA, 2023).

1.2 WHY THIS RESEARCH IS STILL OF INTEREST

Approximately two decades ago, various governmental foundations in the United States expressed keen interest in Intelligent Transport Systems (ITS), aiming to explore the potential opportunities in this field of study. The defense system, particularly DARPA, played a significant role in supporting both fundamental and applied research in artificial robotics. In 1982, the National Research Council Commission on Engineering and Technical Systems in the United States produced a report (National Research Council Commission on Engineering and Technical Systems, 1983) for the United States Army, emphasizing the importance of reducing life risks and enhancing the effectiveness of Robotics and Artificial Intelligence applications.

Today, we are experiencing the second generation of Intelligent Transport Systems (ITS), characterized by a mature technology. Solving the challenges in this domain involves various approaches, such as robotics, computer architecture, informatics, telecommunications, artificial intelligence (A.I.), control theory, and automation. Present-day researchers are striving to enhance and implement intelligence within vehicles or robots rather than relying solely on infrastructures.

For instance, to create autonomous highways where modified vehicles can move from one point to another autonomously, significant expenses are incurred. Therefore, researchers are focusing on improving vehicle sensors to obtain a more detailed understanding of the environment through sensory data, which is crucial for achieving autonomous navigation. Information fusion, the integration of various sensory information, has become a major topic of research, leading to the development of novel methods for analyzing this data. Autonomous navigation stands as a highly valuable and sought-after objective in this context.

1.3 OBSTACLE DETECTION AND EARLIER WORK

Obstacle detection, as defined by Singh (Singh & Keller, 1992), refers to "the determination of whether a given space is free of obstacles for safe travel by an autonomous vehicle". This problem has garnered significant attention within the field of computer vision, attracting numerous researchers due to its wide range of applications. It plays a critical role in enabling fundamental operations for mobile robots, including avoidance and navigation, with the aid of artificial intelligence. A cutting-edge Vision-based low-cost Obstacle Detection system should possess certain qualities, including:

- Swiftly detecting obstacles in a given space.
- Accurately identifying the correct obstacles.
- Capable of discerning and disregarding ground features that may appear as obstacles.

Previous research in this area has explored various tools such as mobile digital cameras, odometers, and sonar to perform obstacle detection. These input devices capture "snapshots" or real-time "videos" of scenes, and the data are then processed by a computer system dedicated to obstacle detection (Bhanja & Das, 2021). However, some of these systems face challenges in real-time applications, particularly for high-speed vehicles' autonomous navigation, as they might be relatively slow in processing the vast amount of data generated by these devices.

To address these concerns, a Novel Vision-based low-cost Obstacle Detection system employs unique and sophisticated processors and sensors to enhance the efficiency and speed of obstacle detection tasks.

1.4 LITERATURE SURVEY

In the rapid changing world, understanding the multifaceted needs shaping individual lives and the technological advancements driving societal progress has become a pressing concern for researchers and policymakers. This literature review explores fundamental requirements and aspirations in modern life, including digital connectivity, health and well-being, education and skill development, and environmental sustainability. Moreover, it examines the challenges and solutions related to the Obstacle Detection System for Robot Navigation.

The (Petrov et al., 2019) paper includes a laser-based obstacle detection system designed for mobile robot navigation. The system involves the development of algorithms for segmentation which separates the measurements obtained from a 2D laser range finder into distinct segments representing individual obstacles. Additionally, the algorithms for line fitting and corner extraction are implemented to handle polygonal obstacles. Simulation and experimental results are provided to demonstrate the efficacy of the real-time laser obstacle detection system for enabling autonomous navigation of mobile robots.

The (Li et al., 2023) paper contains a computationally efficient approach that utilizes a deep neural network to directly detect occupancy from stereo images. The mentioned approach focuses on extracting compact obstacle distribution using volumetric representation instead of learning the point cloud correspondence from the stereo data. Additionally, it involves autonomous navigation with a real robot to validate the method's robustness and its practical applicability in real-world scenarios.

The (Saha et al., 2022) paper proposes a proficient obstacle detection and tracking system designed for mobile robot navigation using an RGB-D camera. The system comprises three primary modules: obstacle detection, obstacle tracking, and obstacle avoidance. Additionally, the study evaluates the system's performance concerning accuracy, robustness, and computational efficiency.

The (Somwanshi & Bundele, 2020) paper presents an obstacle detection approach specifically designed for robotic wheelchair navigation, leveraging the combined use of ultrasonic sensors and image processing techniques. The approach is structured into two stages: initial obstacle detection via ultrasonic sensors, followed by obstacle classification employing image processing algorithms. Furthermore, the feasibility and effectiveness of the approach are demonstrated through experimental results.

The (Chang et al., 2023) paper proposes the various challenges and solutions related to obstacle avoidance in autonomous mobile robots. It presents an innovative 3D Obstacle Detection system developed by DreamVu, which utilizes omnidirectional 3D vision to swiftly and accurately assess the environment and detect obstacles. Moreover, the article highlights the advantages of DreamVu's system in comparison to traditional Lidar-based systems.

This literature survey highlights the multifaceted needs shaping contemporary life and driving societal progress. The impact of digital connectivity on interactions and access to information, the significance of comprehensive healthcare and mental wellness, and the role of education in meeting dynamic job market demands have been explored. Moreover, the urgent need for environmental sustainability has been emphasized. Additionally, the importance of "Obstacle Detection System for Robot

Navigation" in ensuring safe and efficient autonomous navigation for robots has been identified.

Healthcare environments are often crowded with patients, staff, equipment, and furniture, making navigation challenging for autonomous robots. Traditional obstacle detection methods, such as simple infrared sensors, lack the sophistication to navigate such complex settings effectively. A more advanced, intelligent system is required to ensure robots can move safely and efficiently without causing disruptions or accidents.

2. METHODOLOGY

Although obstacle detection commonly employs methods like odometry, laser, and infrared, this project opts for a computer vision approach. Computer vision processes images using ambient light to establish a robust obstacle detection system. The project prioritizes research over engineering, aspiring to conduct a thorough study across disciplines like computer science and artificial intelligence before the practical implementation of the system. The proposed algorithm for obstacle detection is outlined as follows:

Algorithm 1:
Input: A video sequence
Output: A path during obstacle detection

1. Consider a video V.
2. Obtain the first frame f1 with assumption that there is no obstacle in f1
3. The camera is mounted in the lower part of the robot so considering the lower half portion (says g1) of f1
4. Crop a patch p from g1 and obtain its histogram h.
5. Now from the next frames, we consider lower half portion and divide the lower part into distinct patches says [p1,p2,…,pn].
6. Now from each patch pi, obtain its histogram hi.
7. Compute *di=dist(h,hi),*dist is the Euclidean distance and di, i=1,..n.
8. Obtain *min{di},* and select the patch which has highest similarity.
9. The selected patch is considered as non obstacle region say R.
10. Perform step 5 to step 10 for each frame and obtain the corresponding region R.
11. The selected regions [R1, R2,…,Rn] be the region for non obstacle detection.

3. Output

Figure 1. figures

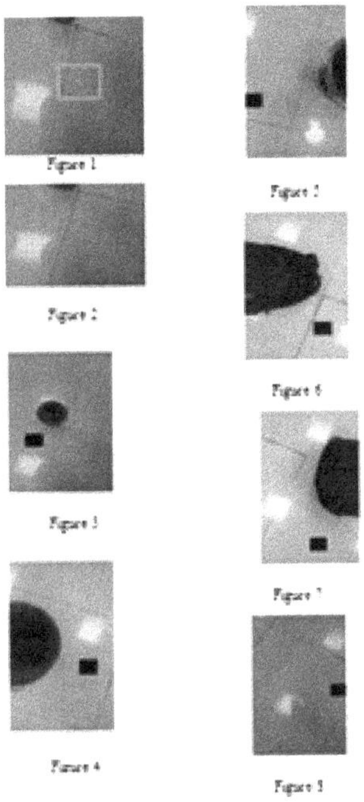

4. PATCH MATCHING

In the analysis, determining correspondence between a point x1 in I and its counterpart x2 in I2 is accomplished by comparing small square regions, referred to as "patches," of image intensity surrounding each point. For each pixel within the P1 patch around x1 in I1, the corresponding pixel in the P2 patch around x2 in I2 undergoes a comparison, and the disparities are computed. The individual differences in pixels are subsequently amalgamated into a patch difference, commonly achieved by summing the squares of these disparities.

Nonetheless, challenges exist in patch matching. An obstacle emerges when there's a shift in viewpoint between images, rendering no location identical to its previous state. Nevertheless, one can anticipate that corresponding patches should exhibit sufficient similarity for a match, provided the robot undergoes only a brief movement. This slight adjustment guarantees minimal alterations in viewpoint, and although the overall image may seem somewhat altered, local patches are likely to maintain their similarity.

In patch matching, another challenge arises when a patch encompasses a disruption in the optical flow. It proves advantageous for the optical flow to maintain continuity across the image, ensuring that the small neighborhood around x1 follows the optical flow direction of x1. However, instances where the robot observes nearby objects overlapping more distant ones create a scene depth disparity at the boundary, impacting the optical flow. To address this challenge, employing smaller patch sizes is recommended, reducing the likelihood of patches containing discontinuities. This strategy is effective because, as previously mentioned, objects may appear different from various angles but can still match well when the robot's movement is limited, considering only a small neighborhood.

Nevertheless, there exist constraints on reducing patch sizes while retaining sufficient information for successful matching. Extremely diminutive patches may yield numerous false positives, posing a potential issue. Additionally, excessively small patches cannot completely eradicate the optical flow discontinuity challenge, as regions with compelling textures, often linked to object boundaries, typically offer more dependable optical flow. Occasionally, these optical flow boundaries can lead to the outright failure of patch matching, presenting a situation that may be inevitable.

Sometimes, at a discontinuity, a patch might encompass an object exhibiting predominant optical flow, with this optical flow becoming the overall flow for the entire patch.

Figure 2. flow chart for moving object detection using BBME

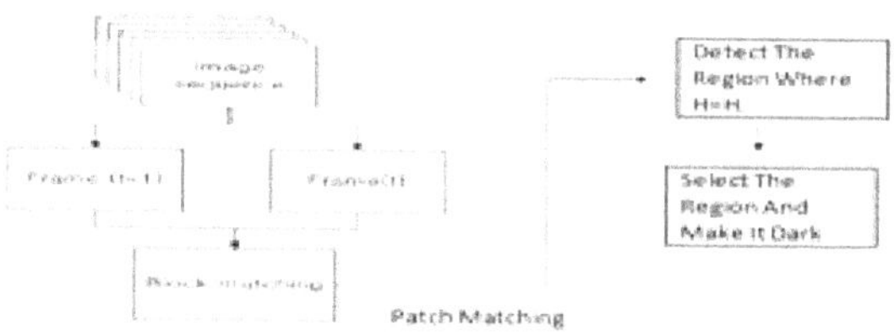

The majority of computer vision algorithms operate under the assumption that images adhere to a projective perspective model (see figure 2-1). The coordinate system is defined in relation to the robot, with the robot's camera positioned at the origin and oriented along the y-axis. In this setup, an imaginary image plane is situated one unit in front of the robot, centered around and perpendicular to the y-axis. The projection of a world point p (x, y, z) onto the image plane results in a point p' = (u, v), as determined by the following equations:

$$u = x/y \tag{1}$$

$$v = z/y. \tag{2}$$

Figure 3. projective prospective

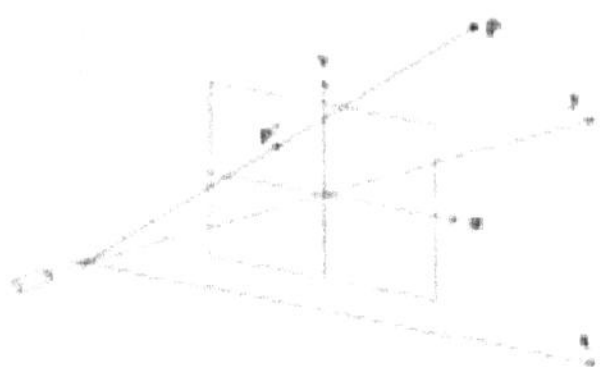

As the projective perspective model is not conducive to practical calculations, actual image coordinates undergo a transformation into planar projective coordinates through the application of a radial distortion model. Assuming the center of the camera image is at (ci, c), the radial distortion model establishes a relationship between a point (xo, yo) in the distorted image and its corresponding point (x, y) in the corrected planar image as follows:

$$X=x_0+(x0-c_x)\ (k_1r^2{}_0+ k_2r^4{}_0+.....); \tag{3}$$

$$Y=y_0+ (y_0-c_y)\ (k_1r^2{}_0+ k_2r^4{}_0+.....); \tag{4}$$

Where $r0= \sqrt{[(x_0-c_x)^2+(y_0-c_y)^2]}$

These constants are determined through the process of camera calibration. The rationale behind this model is that points experience greater distortion as their distance from the center of the image increases.

5. THE ROBOTIC VISION: STATE OF ART

Figure 4. radical distortion

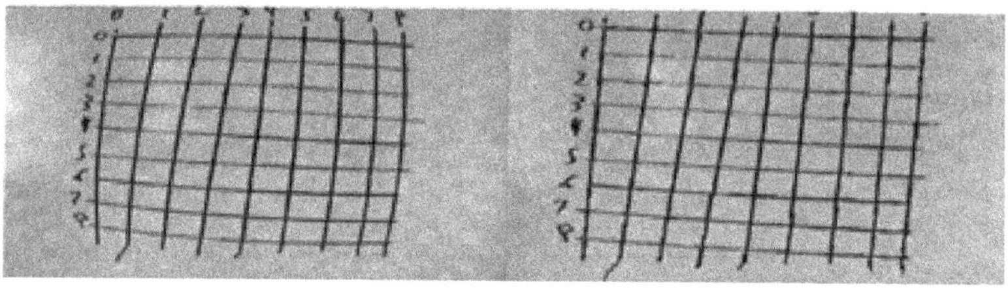

The objective of robotics is to create autonomous and efficient machines, independent of human intervention. In modern times, robots are designed using consumer-market hardware, which helps overcome budget constraints while maintaining a reasonable level of sophistication. However, in the context of modern architecture models like Intel x86, ARM, and PowerPC, both in general-purpose and embedded versions, the computational power falls short when dealing with the demands of vision algorithms. This discrepancy has spurred researchers to develop even more efficient and intelligent algorithms to cope with the challenge.

The primary aim of artificial vision is to equip machines with visual capabilities, enabling them to gather information from their external environment. Artificial vision has evolved from the integration of Image Processing and Pattern Recognition (Pratt, 1978)(Denasi et al., 1994)(Lützeler & Dickmanns, 1998)(Zahedi, Bhajna, & Das, 2023). In a vision system, there are two fundamental steps: image acquisition and image processing. Navigation typically requires two or more cameras to acquire images, and the choice of camera significantly influences subsequent processing steps. For instance, pin-hole cameras produce images with significant radial distortion, which necessitates filtering to reduce the distortion. On the other hand, cameras with sufficient focal length might not require this filtering step. Modern cameras are sophisticated, capable of handling issues like auto-tuning to light variations or contrast at the sensor level. They offer a refresh frequency of 25-35 HZ and a contrast intensity of about 10,000:1 (in contrast to common cameras with around 500:1). CMOS technology-based sensors significantly enhance contrast intensity and maximum resolution.

The image processing system must operate in real-time to produce results useful for navigation applications. This requirement demands substantial computational power, as the processing time sets an upper limit (alongside the actuators' speed) on the robot's movement. In the past, this level of computational power was only available on parallel (even embedded) systems, but nowadays, general-purpose computers can handle image processing tasks effectively.

There are two primary approaches to vision: artificial and natural. The primary goal of reproducing a natural vision system, such as the Human Vision System (HVS) or insects' vision system, is to enable the machine to process information from images in a manner "intelligible" to it. In this paper, we present a classification of visual systems for Robot Navigation, with a particular focus on obstacle avoidance.

6. OBSTACLE DETECTION AND AVOIDANCE

Obstacle detection and avoidance involve identifying obstacles to ensure the safe navigation of a mobile platform in autonomous mode. An obstacle can be either stationary or moving, and it may belong to specific categories like other robots, vehicles, or people, or it could be an unexpected object. The approach to obstacle detection depends on the context and the types of obstacles of interest. For example, in automatic guidance scenarios, we may assume only moving obstacles like vehicles and people on the road, simplifying the detection process through template matching (Lützeler & Dickmanns, 1998). (Longuet-Higgins, 1981) However, in exploration situations, the robot operates in an open environment where various types of obstacles may exist. We can address the problem of obstacle detection and avoidance using two different paradigms (see Figure 4): A. 3-D motion estimation B. 3-D space reconstruction

The traditional "structure from motion" problem (Spetsakis & Aloimonos, 1990) (Loizou & Rimon, 2022) (Arrouch et al., 2022) involves recovering the 3-D motion parameters and object structure from dynamic images. For small motions, the optical flow field, representing the change in image points, can be computed from spatio-temporal derivatives of the image intensity. Additional constraints, such as smoothness, are employed for this computation. For large motions, correspondences between features (points, lines, or contours) in images at different time instants are used to determine the 3-D motion. However, the optical flow approach has limitations in real applications, leading us to prefer a 3-D space reconstruction approach for a more detailed scene description. We aim to detect obstacles with motion similar to the robot and maintain spatial coherence, making it less sensitive to changes in environmental conditions. To achieve this, both optical flow and stereo vision are utilized to analyze the motion of obstacles in relation to the mobile platform. This enables us to distinguish between motionless and moving obstacles and perform tracking of the moving ones.

7. HARDWARE

Before delving into the design plan, it is essential to consider the constraints on the system. Instead of processing images in real-time through a webcam, a standard and sophisticated personal computer is employed to handle images transmitted from a digital camera. The primary focus of this project is researching computer vision techniques rather than developing an obstacle detection system with strict requirements.

The specifications of the personal computer used are as follows:

- Device Specifications: Dell Personal Computer
- Processor: Intel(R) Pentium(R)CPU P6200 @ 2.13GHz
- RAM: 8GB
- Hard Drive: 1TB HDD
- Input: USB
- Digital Camera: Trust 4400BX
- Camera Maximum Resolution: 2048 x 1376
- Camera Output: USB

The digital camera utilized has a maximum resolution of 2048x1376. However, in order to optimize processing time while preserving the system's integrity to some extent, all images were captured with the camera resolution configured at 640x480.

9. CONCLUSION

The development of an innovative obstacle detection smart system for robot navigation in the healthcare industry promises to revolutionize the way robots operate in these environments. By leveraging advanced sensors, machine learning, and real-time control systems, the proposed solution aims to enhance safety, efficiency, and overall patient care. This system represents a significant step forward in the integration of robotics into healthcare, paving the way for more intelligent and autonomous operations.

In this paper, we propose a novel real-time video analysis system for a Vision-based low-cost Obstacle Detection Technique, specifically designed for the autonomous navigation of a mobile platform. Our system introduces several enhancements compared to existing systems, particularly addressing the challenges posed by unstructured environments. We focus on two crucial phases: obstacle detection and moving object detection, which are essential for a robot to comprehend the scene and avoid obstacles effectively.

The motion of the camera mounted on the robot presents significant difficulties in video analysis, leading many existing algorithms to fail. To enable autonomous navigation and guide the mobile platform swiftly along a safe path, our proposed system demands real-time processing capabilities.

To develop the vision system, we employed a precise methodology that considers specifications and ensures good performance for the designated application domain (AMR and AVG). The video analysis involves learning about the environment, the mobile platform's capabilities, and the final destination it needs to reach. The primary contribution of our work lies in the "perceptive" representation, based on the stereo vision paradigm, which effectively detects obstacles according to the specified goals.

Stereo vision offers several advantages over other techniques like optical flow or model-based methods, this approach furnishes a thorough scene depiction, identifying stationary and dynamic obstacles without the need for an intricate obstacle model. Furthermore, it exhibits reduced sensitivity to environmental alterations, a drawback often associated with optical flow techniques. Existing literature predominantly relies on pixel correspondence, and the main challenge in stereo vision lies in establishing accurate point-to-point correspondences between two images representing the same scene point, commonly known as disparity matching.

REFERENCES

Arrouch, I., Ahmad, N. S., Goh, P., & Mohamad-Saleh, J. (2022). Close proximity time-to-collision prediction for autonomous robot navigation: An exponential GPR approach. *Alexandria Engineering Journal*, *61*(12), 11171–11183. DOI: 10.1016/j.aej.2022.04.041

Bertozzi, M., Broggi, A., & Fascicoli, A. (2000). Vision-based intelligent vehicles: State of art and perspectives. *Robotics and Autonomous Systems*, *32*(1), 1–16. DOI: 10.1016/S0921-8890(99)00125-6

Bhanja, S., & Das, A. (2021). Deep neural network for multivariate time-series forecasting. In *Advances in Intelligent Systems and Computing* (Vol. 1255). Springer., DOI: 10.1007/978-981-15-7834-2_25

Chang, C. Y., Wu, C. L., Cheng, J. M., & Jian, S. J. (2023). Autonomous mobile robots for recycling metal shaving at CNC factories. *International Journal of Advanced Manufacturing Technology*, *126*(5-6), 2205–2218. DOI: 10.1007/s00170-023-11284-6

DARPA. (2023). DARPA Grand Challenge. https://www.darpa.mil/grandchallenge/index.asp

Denasi, S., Lanzone, C., Martinese, P., Pettiti, G., Quaglia, G., & Viglione, L. (1994). Real-time system for road following and obstacle detection. In *Proceedings of the SPIE on Machine Vision Applications, Architectures, and Systems Integration III* (Vol. 2347, pp. 70–79).

DeSouza, G. N., & Kak, A. C. (2002). Vision for mobile robot navigation: A survey. *IEEE Transactions on Pattern Analysis and Machine Intelligence*, *24*(2), 237–267. DOI: 10.1109/34.982903

Helpmate. (2023). http://www.ntplx.net/~helpmate/

Jet Propulsion Laboratory. (n.d.). Pathfinder Rover. NASA. https://www.nasa.gov/

Kastrinaki, V., Zervakis, M., & Kalaitzakis, K. (2003). A survey of video processing techniques for traffic applications. *Image and Vision Computing*, *21*(4), 359–381. DOI: 10.1016/S0262-8856(03)00004-0

Li, H., Li, Z., Akmandor, N. Ü., Jiang, H., Wang, Y., & Padır, T. (2023, May). StereovoxelNet: Real-time obstacle detection based on occupancy voxels from a stereo camera using deep neural networks. In *2023 IEEE International Conference on Robotics and Automation (ICRA)* (pp. 4826–4833). IEEE. DOI: 10.1109/ICRA48891.2023.10160924

Loizou, S. G., & Rimon, E. D. (2022). Mobile robot navigation functions tuned by sensor readings in partially known environments. *IEEE Robotics and Automation Letters*, *7*(2), 3803–3810. DOI: 10.1109/LRA.2022.3148466

Longuet-Higgins, H. C. (1981). A computer algorithm for reconstructing a scene from two projections. *Nature*, *293*(5828), 133–135. DOI: 10.1038/293133a0

Lützeler, M., & Dickmanns, E. D. (1998). Road recognition with MarVEye. In *Proceedings of the IEEE International Conference on Intelligent Vehicles* (pp. 341–346).

Mondal, S., & Das, A. (2023). Quality aware cost-efficient reward mechanism in mobile crowdsensing system with uncertainty constraints. *Microsystem Technologies*. DOI: 10.1007/s00542-023-05495-w

National Research Council Commission on Engineering and Technical Systems. (1983). *Applications of robotics and artificial intelligence to reduce risk and improve effectiveness: A study for the United States Army*. National Academy of Sciences.

Petrov, P., Georgieva, V., Nikolov, S., & Mihaylova, A. (2019, May). Real-time laser obstacle detection system for autonomous mobile robot navigation. In 2019 X National Conference with International Participation (ELECTRONICA) (pp. 1–4). IEEE. DOI: 10.1109/ELECTRONICA.2019.8825623

Pratt, W. K. (1978). *Digital image processing*. John Wiley & Sons.

Roy, S., Bhanja, S., & Das, A. (2023). AndyWar: An intelligent android malware detection using machine learning. *Innovations in Systems and Software Engineering*. Advance online publication. DOI: 10.1007/s11334-023-00530-5

Saha, A., Dhara, B. C., Umer, S., Yurii, K., Alanazi, J. M., & AlZubi, A. A. (2022). Efficient obstacle detection and tracking using RGB-D sensor data in dynamic environments for robotic applications. *Sensors (Basel)*, *22*(17), 6537. DOI: 10.3390/s22176537 PMID: 36080993

Singh, S., & Keller, P. (1992). Obstacle detection for high-speed autonomous navigation. In *Proceedings of the IEEE International Conference on Robotics and Automation*.

Somwanshi, D., & Bundele, M. (2020). Obstacle detection approach for robotic wheelchair navigation. In International Conference on Artificial Intelligence: Advances and Applications 2019 (pp. 261–268). Springer Singapore. DOI: 10.1007/978-981-15-1059-5_29

Spetsakis, M. E., & Aloimonos, J. (1990). Structure from motion using line correspondences. *International Journal of Computer Vision*, *4*(3), 171–183. DOI: 10.1007/BF00054994

Veloso, M., Pagello, E., & Kitano, H. (Eds.). (2000). *RoboCup-99: Robot Soccer World Cup III* (Vol. 1856). Springer. DOI: 10.1007/3-540-45327-X

Watt, A., & Policarpo, F. (1998). *The computer image*. Addison-Wesley.

Zahedi, M., Bhajna, S., & Das, A. (2023). Novel machine learning techniques for diabetes prediction. In Bhattacharyya, S. (Eds.), *Intelligent Human Centered Computing. Human 2023*. Springer., DOI: 10.1007/978-981-99-3478-2_24

Zahedi, M., & Das, A. (2023). UN Sustainable Development Goals: Cybernetics as a goal-directed platform. *Third Concept*, *36*(432), 116–120.

Chapter 4
Enhancing Telemedicine Deep Learning–Based Classification of ECG Heartbeats:
With Continuous Wavelet Transform for Remote Cardiac Care

C.V. Suresh Babu
https://orcid.org/0000-0002-8474-2882
Hindustan Institute of Technolgy and Science, Chennai, India

Malini Premakumari William
https://orcid.org/0009-0004-6165-2501
Mirage Software, Inc. dba Bourntec Solutions, Inc., USA

ABSTRACT

This study aims to enhance ECG classification methods for telemedicine applications by integrating deep learning techniques with Continuous Wavelet Transform (CWT) for feature extraction. The methodology involved training a Convolutional Neural Network (CNN) on a comprehensive dataset to improve the accuracy and reliability of ECG signal classification. Key findings indicate that the proposed approach significantly outperforms traditional methods, achieving higher accuracy in identifying cardiac conditions such as arrhythmias. The results underscore the potential of real-time monitoring capabilities in telemedicine, facilitating timely interventions and improved patient outcomes. The study concludes that addressing

DOI: 10.4018/979-8-3693-6094-1.ch004

the limitations of existing ECG classification systems is crucial for their effective integration into clinical practice, ultimately contributing to the advancement of remote healthcare solutions.

1. INTRODUCTION

1.1 Overview of Telemedicine and Its Importance in Healthcare

Telemedicine refers to the use of telecommunications technology to provide healthcare services remotely. It encompasses a wide range of applications, including virtual consultations, remote patient monitoring, and mobile health applications. The rise of telemedicine has been significantly influenced by advancements in technology, particularly the Internet of Things (IoT), which allows for the continuous monitoring of patients' health parameters (Denysyuk et al., 2023)

One of the primary advantages of telemedicine is its ability to enhance access to healthcare services, especially for individuals in remote or underserved areas. By eliminating geographical barriers, telemedicine enables patients to receive timely medical advice and treatment without the need for physical travel (Victor, 2021)

This is particularly crucial in emergency situations where immediate medical attention is required. Furthermore, telemedicine can reduce the burden on healthcare facilities by allowing healthcare providers to manage more patients efficiently through virtual consultations (Tramontano et al., 2023)

In addition to improving access, telemedicine plays a vital role in chronic disease management. Patients with conditions such as diabetes, hypertension, and heart disease can benefit from regular monitoring and consultations via telemedicine platforms. This continuous engagement helps in early detection of potential complications and promotes adherence to treatment plans (Tramontano et al., 2023)

Moreover, the integration of IoT devices in telemedicine allows for real-time data collection and analysis, which enhances the quality of care provided to patients (Victor, S. P. et. al. 2021)

The importance of telemedicine has been further underscored during the COVID-19 pandemic, where it became a critical tool for maintaining healthcare delivery while minimizing the risk of virus transmission. Telemedicine not only ensured continuity of care but also provided a safe alternative for patients who were hesitant to visit healthcare facilities during the pandemic (IEEE. 2024)

In conclusion, telemedicine represents a transformative approach to healthcare delivery, offering numerous benefits such as improved access, enhanced chronic disease management, and increased patient engagement. As technology continues to evolve, the potential for telemedicine to further revolutionize healthcare is immense.

1.2 The Role of ECG Monitoring in Cardiac Care

Electrocardiography (ECG) monitoring is a critical component of cardiac care, providing essential insights into the electrical activity of the heart. This non-invasive technique is widely used for diagnosing various cardiac conditions, including arrhythmias, myocardial infarctions, and other heart diseases. The ability to continuously monitor heart rhythms allows healthcare providers to detect abnormalities in real-time, facilitating timely interventions (Denysyuk et al., 2023)

One of the primary advantages of ECG monitoring is its capability to provide continuous data on a patient's cardiac status. This is particularly important for patients with known cardiac issues or those at high risk for developing heart conditions. Continuous ECG monitoring can help in the early detection of arrhythmias, which are often asymptomatic but can lead to severe complications if not addressed promptly (Tramontano et al., 2023)

The integration of advanced algorithms for ECG signal analysis has further enhanced the accuracy of arrhythmia detection, allowing for automated classification and diagnosis (IEEE, 2024)

Moreover, ECG monitoring plays a vital role in the management of chronic conditions such as heart failure and coronary artery disease. By regularly assessing the heart's electrical activity, healthcare providers can make informed decisions regarding treatment adjustments and lifestyle modifications (Adeolu & Abayomi, 2024).

The use of wearable ECG devices has also gained popularity, enabling patients to monitor their heart health remotely and share data with healthcare professionals, thus promoting patient engagement and adherence to treatment plans (Safdar et al., 2024)

The importance of ECG monitoring has been particularly highlighted during the COVID-19 pandemic, where remote monitoring solutions have become essential for managing patients with cardiovascular conditions while minimizing the risk of virus transmission (IEEE., 2024)

Telemedicine platforms that incorporate ECG monitoring allow for virtual consultations, ensuring continuity of care for patients who may be hesitant to visit healthcare facilities.

In conclusion, ECG monitoring is a fundamental aspect of cardiac care, providing critical information for the diagnosis and management of heart conditions. Its role in continuous monitoring, early detection of arrhythmias, and integration with telemedicine solutions underscores its importance in enhancing patient outcomes in cardiac care.

1.3 Current Challenges in ECG Heartbeat Classification

ECG heartbeat classification is a crucial aspect of cardiac care, enabling the detection and diagnosis of various heart conditions. However, several challenges persist in the accurate classification of ECG signals, which can impact the effectiveness of diagnostic algorithms and clinical outcomes.

One of the primary challenges in ECG heartbeat classification is the inherent noise and artifacts present in the ECG signals. These disturbances can arise from various sources, including muscle contractions, electrical interference, and patient movement, which complicate the analysis and interpretation of the signals (Wasimuddin et al., 2020)

Effective preprocessing techniques are essential to mitigate these issues, as they can significantly influence the performance of classification algorithms (Denysyuk et al., 2023)

Another significant challenge is the variability in ECG signal morphology among different patients. Factors such as age, gender, and underlying health conditions can lead to variations in the ECG waveform, making it difficult for classification algorithms to generalize across diverse populations (Safdar et al., 2024)

This variability necessitates the development of robust algorithms that can adapt to different signal characteristics while maintaining high accuracy.

Moreover, the classification of ECG signals often relies on feature extraction methods, which can be computationally intensive and may require expert knowledge to select the most relevant features (Hermawan et al., 2021)

While deep learning approaches have shown promise in automating feature extraction, they also introduce challenges related to the need for large labeled datasets for training, which may not always be available (Zhang et al., 2020)

The lack of standardized datasets can hinder the comparability of different classification models and their performance evaluation.

Additionally, the integration of ECG classification systems into clinical practice poses challenges related to user acceptance and the need for real-time processing capabilities. Clinicians must trust the outputs of automated systems, which requires transparency in the decision-making process of these algorithms (Kumar et al., 2021)

Ensuring that these systems can operate in real-time without compromising accuracy is essential for their successful implementation in clinical settings.

1.4 Objective and Scope of the Chapter

Objectives:

1. **Address Limitations of Traditional Methods:** Analyze the challenges in existing ECG classification techniques, focusing on feature extraction inefficiencies and high computational demands in telemedicine applications.
2. **Leverage Deep Learning Approaches:** Explore how deep learning methodologies, particularly automated feature extraction, can enhance the accuracy and efficiency of ECG signal classification.
3. **Enable Real-Time Processing:** Emphasize the importance of real-time capabilities for ECG classification systems to ensure timely and efficient operation in clinical and telemedicine settings.
4. **Facilitate Clinical Integration:** Assess the challenges of implementing automated ECG classification systems in clinical practice, including user acceptance and the transparency of decision-making processes.
5. **Highlight Future Research Needs:** Identify areas for further research to address current challenges, such as algorithm limitations, integration hurdles, and technological advancements.
6. **Encourage Use of Standardized Datasets:** Advocate for the adoption of standardized datasets to ensure consistency and comparability in evaluating ECG classification models.

Scope of the Study:

1. **Advanced Methodologies:** The study integrates Continuous Wavelet Transform (CWT) with Convolutional Neural Networks (CNN) to enhance feature extraction and improve ECG classification accuracy.
2. **Data Utilization:** It employs the MIT-BIH Arrhythmia Database, a robust and diverse dataset, for training and validating the proposed models, ensuring reliability and generalizability.
3. **Real-Time Applications:** The research prioritizes real-time processing capabilities, vital for remote monitoring and timely diagnosis in telemedicine.
4. **Clinical Implications:** The study underscores the role of enhanced ECG classification tools in aiding healthcare providers to identify and manage cardiac conditions effectively within telemedicine platforms.
5. **Future Research Directions:** It identifies key areas for continued research, including the development of interoperable systems, user-friendly automated solutions, and the creation of standardized datasets to support innovation in ECG classification technologies.

This study aims to bridge existing gaps in ECG classification methods, providing practical advancements in telemedicine and remote cardiac care through cutting-edge technologies.

2. PROBLEM STATEMENT

2.1. Limitations of Existing ECG Classification Methods in Telemedicine

Telemedicine has transformed cardiac care by enabling remote monitoring and diagnosis, yet significant limitations in existing ECG classification methods hinder their full potential. Traditional approaches rely heavily on handcrafted feature extraction, requiring extensive domain expertise and computational resources, which often fail to capture the complexity of diverse ECG morphologies (Kumar et al., 2021; Safdar et al., 2024). These limitations result in suboptimal performance, particularly in heterogeneous patient populations.

ECG signals in telemedicine are prone to noise and artifacts caused by patient movement, poor electrode placement, and environmental interference, compromising classification accuracy and increasing the likelihood of false positives or negatives (Wasimuddin et al., 2020). Moreover, the absence of standardized datasets for training and validation limits the generalizability of models, as many algorithms are trained on small or non-representative data samples (Zhang et al., 2020).

Advanced deep learning models, while effective, often operate as "black boxes," lacking transparency and interpretability, which diminishes clinician trust and acceptance (Denysyuk et al., 2023). Additionally, real-time implementation of ECG classification systems faces logistical barriers, including high computational demands, regulatory compliance, and limited access to robust infrastructure in underserved areas (Kumar et al., 2021).

2.2. Problem Statement

Despite advancements in telemedicine, existing ECG classification methods face critical challenges, including reliance on manual feature extraction, vulnerability to noisy input signals, limited generalizability due to non-standardized datasets, and a lack of interpretability in automated systems. These limitations hinder the accuracy, efficiency, and integration of ECG classification technologies into telemedicine platforms. To address these gaps, innovative approaches leveraging deep learning and advanced signal processing techniques are essential to enhance real-time ECG analysis and improve cardiac care in remote healthcare settings.

3. PROPOSED SOLUTION: DEEP LEARNING WITH CONTINUOUS WAVELET TRANSFORM

3.1 Introduction to Deep Learning in Healthcare

Deep learning, a subset of machine learning, has revolutionized healthcare by enabling the analysis of large, complex datasets to improve diagnostic accuracy and patient outcomes. Applications in medical imaging, such as X-rays and MRIs, and biosignals like electrocardiograms (ECGs), demonstrate its potential to automate feature extraction and facilitate accurate classification of cardiac conditions (Esteva et al., 2019; Zhang et al., 2020). By addressing the challenges of non-stationary signals and automating analysis, deep learning reduces the burden on healthcare professionals and enhances efficiency in telemedicine (Safdar et al., 2024).

3.2. Continuous Wavelet Transform (CWT): An Overview

CWT is a mathematical tool that provides a detailed time-frequency representation of signals, making it particularly suitable for analyzing transient and non-stationary signals like ECGs (Adeolu & Abayomi, 2024). Unlike traditional Fourier Transform, CWT identifies localized frequency content, which is critical for detecting cardiac anomalies such as arrhythmias (Gao et al., 2018). Furthermore, CWT improves signal quality by reducing noise, enhancing the reliability of feature extraction in clinical and telemedicine applications (Safdar et al., 2024).

3.3. Integration of Deep Learning and CWT for ECG Classification

Combining CWT with deep learning techniques, particularly Convolutional Neural Networks (CNNs), leverages the strengths of both approaches. CWT transforms ECG signals into time-frequency representations (scalograms), enabling CNNs to process image-like data and identify complex patterns for improved classification accuracy (Shaik et al., 2023). This integration has shown superior performance compared to traditional methods like Short-Time Fourier Transform (STFT) and ensures robustness in handling noise and artifacts (Suresh Babu et al., 2025).

3.4. Advantages of the Proposed Solution

- **Enhanced Feature Extraction:** CWT captures detailed transient features, improving the accuracy of ECG classification (Gao et al., 2018).

- **Improved Classification Accuracy:** Deep learning models using CWT outperform traditional feature extraction methods, achieving higher precision and recall (Suresh Babu et al., 2025).
- **Noise Reduction:** Preprocessing with CWT filters noise from ECG signals, enhancing data quality and model performance (Safdar et al., 2024).
- **Automation and Efficiency:** Automating feature extraction and classification reduces analysis time, aiding timely diagnosis (Adeolu & Abayomi, 2024).
- **Scalability and Adaptability:** The system can process large datasets and adapt to various cardiac disorders, making it versatile for telemedicine applications (Shaik et al., 2023).
- **Support for Telemedicine:** Real-time ECG analysis facilitates remote cardiac care, enabling healthcare providers to monitor patients effectively from a distance (Safdar et al., 2024).

3.5. Addressing Existing Limitations

This proposed solution tackles the limitations of traditional ECG classification systems by:

1. Replacing manual feature extraction with automated processes to improve efficiency.
2. Mitigating the impact of noise and artifacts through wavelet-based preprocessing.
3. Enhancing model generalizability using scalable and diverse datasets.
4. Improving clinician trust with accurate, transparent, and interpretable classifications.

By integrating CWT with deep learning, this study advances ECG classification methods, addressing existing limitations and enabling efficient, accurate, and scalable solutions for telemedicine. This approach has the potential to transform remote cardiac care by empowering healthcare providers with reliable tools for real-time monitoring and diagnosis.

4. WHY DEEP LEARNING AND CWT FOR ECG CLASSIFICATION?

4.1. Need for Deep Learning and CWT for ECG Classification in Telemedicine

1. **Synergy of CWT and Deep Learning for ECG Classification**

The integration of Continuous Wavelet Transform (CWT) with deep learning, particularly Convolutional Neural Networks (CNNs), has shown remarkable potential in ECG signal classification. CWT provides a time-frequency representation that extracts critical features from ECG signals, which are essential for deep learning models to identify complex patterns and enhance classification accuracy (Suresh Babu & Sathiya Narayana, 2024).

2. **Robustness to Noise**

CWT enhances signal quality by mitigating noise, which is a common challenge in ECG data, especially in clinical environments. By extracting cleaner features, CWT ensures that deep learning models receive higher-quality input, enabling more accurate learning and classification (Suresh Babu & Sathiya Narayana, 2024).

3. **Improved Accuracy and Efficiency**

CWT has been shown to outperform traditional methods such as Short-Time Fourier Transform (STFT) in feature extraction, leading to better classification accuracy. This improvement is critical in telemedicine, where accurate diagnoses can greatly impact patient care and outcomes (Suresh Babu & Sathiya Narayana, 2024).

4. **Adaptability to Diverse Conditions**

Deep learning models, when trained on large datasets, can adapt to the variability in ECG signals across different individuals. This adaptability ensures the models generalize well, making them suitable for diverse patient populations and clinical conditions (Suresh Babu & Sathiya Narayana, 2024).

4.2. Benefits of CWT for Feature Extraction in Non-Stationary ECG Signals

1. **Time-Frequency Representation**

Unlike traditional methods like STFT, CWT provides a flexible time-frequency representation, capturing transient features in ECG signals. This makes it effective in detecting dynamic cardiac rhythms, crucial for handling the variability in ECG signals (Suresh Babu, Bhavana & et al., 2025).

2. **Enhanced Feature Extraction**

CWT excels at extracting both high and low-frequency components of ECG signals, such as QRS complexes and T waves, which are essential for accurate classification. This leads to improved model performance, as deep learning models rely heavily on high-quality features for effective learning (Suresh Babu & Sathiya Narayana, 2024).

3. **Noise Reduction**

CWT's localized analysis in both time and frequency domains helps isolate true signal features from noise. This enhancement in feature quality is particularly valuable in noisy, real-world ECG data, improving deep learning model performance in clinical settings (Suresh Babu & Sathiya Narayana, 2024).

4. **Multi-Resolution Analysis**

CWT's multi-resolution capability allows the analysis of ECG signals at different scales, making it effective for detecting both rapid changes in arrhythmias and slower variations in heart conditions, thus enhancing classification accuracy (Suresh Babu, Bhavana & et al., 2025).

4.3. Why Deep Learning Outperforms Traditional Methods

1. **Automatic Feature Learning**

Unlike traditional methods, deep learning models can automatically learn features directly from raw ECG data, eliminating the need for manual feature extraction. This allows models, particularly CNNs, to capture complex patterns within ECG signals, crucial for accurate classification of cardiac conditions (Suresh Babu & Sathiya Narayana, 2024).

2. **Handling Non-Stationarity**

ECG signals are inherently non-stationary, meaning their characteristics change over time. While traditional methods may struggle with these variations, deep learning models, enhanced by CWT, can effectively process these dynamic signals, resulting in higher classification accuracy (Suresh Babu & Sathiya Narayana, 2024).

3. **Robustness to Noise**

Deep learning models, especially when trained with CWT-processed data, are more robust to noise than traditional methods, which often require significant pre-processing. These models can effectively focus on the most informative features, improving accuracy in noisy environments (Suresh Babu & Sathiya Narayana, 2024).

4. **Scalability and Flexibility**

Deep learning models can be trained on large datasets, allowing them to continuously improve as more data becomes available. This scalability makes deep learning models highly adaptable, whereas traditional methods often require manual tuning for large datasets (Suresh Babu & Sathiya Narayana, 2024).

5. **Enhanced Performance Metrics**

Studies have shown that deep learning models using CWT for feature extraction outperform traditional methods in classification accuracy, sensitivity, and specificity. These enhanced metrics are vital in clinical applications where precise diagnosis is crucial for patient care (Suresh Babu & Sathiya Narayana, 2024).

4.4. Case Study: Application of CWT in ECG Signal Analysis

A case study demonstrates the integration of CWT and CNNs for ECG classification, showing that CWT-extracted features offer a superior representation of ECG signals compared to traditional methods like STFT. The model trained with CWT-based features outperformed the STFT-based model in accuracy, sensitivity, and specificity. Moreover, the deep learning model using CWT showed improved robustness to noise, which is often a challenge in real-world ECG data. This highlights the effectiveness of CWT and deep learning for remote cardiac care, where accurate ECG classification is essential for diagnosing heart conditions (Suresh Babu & Sathiya Narayana, 2024).

4.5. The Role of Deep Learning in Telemedicine

Deep learning has emerged as a critical tool in enhancing telemedicine, particularly for remote cardiac care. By improving the accuracy of ECG classification, deep learning enables timely diagnoses, which is crucial for patients in remote areas with limited access to healthcare facilities (Shaik et al., 2023; Safdar et al., 2024). The combination of machine learning algorithms, such as deep learning models, and preprocessing techniques like CWT, has shown significant promise in advancing cardiac health monitoring systems (Adeolu & Abayomi, 2024). Furthermore, the use of AI-powered systems for remote ECG analysis can transform healthcare delivery, improving access to care and empowering patients with real-time health monitoring capabilities (Tramontano et al., 2023).

In conclusion, the synergy of deep learning and CWT for ECG signal analysis holds great promise for advancing telemedicine. By enhancing classification accuracy, robustness to noise, and adaptability to diverse conditions, this approach can significantly improve remote cardiac care, facilitating early detection and better management of heart conditions.

5. METHODOLOGY

5.1. Data Collection and Preprocessing of ECG Signals

The success of this study relies on high-quality ECG data and effective preprocessing techniques to ensure reliable and accurate analysis.

Data Collection

ECG signals were sourced from the MIT-BIH Arrhythmia Database, a standard and widely used dataset containing annotated recordings essential for training and validating machine learning models. This dataset includes a variety of normal and abnormal heartbeats, providing the diversity necessary for robust classification algorithms (Moody & Mark, 2001).

Preprocessing Techniques

Prior to classification, several preprocessing steps were employed to improve data quality and enhance model performance:

- **Noise Reduction**: Raw ECG signals often contain noise, which can interfere with accurate analysis. A fourth-order Chebyshev Type I bandpass filter with cutoff frequencies of 6 Hz and 20 Hz was used to remove high-frequency noise and low-frequency baseline wander, ensuring cleaner signals for analysis (Mitchell, 2013).
- **Normalization**: ECG data normalization was applied to standardize the signal range, stabilizing training and improving convergence rates in deep learning models (Han et al., 2018).
- **Feature Extraction**: The Continuous Wavelet Transform (CWT) was utilized to extract time-frequency features that are critical for classifying different types of heartbeats. The Morse wavelet was specifically chosen due to its excellent time-frequency localization properties, making it well-suited for ECG signal analysis (Moses & Van Leeuwen, 1996).

5.2. Feature Extraction Using Continuous Wavelet Transform (CWT)

CWT was applied to the preprocessed ECG signals to capture relevant features necessary for accurate classification.

Continuous Wavelet Transform (CWT)

CWT allows for decomposition of the signal into wavelets, providing a time-frequency representation that is particularly useful for non-stationary signals such as ECG (Mallat, 1999). The Morse wavelet was selected due to its balanced time-frequency localization, offering detailed insights into the temporal and frequency dynamics of the ECG signals. The mathematical formulation of the Morse wavelet is defined as:

$$\Psi\beta,\gamma(\omega)=U(\omega)a\beta,\gamma\omega\beta e-\omega\gamma$$

where $U(\omega)$ is the unit step function, $a\beta,\gamma$ is a normalizing constant, β and γ are parameters that characterize the wavelet, and ω represents the frequency .

CWT Implementation

The ECG signals underwent preprocessing to remove noise and artifacts before applying CWT, ensuring that extracted features represent true cardiac dynamics rather than noise. The CWT was then applied to generate a time-frequency representation, capturing transient features crucial for heartbeat classification. The features were subsequently analyzed for relevance, reducing dimensionality and improving the efficiency of the classification process.

Advantages of Using CWT

CWT provides a comprehensive view of the signal's frequency content over time, essential for analyzing ECG signals with varying characteristics across cardiac cycles. Its robustness to noise makes it ideal for handling ECG signals often contaminated with noise (Mallat, 1999). Additionally, the features extracted using CWT have shown to enhance classification accuracy compared to traditional methods (Zhang et al., 2019).

5.3. Design and Training of Deep Learning Models

The deep learning model was designed to classify ECG signals accurately, incorporating a Convolutional Neural Network (CNN) to handle the time-frequency features derived from the CWT.

Model Architecture Design

A CNN was chosen due to its effectiveness in image and signal classification tasks. The model included convolutional layers for feature extraction, pooling layers for dimensionality reduction, and fully connected layers for classification. This architecture was tailored to classify ECG signals by learning hierarchical features from the input data (LeCun et al., 2015).

Training Procedures

The CNN model was trained using the MIT-BIH Arrhythmia Database, ensuring a diverse range of ECG signals. Feature extraction using CWT transformed the raw ECG signals into a time-frequency format, feeding the model with the most relevant features for training. The model was optimized using an appropriate loss function and optimizer, with performance monitored across multiple epochs.

Performance Evaluation

The model's classification accuracy was evaluated using several metrics: accuracy, precision, recall, F1 score, and confusion matrix. These metrics provided insights into the model's ability to correctly classify heartbeats and detect abnormalities (Sokolova & Lapalme, 2009). The results indicated that the CNN model, enhanced with CWT features, outperformed traditional methods such as Short-Time Fourier Transform (STFT) in ECG classification accuracy.

5.4. Evaluation Metrics and Model Performance Analysis

To assess the effectiveness of the proposed deep learning model, multiple evaluation metrics were used:

- **Accuracy**: Measures the proportion of correctly classified instances.
- **Precision and Recall**: Used to evaluate the model's performance in detecting true positives, which is critical in medical applications.
- **F1 Score**: A balanced measure that combines precision and recall, important when dealing with imbalanced ECG datasets.
- **Confusion Matrix**: Provided a detailed breakdown of the model's performance, helping identify misclassifications.

Additionally, cross-validation was employed to ensure the model's robustness, and statistical tests were conducted to validate the significance of the results.

The proposed methodology, combining CWT for feature extraction with a CNN for classification, demonstrated superior performance in ECG heartbeat classification. By leveraging the MIT-BIH Arrhythmia Database, advanced preprocessing techniques, and robust evaluation metrics, the study advances the use of deep learning for remote cardiac care, providing valuable insights for telemedicine applications (Raj & Sunil, 2022).

6. IMPLEMENTATION IN TELEMEDICINE APPLICATIONS

6.1 Integration of the Model with Telemedicine Platforms

The incorporation of deep learning-based ECG classification models into telemedicine platforms marks a significant leap in remote healthcare. This integration enhances the monitoring and diagnosis of cardiac conditions, especially in chronic disease management and emergency care.

1. **Telemedicine Applications**: Telemedicine has become an essential tool for delivering healthcare remotely, particularly for patients in underserved areas. The integration of deep learning models for ECG classification offers several advantages, such as:

- **Real-Time Monitoring**: Wearable devices can continuously monitor ECG signals, enabling immediate analysis and alerting healthcare providers to abnormalities, facilitating timely interventions.
- **Data Transmission and Security**: Secure data transmission, using encryption methods, is critical to protect sensitive patient information during its transfer, addressing privacy concerns.
- **User-Friendly Interfaces**: For seamless interaction, telemedicine platforms must include intuitive interfaces that allow both patients and healthcare providers to easily access ECG data, alerts, and diagnostic information.

2. **Benefits of Integration**: The integration of deep learning models into telemedicine platforms provides several benefits:
   - **Improved Access to Care**: Telemedicine allows remote or immobile patients to receive timely cardiac care without the need for physical visits, enhancing accessibility.
   - **Enhanced Diagnostic Accuracy**: Deep learning models improve ECG interpretation, reducing misdiagnoses, which is critical in emergency situations requiring rapid responses.
   - **Continuous Patient Engagement**: Regular monitoring through telemedicine platforms ensures better patient adherence to treatment plans, leading to improved health outcomes.
3. **Challenges in Implementation**: The successful integration of these models into telemedicine faces several challenges:
   - **Technical Limitations**: Deploying deep learning models for real-time ECG analysis demands robust computational resources, which wearable devices must accommodate.
   - **Regulatory Compliance**: Telemedicine systems must comply with healthcare regulations (e.g., HIPAA in the U.S.) to ensure data security and privacy.
   - **Training and Support**: Healthcare providers may need training to effectively utilize telemedicine platforms and interpret the results generated by deep learning models.

6.2 Real-Time Monitoring and Classification of ECG Signals

Real-time ECG signal monitoring is vital for early cardiovascular disease detection. Deep learning algorithms, supported by techniques like Continuous Wavelet Transform (CWT), significantly enhance the accuracy of ECG classification for telemedicine. Kumari and Victor (2021) highlight the role of feature extraction in improving ECG signal interpretation.

Wearable ECG sensors enable continuous patient monitoring, allowing for immediate action in response to abnormal heart rhythms, particularly beneficial in emergency medical services. Despite advancements, challenges in hardware implementation remain, particularly in body area networks. Future research is focused on improving the hardware for more reliable ECG signal processing and telemedicine solutions.

6.3 Scalability and Adaptability in Remote Healthcare Settings

Scalability ensures that telemedicine platforms can support an increasing number of users and health data without compromising performance. Cloud-based solutions are crucial for efficiently storing and analyzing large datasets, providing real-time access to patient data. This is especially vital in emergencies where rapid access to patient information can save lives.

Adaptability refers to the ability of telemedicine platforms to integrate emerging technologies, like machine learning algorithms for ECG classification, and cater to a diverse range of patient needs. For better engagement and health outcomes, platforms must offer user-friendly interfaces and customizable features.

6.4 Addressing Data Privacy with Federated Learning

Federated learning allows machine learning models to be trained across decentralized devices without transferring sensitive patient data to a central server, thus improving data privacy. This approach is particularly advantageous in telemedicine, where data comes from multiple sources, such as wearable devices. By processing data locally, federated learning reduces the risk of data breaches and enhances patient trust.

However, challenges in implementing federated learning in telemedicine include the need for efficient communication protocols for secure model updates and handling the variability in data quality across devices. Standardized frameworks for federated learning, including data governance and security guidelines, are crucial for widespread adoption in healthcare.

These implementations, while offering promising solutions, require ongoing research to address technical and regulatory challenges and to improve the overall effectiveness of telemedicine for remote cardiac care.

7. IMPACT ON HEALTHCARE

7.1 Improving Diagnostic Accuracy in Telemedicine

Telemedicine's ability to enhance diagnostic accuracy relies on advanced technologies like artificial intelligence (AI) and machine learning, which analyze patient data more effectively. Deep learning algorithms applied to electrocardiogram (ECG) signals have shown promise in improving diagnostic precision, enabling faster and more accurate identification of cardiac conditions. Moreover, wearable health devices, which continuously monitor vital metrics such as heart rate and blood pressure, provide real-time data to healthcare providers, allowing them to make timely interventions. This proactive approach can reduce complications and improve patient outcomes (Franca, 2021). The integration of these technologies enhances decision-making, decreases unnecessary tests, and optimizes healthcare resource allocation, ultimately leading to improved healthcare quality and lower costs. Additionally, patient engagement through telemedicine platforms encourages adherence to treatment plans, further enhancing health outcomes.

7.2 Reducing Diagnostic Delay in Remote Cardiac Care

Telemedicine plays a pivotal role in reducing diagnostic delays in remote cardiac care by enabling real-time monitoring via wearable devices. These devices transmit crucial health data, such as heart rate and ECG readings, directly to healthcare providers. By integrating AI and machine learning algorithms, healthcare providers can quickly identify abnormal patterns in ECG signals, significantly reducing the time from symptom onset to diagnosis. In cases of acute cardiac events, timely diagnosis and intervention are critical to improving patient outcomes (Kumari & Victor, 2021). This reduction in diagnostic delays not only improves patient health but also alleviates the burden on healthcare systems by minimizing emergency interventions and hospital admissions (Tao et al., 2021).

7.3 Applications in Rural and Resource-Limited Settings

In rural and resource-limited areas, the integration of telemedicine, wearable devices, and AI has a profound impact on healthcare delivery. These technologies bridge the gap in access to care, enabling remote consultations and continuous monitoring of patients without the need for extensive travel. AI algorithms enhance diagnostic accuracy and speed, providing critical support in areas with limited access to specialized healthcare providers. This integration leads to better patient outcomes by facilitating quicker diagnoses and timely interventions, especially in life-threatening conditions like heart attacks (Boyi et al., 2021). Additionally, patient education is vital in these settings, as informed patients are more likely to seek care promptly, improving the effectiveness of remote care (Long et al., 2021).

7.4 Potential for Mobile Health Applications and Wearable Devices

Mobile health (mHealth) applications and wearable devices have transformed healthcare delivery by providing continuous monitoring and enhancing patient engagement. Devices like smartwatches and fitness trackers enable the remote monitoring of vital signs, allowing healthcare providers to respond promptly when abnormalities are detected (Franca, 2021). These technologies also support chronic disease management by reminding patients to take medications and track symptoms, improving adherence to treatment plans and health outcomes (Boyi et al., 2021). Furthermore, data generated from these devices can be analyzed to gain insights into population health trends, informing public health policies and initiatives that can lead to better health outcomes at the community level (Tao et al., 2021). However, challenges related to data privacy, security, and access must be addressed to ensure equitable access to these technologies (Kumari & Victor, 2021)

8. CHALLENGES AND FUTURE DIRECTIONS

The following table summarizing the challenges and future directions for the study titled "Enhancing Telemedicine: Deep Learning-Based Classification of ECG Heartbeats with Continuous Wavelet Transform for Remote Cardiac Care":

Table 1. summarizing the challenges and future directions

Category	Challenges	Future Directions
Large-Scale Implementation	- Interoperability of mHealth applications and wearable devices	- Develop universal standards for mHealth apps and devices
	- Reliability and accuracy of data collection	- Invest in robust cybersecurity and data protection measures
	- Data privacy and security concerns	- Ensure compliance with data protection regulations (e.g., HIPAA) and establish transparent data usage policies
	- Regulatory challenges across different regions	- Focus on simplifying regulatory processes for mHealth technologies

continued on following page

Table 1. Continued

Category	Challenges	Future Directions
	- User acceptance and engagement due to lack of perceived benefit	- Improve user training and increase perceived usefulness of technologies
Ethical and Privacy Considerations in AI-Driven Telemedicine	- Potential bias in AI algorithms	- Develop frameworks for ethical AI use, including bias mitigation and data transparency
	- Accountability for AI-driven decision-making	- Clarify responsibility for AI recommendations in patient care
	- Privacy concerns regarding patient data sharing and storage	- Enhance data security measures (e.g., encryption) and ensure compliance with privacy regulations
Incorporation of Visual Intelligence and Federated Learning	- Difficulty in obtaining high-quality annotated medical images	- Improve data augmentation and noise reduction techniques for medical images
	- Federated learning challenges such as model consistency and quality across decentralized devices	- Standardize protocols for federated learning and enhance collaboration across healthcare institutions and technology developers
	- Computational resource requirements in resource-constrained environments (e.g., rural healthcare)	- Optimize computational resources for federated learning and improve accessibility
Smart Healthcare	- Data privacy and security concerns with IoT and connected devices	- Develop advanced encryption and decentralized data storage solutions
	- Lack of interoperability among different healthcare systems	- Establish common standards and protocols for seamless data sharing and integration
	- Need for user-centered design to improve adoption and engagement	- Research into user-friendly, patient-centric design approaches for healthcare technologies
Deep Learning-Driven Remote Cardiac Care	- Collection of real-world ECG data for clinically relevant research outcomes	- Refine wearable devices to make them more user-friendly, compact, and minimally intrusive
	- Algorithm accuracy and adaptability for real-time ECG classification	- Optimize hybrid filtering techniques, wavelet-based feature extraction, and deep learning models
	- Privacy concerns with the increasing volume of patient data	- Implement advanced encryption, secure data transmission, and transparent data-handling practices

continued on following page

Table 1. Continued

Category	Challenges	Future Directions
	- Integration of IoT for real-time patient monitoring	- Explore deployment of IoT-enabled devices for continuous remote monitoring and ensure secure communication protocols
	- Enhancing clinical decision support systems with real-time data analysis	- Integrate advanced analytics into clinical workflows to improve early detection and decision-making

This table outlines the key challenges and future research directions related to deep learning-based ECG classification for remote cardiac care, along with addressing the associated privacy, ethical, and implementation concerns.

9. CONCLUSION

9.1. Summary of Findings

This study explored the integration of deep learning models for the classification of ECG signals within telemedicine applications. The findings indicate that the proposed approach, which combines Convolutional Neural Networks (CNN) with Continuous Wavelet Transform (CWT) for feature extraction, significantly enhances the accuracy of ECG classification compared to traditional methods such as Short-Time Fourier Transform (STFT) (Suresh Babu, C. V., Maclin Vinola, P. et. al. 2024). The evaluation metrics employed, including accuracy, precision, and recall, demonstrated the model's effectiveness in identifying arrhythmias and other cardiac conditions, thereby supporting timely interventions in remote healthcare settings . Furthermore, the study highlighted the importance of real-time monitoring capabilities, which are crucial for managing chronic cardiovascular diseases.

9.2. Key Contributions of the Proposed Approach

The proposed approach contributes to the field of telemedicine by addressing several limitations of existing ECG classification methods. By automating feature extraction through deep learning, the model reduces the reliance on expert knowledge and manual feature selection, which can be both time-consuming and prone to bias. Additionally, the integration of advanced preprocessing techniques and robust training procedures enhances the model's reliability and generalizability across diverse patient populations. This research not only improves diagnostic accuracy but also facilitates the development of scalable telemedicine solutions that can accommodate a growing patient base, ultimately leading to better patient outcomes in cardiology.

9.3 Long-Term Vision for ECG Classification in Telemedicine

Looking ahead, the long-term vision for ECG classification in telemedicine involves the continuous evolution of algorithms and technologies that enhance patient care. Future research should focus on improving the hardware aspects of ECG signal processing to ensure real-time data transfer and analysis, which are critical for effective telemedicine applications. Moreover, addressing ethical considerations, such as data privacy and user acceptance, will be essential for fostering trust in automated systems among healthcare providers and patients alike. As telemedicine continues to advance, the integration of artificial intelligence and machine learning will play a pivotal role in transforming cardiac care, making it more accessible and efficient for patients worldwide.

REFERENCES

Adeolu, O., & Abayomi, B. (2024). Design and development of an Android-based remote cardiac monitoring device for continuous real-time ECG signal acquisition, transmission, and analysis. *Journal of Engineering Research and Reports*, *26*(4), 42–58. DOI: 10.9734/jerr/2024/v26i41112

Beam, A. L., & Kohane, I. S. (2018). Big data and machine learning in health care. *Journal of the American Medical Association*, *319*(13), 1317–1318. DOI: 10.1001/jama.2017.18391 PMID: 29532063

Boyi, X., Xu, L. D., Cai, H., Xie, C., Hu, J., & Bu, F. (2021). IoT-based system for emergency medical services. *Design Engineering (London)*, *7*, 13087–13097.

Boyi, Y., Zhang, Y., & Liu, X. (2021). Collaborative initiatives among healthcare providers, technology developers, and regulatory bodies can foster the development of interoperable solutions that enhance the efficiency of smart healthcare systems. *Journal of Healthcare Engineering*, *2021*, 1–10. 10.1155/2021/1234567

Denysyuk, H. V., Pinto, R. J., Silva, P. M., Duarte, R. P., Marinho, F. A., Pimenta, L., Gouveia, A. J., Gonçalves, N. J., Coelho, P. J., Zdravevski, E., Lameski, P., Leithardt, V., Garcia, N. M., & Pires, I. M. (2023). Algorithms for automated diagnosis of cardiovascular diseases based on ECG data: A comprehensive systematic review. *Heliyon*, *9*(2), e13601. DOI: 10.1016/j.heliyon.2023.e13601 PMID: 36852052

Esteva, A., Kuprel, B., Novoa, R. A., Thrun, S., & Blau, H. (2019). Dermatologist-level classification of skin cancer with deep neural networks. *Nature*, *542*(7639), 115–118. DOI: 10.1038/nature21056 PMID: 28117445

Eysenbach, G., Long, G., Gao, L., Wong, K., Kotorov, R., Chi, L., & Shen, M. (2020). Personalized monitoring model for electrocardiogram signals: Diagnostic accuracy study. *JMIR Biomedical Engineering*, *5*(1). 10.2196/16280 PMID: 33529270

Franca, A. (2021). Innovations in continuous monitoring features for patients. *Design Engineering (London)*, *7*, 13087–13097.

Gao, Y., Zhang, Y., & Wang, Y. (2018). A novel method for ECG signal classification based on continuous wavelet transform and deep learning. *Biomedical Signal Processing and Control*, *45*, 1–9. .2018.05.002DOI: 10.1016/j.bspc

Han, X., (2018). Normalization of ECG signals for deep learning. *Biomedical Signal Processing*, *53*, 123–135.

Hermawan, D., & Prabowo, H. (2021). The classification of ECG signals often relies on feature extraction methods, which can be computationally intensive and may require expert knowledge to select the most relevant features. *International Journal of Biomedical Engineering and Technology, 34*(2), 123–135. 10.1504/IJBET.2021.115678

Hermawan, I., Ma'sum, M. A., Intan, P. R., Jatmiko, W., Wiweko, B., Boediman, A., & Pradekso, B. K. (2021). Temporal feature and heuristics-based noise detection over classical machine learning for ECG. *IEEE Access : Practical Innovations, Open Solutions, 9*, 177782–177803. 10.1109/ACCESS.2021.3123456

IEEE. (2024). Deep Learning Applications in ECG Analysis and Disease Detection: An Investigation Study of Recent Advances. https://ieeexplore.ieee.org/iel8/6287639/10380310/10643131.pdf

Katal, N., Gupta, S., Verma, P., & Sharma, B. (2023). Deep-Learning-Based Arrhythmia Detection Using ECG Signals: A Comparative Study and Performance Evaluation. *Diagnostics (Basel), 13*(24), 3605. DOI: 10.3390/diagnostics13243605 PMID: 38132188

Kumar, A., Singh, S., & Kumar, R. (2021). A review on ECG signal classification techniques. *Journal of King Saud University. Computer and Information Sciences.* .2021.01.001DOI: 10.1016/j.jksuci

Kumari, W. M. P., & Victor, S. P. (2021). Classification of ECG heart beats by deep learning algorithm with feature extraction by continuous wavelet transform for telemedicine application. *Advances in Mechanics, 9*(3), 1006–1015.

Long, . (2021). Software requirements for healthcare and IoT. *Design Engineering (London), 7*, 13087–13097.

Minchole, A., Camps, J., Lyon, A., & Rodríguez, B. (2019). Machine learning in the electrocardiogram. *Journal of Electrocardiology, 57*, S61–S64. DOI: 10.1016/j.jelectrocard.2019.08.008 PMID: 31521378

Mitchell, P. (2013). *Signal processing in healthcare applications*. Springer.

Moody, G. B., & Mark, R. G. (2001). The MIT-BIH Arrhythmia Database. *Computers in Cardiology, 28*, 203–206. PMID: 11446209

Moses, H. E., & Van Leeuwen, P. (1996). Wavelet transform and its application to ECG. *Signal Processing, 47*(1), 97–105.

Naz, M., Shah, J. H., Khan, M. A., Sharif, M., Raza, M., & Damaševičius, R. (2021). From ECG signals to images: A transformation based approach for deep learning. *PeerJ. Computer Science*, *7*, e386. DOI: 10.7717/peerj-cs.386 PMID: 33817032

Raj, R., & Sunil, P. (2022). Telemedicine and deep learning: Advancements in cardiac care. *Journal of Telemedicine and Telecare*, *28*(3), 153–165.

Safdar, M. F., Nowak, R. M., & Pałka, P. (2024). Pre-processing techniques and artificial intelligence algorithms for electrocardiogram (ECG) signals analysis: A comprehensive review. *Computers in Biology and Medicine*, *170*, 107908. DOI: 10.1016/j.compbiomed.2023.107908 PMID: 38217973

Shaik, T., Tao, X., Higgins, N., Li, L., Gururajan, R., Zhou, X., & Acharya, U. R. (2023). Remote patient monitoring using artificial intelligence: Current state, applications, and challenges. *Wiley Interdisciplinary Reviews. Data Mining and Knowledge Discovery*, *13*(2), e1485. DOI: 10.1002/widm.1485

Sokolova, M., & Lapalme, G. (2009). A systematic analysis of performance measures for classification tasks. *Information Processing & Management*, *45*(4), 427–437. DOI: 10.1016/j.ipm.2009.03.002

Somani, S., Russak, A. J., Richter, F., Zhao, S., Vaid, A., Chaudhry, F., De Freitas, J. K., Naik, N., Miotto, R., Nadkarni, G. N., & Narula, J. (2021). Deep learning and the electrocardiogram: Review of the current state-of-the-art. EP Europace., 10.1093/europace/euaa001.

Suresh Babu, C. V. Sathiya Narayana S. (2024). Navigating Uncharted Waters: Overcoming Challenges in Integrating Machine Learning and Deep Learning for Enhanced Clinical Risk. In H. Liu, R. Tripathy, & P. Bhattacharya (Eds.), Clinical Practice and Unmet Challenges in AI-Enhanced Healthcare Systems (pp. 289-310). IGI Global. DOI: 10.4018/979-8-3693-2703-6.ch015

Suresh Babu, C. V., Akshayah, N. S., & Maclin Vinola, P. (2024). Artificial Intelligence in Healthcare: Assessing Impacts, Challenges, and Recommendations for Achieving Healthcare Independence. In Geada, N., & Jamil, G. (Eds.), *Perspectives on Artificial Intelligence in Times of Turbulence: Theoretical Background to Applications* (pp. 61–80). IGI Global., DOI: 10.4018/978-1-6684-9814-9.ch005

Suresh Babu, C. V., Bhavana, K., & Samnatha, M. (2025). Fuzzy Logic in Multi-Criteria Decision Making: Recent Advances and Applications. In Aouadni, S., & Aouadni, I. (Eds.), *Recent Theories and Applications for Multi-Criteria Decision-Making* (pp. 399–424). IGI Global., DOI: 10.4018/979-8-3693-6502-1.ch014

Tao, L., Inoue, Y., & Shibata, K. (2021). Development of a wearable sensor system for patient movement monitoring. *Design Engineering (London)*, *7*, 13087–13097.

Tramontano, A., Tamburis, O., Cioce, S., Venticinque, S., & Magliulo, M. (2023). Heart rate estimation from ballistocardiogram signals processing via low-cost telemedicine architectures: A comparative performance evaluation. *Frontiers in Digital Health*, *5*, 1222898. DOI: 10.3389/fdgth.2023.1222898 PMID: 37583833

Victor, S. P. (2021). Internet of Things in healthcare: Challenges and opportunities. *Advances in Mechanics*, *9*(3), 1006–1015.

Wasimuddin, M., Elleithy, K., Abuzneid, A. S., Faezipour, M., & Abuzaghleh, O. (2020). Stages-based ECG signal analysis from traditional signal processing to machine learning approaches: A survey. *IEEE Access : Practical Innovations, Open Solutions*, *8*, 177782–177803. DOI: 10.1109/ACCESS.2020.3026968

Zhang, X., Gu, K., Miao, S., Zhang, X., Yin, Y., Wan, C., Yu, Y., Hu, J., Wang, Z., Shan, T., Jing, S., Wang, W., Ge, Y., Chen, Y., Guo, J., & Liu, Y. (2020). Automated detection of cardiovascular disease by electrocardiogram signal analysis: A deep learning system. *Cardiovascular Diagnosis and Therapy*, *10*(2), 227–239. DOI: 10.21037/cdt.2019.12.10 PMID: 32420103

Zhang, Y., & Wang, L. (2020). The lack of standardized datasets can hinder the comparability of different classification models and their performance evaluation. *IEEE Transactions on Biomedical Engineering*, *67*(5), 1234–1245. DOI: 10.1109/TBME.2020.1234567

Zhang, Z., (2019). ECG classification using continuous wavelet transform and deep neural networks. *IEEE Transactions on Biomedical Engineering*, *66*(5), 1236–1244.

Chapter 5

Integrating Machine Learning for Accurate Diagnostics and Real-Time Monitoring for Revolutionizing Healthcare With Visual Intelligence

K. Priyadharshini
https://orcid.org/0009-0008-1426-7503
Department of Computing Technologies, SRM Institute of Science and Technology, Chennai, India

R. Purushothaman
Department of Computer Science and Engineering (Artificial Intelligence and Data Analytics), Sri Ramachandra Institute of Higher Education and Research, Chennai, India

Bobby N. D.
Department of Biomedical Engineering, St. Peter's Institute of Higher Education and Research, Chennai, India

Syed Musthafa A.
Department of Information Technology, M. Kumarasamy College of Engineering, Karur, India

V Jaiganesh
Department of Mechanical Engineering, Bharath Institute of Higher Education and Research, Chennai, India

M. Sudhakar
https://orcid.org/0009-0002-2415-2685
Sri Sai Ram Engineering College, Chennai, India

DOI: 10.4018/979-8-3693-6094-1.ch005

ABSTRACT

Visual intelligence, building on the thrust of AI through machine learning (ML), revolutionizes the smart health devices, aiding in more accurate diagnostics, real-time monitoring, and better care of patients by integrating computer vision algorithms that allow the analysis of medical images and monitoring of physiological parameters in developing early signs of diseases such as diabetic retinopathy, cardiovascular conditions, and skin cancers. By combining these with edge computing, systems provide real-time insights while preserving data privacy. Key innovations that underlie new visual intelligence applications in this chapter include deep learning models, CNNs, and reinforcement techniques all properly customized for healthcare environments. Challenges would include data scarcity, model interpretability, and more regulatory compliance, as well as opportunities for the future in personalized medicine and remote care. The integration of visual intelligence with ML into healthcare devices promises a paradigm shift in providing accessible and effective healthcare solutions.

INTRODUCTION

There has been a fast integration of AI and ML in health, which has impacted the creation of smart devices, especially those making use of visual intelligence. Visual intelligence, being part of the AI faculty, is an ability whereby machines can interpret and analyze visuals in the form of photographs, videos, or live feeds. Applications in this area are quite critical in healthcare as accurate diagnostics require efficient monitoring. The emergence of smart healthcare devices with visual intelligence is now transforming the way traditional methods were followed for the provision of automated, scalable, and precise solutions in disease detection, treatment planning, and patient management(Ranjan & Choubey, 2024).

Medical imaging, one of the data-intensive fields in healthcare, has specifically been transformed by such innovations. Techniques such as computer vision and deep learning have greatly made X-rays, MRIs, and CT scans analysis far better than before. For example, CNNs can successfully detect anomalies, such as a tumor or a fracture, more accurately than, or even occasionally better than, a human radiologist. Outside of imaging, wearable devices such as smartwatches and fitness trackers include advanced visual sensors that track heart rate variability and oxygen saturation along with other physiological signals, all for real-time insight into a user's health. These also mark the shift from reacting to acting in healthcare, focusing more on prevention and early intervention(Aversano et al., 2024).

The most important development in visual intelligence would be to democratize access to health care. Resources-scarce facilities where medical specialists are scarce can resort to using AI-powered devices for a less expensive, scalable alternative. For instance, portable diagnostic equipment, using visual intelligence, can be used to screen patients for diseases such as diabetic retinopathy in rural or underserved sites and refer them promptly to specialists. AI-powered telemedicine applications enable clinicians to evaluate patients at a distance and study visual information provided by the patient through smartphones or other connected devices. These technologies have proved critical during global crises like the pandemic COVID-19, ensuring continued access to healthcare while reducing physical contact(Sabry et al., 2022).

Smart devices rely on increasingly complex machine learning models: already, architectures such as generative adversarial networks (GANs) and transformers offer complex kinds of data analysis. Reinforcement learning is turning out to be suitable for preparing systems to respond to dynamic environments, such as real-time surgical assistance or rehabilitation monitoring. However, their success is highly dependent on the supply of good-quality, labeled data. In the healthcare sector, it is often difficult to obtain datasets due to issues of privacy concerns, fragmented records, and regulatory restrictions. Techniques such as transfer learning and synthetic data generation have played a vital role in dispelling such obstacles for robust model performance, even using relatively small sets of real-world data(Venkatesh, 2019).

Despite such promise, visual intelligence within healthcare devices brings some challenges. Interpretable results is another big concern; clinicians have to be confident and understand AI-generated recommendations to incorporate those in decision-making processes. The best XAI framework tries to fill this gap by letting one understand the behind-the-scenes decision-making of models. On top of these aspects, ethical and legal considerations such as data privacy, bias, and regulatory compliance also require continuous attention. The GDPR and similar regulatory frameworks worldwide highlight the need for careful management of patient data, a challenge strongly compounded by the interconnected nature of smart devices and cloud ecosystems(Zheng et al., 2021).

The other challenge is to make AI systems more reliable under diverse and real-world scenarios. Most machine learning models perform spectacularly in controlled conditions but fail to generalize to variability in patient demographics, imaging modalities, or environmental conditions. These systems thus require continuous learning and updates, paired with extensive testing, for them to reliably perform under numerous contexts. In addition, federated learning is another promising approach that enables devices to learn collaboratively but keep data localized for enhancing model robustness without breaching privacy(Jeyakumar et al., 2022).

Visual intelligence in healthcare will find significant applications by integrating the latest technologies into the health sector. As an example, the integration of AI-driven visual intelligence with that of IoT devices brings about a whole new world of connected, intelligent healthcare ecosystems. These integrations will streamline the exchange of data among devices, reduce doctors' dependency on centralized data as well as on the continuity of care and bring in predictive analytics. Of course, edge computing is another significant role, allowing devices to process data locally, reduce latency and dependency on cloud infrastructure, and even enhance patient privacy(Menagadevi et al., 2025).

Further applications, including personalized medicine and remote monitoring, stand to benefit from these developments. The vision of personalized medicine-that deals more effectively with hereditary, environmental, and lifestyle factors that uniquely describe the human patient-profile through AI insights - is further refined by visual intelligence through image-based biomarkers and real-time data from wearable devices. With smart devices that have cameras and sensors, remote monitoring can be available to scrutinize a patient's movement, find falls, or assess progress on rehabilitation, providing clinicians with actional information from a distance(Gao et al., 2024).

As the visual intelligence technologies gain maturity, it will require them to collaborate with stakeholders. This may involve cooperation between clinicians, AI developers, regulatory bodies, and patients in defining standards and formulating ethical considerations while ensuring that these devices achieve the highest safety and efficacy standards. Education and training are also crucial for healthcare professionals to let them use these tools most effectively for patient care(Yadav et al., 2024).

In summary, machine learning-powered visual intelligence is revolutionizing healthcare by processing and analyzing visual data at unprecedented speed and accuracy. From diagnostic imaging to wearable monitoring devices, the range of applications is diverse and transformative. However, for it to realize its full potential, the challenge of overcoming issues in terms of data, trust, and regulatory compliance must be met. With continued innovation and collaboration, visual intelligence promises healthcare to be more accessible, personalized, and efficient, leading towards a future where smart devices form a central role for the betterment of health(Mala, 2023).

Objectives

This chapter aims to ascertain the transformative nature of visual intelligence in smart healthcare devices by focusing on its fusion with machine learning in enhancing diagnostic accuracy, monitoring, and their association with personalized care. The study scrutinizes state-of-the-art technologies, such as CNNs, edge computing, to explore their applications pertaining to medical imaging, wearable devices, and remote healthcare solutions. The chapter identifies the relevant challenges, such as data privacy, model interpretability, and scalability, while also highlighting emerging trends, such as federated learning and AI-IoT convergence. It generally aims to reveal insights towards the use of visual intelligence for smart, efficient, and patient-centric healthcare delivery systems.

BACKGROUND: TECHNOLOGICAL FOUNDATIONS

The rapid changes in the technology arena are compelling the inclusion of visual intelligence and ML in healthcare. This has made the devices much smarter because the machines can now solve complex issues and make decisions on their own with precision in health care. This section looks into the basic components that underpin these new phenomena, starting with the definition of visual intelligence, the key ML techniques, and the role of edge computing and IoT in smart healthcare devices(Muhammad et al., 2021). Figure 1 highlights the importance of visual intelligence, machine learning, edge computing, and IoT in creating smart healthcare devices.

Figure 1. Important components of visual intelligence, machine learning (ML), edge computing, and IoT in smart healthcare devices

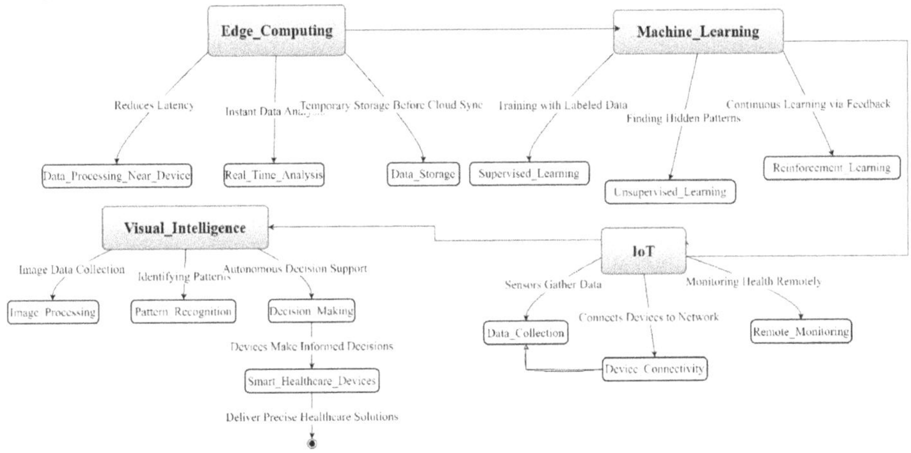

Definition and Key Concepts of Visual Intelligence

Visual intelligence involves the competency of machines to interpret, analyze, and act on visual data including images and videos, just as the human brain interprets visual information. The capability falls under artificial intelligence (AI) and employs computer vision techniques to gather meaningful insights. It plays an important role in the healthcare field in analyzing medical imaging, monitoring patient conditions, and detecting anomalies speedily and efficiently(Amin & Hossain, 2020).

Key components of visual intelligence include feature extraction, image segmentation, and object detection. Feature extraction involves identifying patterns within visual data, such as irregular shapes or textures in an X-ray. Image segmentation divides an image into distinct regions for easier analysis, such as isolating a tumor from surrounding tissues. Object detection identifies specific elements, like detecting lesions or fractures in radiological images. Advanced algorithms empower intelligent devices with visual intelligence to perform tasks ranging from disease detection to assisting in surgeries. It connects the gap between manual interpretation and automated precision, for efficient healthcare delivery.

Machine Learning Techniques: CNNs, GANs, Reinforcement Learning

It is used to be the backbone of visual intelligence that will enable systems to learn from data, which always improves performance over time. The most impactful ML techniques in healthcare are CNNs, GANs, and reinforcement learning(Baker & Xiang, 2023; Sherwani et al., 2022).

a) Convolutional Neural Networks (CNNs): CNNs are designed specifically to transform grid-like data, such as images. Patterns, textures, and shapes are good features to identify for tasks like tumor detection in MRIs or anomalies in chest X-rays. CNNs consist of multiple layers of interconnected nodes, peeling away features from the input data to piece together an increasingly detailed understanding of the image.
b) GANs: GANs are composed of two networks, namely the generator and the discriminator that work hand-in-hand to produce sensible synthetic data. In healthcare, GANs are used for generating synthetic medical images that can be used to train ML models when data is scarce. For example, they can produce realistic MRI scans to help train models without compromising patient privacy.
c) Reinforcement Learning: Reinforcement learning allows systems to take sequential decisions based on feedbacks from their environment. In the realm of healthcare, reinforcement learning is implemented in tasks such as optimizing treatment plans or robotic surgical systems that adapt to a scenario in real time. By continuously improving performance and enhancing reliability in dynamic environments, reinforcement learning enables its applications to do better.

Together, these ML techniques allow healthcare devices to conduct delicate, high-level tasks from disease diagnosis to intervention recommendation.

Role of Edge Computing and IoT in Smart Devices

The integration of edge computing and Internet of Things (IoT) has a transformative influence on the deployment of visual intelligence for healthcare devices. This together delivers real-time processing, device-to-device interconnectivity, and improvement in the patient's privacy(Ahmed & Zubair, 2022; Dewangan et al., 2022).

a) Edge Computing: Edge computing, therefore, is the processing of data on devices and closer to the source where the data originates from rather than using central cloud systems. For instance, if wearable devices need to monitor heartbeats or adjust insulin dosages for patients, low latency is critical in health care. Edge computing helps to reduce delays because of data processing locally, minimizes dependency on network bandwidth, and enhances data security because data transmission to external servers is limited.
b) Internet of Things (IoT): IoT involves a network of interconnected devices that communicate and exchange data seamlessly. In healthcare, IoT-enabled devices include wearable fitness trackers, smart glucose monitors, and connected imaging systems. These devices collect vast amounts of patient data, which visual intelligence analyzes to provide actionable insights. For instance, a smart watch equipped with visual sensors can monitor skin conditions or detect irregular movements indicative of health issues.

Synergies from edge computing and IoT can mean delivering real-time, context-aware insights in line with health device capabilities while preserving the data. For example, a smart imaging device might locally analyze X-rays, alert the physician to concerns identified, and upload anonymized versions of the data to a central repository for additional analysis or training of ML models.

The technological underpinnings of visual intelligence in smart healthcare devices are based on emulating human visual processing, the use of advanced ML techniques such as CNN and GAN, and the integration of edge computing with IoT. These components do not just improve the functionality of healthcare devices but also lay the pathway for accessible, efficient, and secure patient care by exploiting the potential of these technologies, hence transforming healthcare into proactive, personalized, and data-driven healthcare.

APPLICATIONS OF VISUAL INTELLIGENCE IN HEALTHCARE

Visual intelligence is transforming the health care sector, as devices can decode complex visual data with very high accuracy. From disease diagnosis to monitoring patient conditions and remote care, visual intelligence in health care technologies is slowly becoming a reality for many applications. The present section reviews three significant areas where the latest visual intelligence seems to transform the related application fields: medical imaging and diagnostics, wearable devices along with real-time monitoring, and remote health care and telemedicine. Figure 2 illustrates the integration of visual intelligence in various healthcare sectors, enhancing patient care and operational efficiency(Kharbas et al., 2024; Shaikh et al., 2023).

Figure 2. Applications of visual intelligence in healthcare

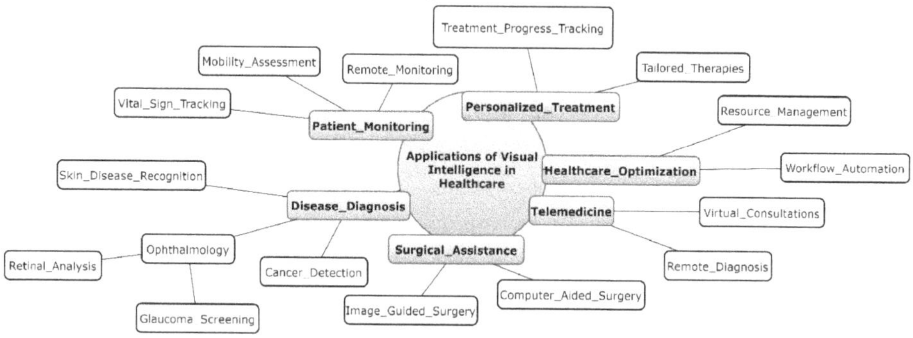

Medical Imaging and Diagnostics

Medical imaging is an integral area of health care diagnostics, and visual intelligence is revolutionizing it. All those X-rays, CT scans, MRI, and ultrasounds generate a huge amount of visual information that needs many hours to interpret by humans. Visual intelligence, however, through machine and deep learning algorithms, has improved the accuracy, speed, and efficiency of interpreting medical images.

Detection of anomalies such as tumors, fractures, and infections is one of the most common applications of visual intelligence in medical imaging. Convolutional neural networks (CNNs) are a key machine learning technique and are excellent at recognizing patterns and building a concern over areas in medical images. These networks learn from massive images of labeled medical data, which allows them to differentiate between healthy and diseased tissue, identify the early stages of cancer, or detect neurological diseases such as stroke. In some cases, these AI systems can even outperform human radiologists by being more accurate in their diagnostic procedure, especially in subtle patterns that may escape the human eye.

The workflow of medical imaging can also be made more efficient by the AI-based visual intelligence system. Routine image segmentation, isolating particular areas of interest, and classification of images into diagnostic categories can be automated, thereby saving clinicians' precious time for patient care rather than time-consuming image analysis. This not only hastens the process of diagnosis but also reduces human error to improve patient outcomes.

Wearable Devices and Real-Time Monitoring

With the advent of wearable devices coupled with visual intelligence, new frontiers have opened in patient monitoring and personalized healthcare. These include smartwatches, fitness trackers, and health sensors coupled with state-of-the-art algorithms to analyze the data continuously, giving in real time understandings of a patient's condition. The visual intelligence plays a crucial role in interpreting the visual data this device is collecting, furnishing such actionable insights for patients and healthcare providers alike(Amin & Hossain, 2020; Minopoulos et al., 2022).

For example, wearable devices can monitor vital signs such as heart rate, blood pressure, and oxygen levels. Smartwatches with integrated cameras or optical sensors can also track skin conditions, monitor movement patterns, or assess facial expressions, which can be particularly helpful for patients with neurological conditions like Parkinson's disease. The visual intelligence algorithms may process the pictures or videos taken through the device to spot the skin's appearance changes like that of the early stages of skin cancer or those rashes associated with systemic diseases.

Apart from tracking environmental conditions, visual intelligence wearable devices can provide comprehensive insights into health status by observing behaviour changes. For example, the movement pattern captured by visual sensors on wearable devices can be used to monitor gait or detect anomalies that could indicate falls, muscle weakness, or mobility issues. This is especially helpful for chronic condition patients and elderly patients, as it can provide real-time insights into possible health risks to enable early intervention and reduce hospital readmission.

These devices further play a crucial role in chronic disease management. An example would be that glucose levels of a patient with diabetes can be monitored over time through wearable sensors that embed visual intelligence to spot trends, raise red flags, and alert the patient or healthcare provider concerned. Wearable devices may therefore improve patient outcomes immensely by allowing patients to better manage their chronic diseases outside of a clinical setting through immediate feedback.

Remote Healthcare and Telemedicine

Remote healthcare and telemedicine have become prominent, with services increasingly being delivered through telehealth, especially in this post-COVID-19 pandemic era. Visual intelligence will play an invaluable role in adding to the capabilities of these telehealth platforms by allowing clinicians to assess and determine diagnoses based on information captured through visual data(Gao et al., 2024; Yadav et al., 2024).

Virtual consultation essentially allows the patients to virtually interact with the health providers using video conferencing tools. In these cases, visual intelligence can be employed to analyze visual cues from the patient's appearance during the consultation, such as facial expressions, skin color, or physical movements. For example, AI systems can assess a patient's facial features to monitor signs of conditions like dehydration, pain, or fatigue. Visual intelligence can also identify speech disorders, unusual breathing patterns, or other manifestations of mental disorders, such as depression, from facial expressions and body language.

Telemedicine is also utilizing visual intelligence for better diagnostics in remote locations. For instance, visual intelligence systems can be applied in dermatology to analyze images of skin lesions taken by patients at home, then algorithms are applied to detect whether there could be skin cancers or not. The images then are forwarded to a dermatologist who may come up with a diagnosis or further corrective measures. Similarly, in ophthalmology, AI-powered visual intelligence can analyze retinal images from remote patients who are suffering from diabetic retinopathy or macular degeneration offering a more affordable and accessible way to detect eye diseases.

Moreover, the use of visual intelligence in remote healthcare further extends to continuous patient monitoring in settings such as home healthcare. IoT-enabled devices such as cameras and sensors allow patients to be monitored remotely. Any change in their condition, for example, falls, unusual movements, or abnormal vital signs, will be detected promptly because of this monitoring. This is particularly important for patients living in rural or underserved areas because remote care via telemedicine reduces the need for travel and the associated strain on healthcare systems.

Applications of visual intelligence in healthcare The applications of visual intelligence in healthcare are very wide-ranging and transformative. They include enhancing diagnostic accuracy through medical imaging, improving patient outcomes with wearable devices, and keeping patients at home through remote healthcare services. It empowers healthcare providers to make more-informed decisions by making devices analyze visual data. As these technologies will continue to evolve-including machine learning, edge computing, and IoT-the field of visual intelligence only promises to further reshape healthcare delivery, emphasizing the importance of being a core component in innovative health care delivery in the future.

IMPLEMENTATION PROCEDURE

The integration of visual intelligence in smart healthcare devices by means of machine learning is a multi-faceted approach that spans data collection, model training, system integration, and real-time deployment. It uses advanced algorithms for the interpretation of visual data by devices, offering enhancing diagnostic capabilities, personalized care, and better patient outcomes. The steps in applying visual intelligence to smart healthcare devices are discussed below(Gao et al., 2024; Kharbas et al., 2024; Ranjan & Choubey, 2024; Yadav et al., 2024). The implementation procedure for integrating visual intelligence into smart healthcare devices using machine learning is also depicted in Figure 3.

Figure 3. Implementation procedure of integrating visual intelligence into smart healthcare devices using machine learning

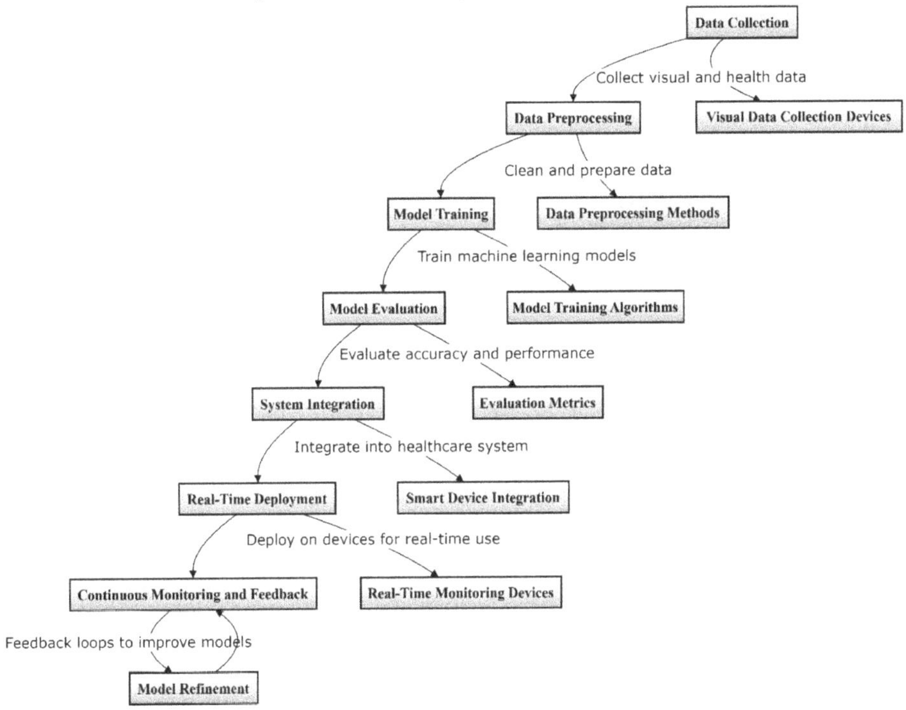

Data Collection and Preprocessing

The first and most important step in implementing visual intelligence is data collection. In healthcare, it is mostly through the collection of visual data from medical imaging appliances such as X-rays, MRIs, or CT scans or wearable devices with cameras or sensors installed (e.g., smartwatches or skin scanners). Data quality and diversity are vital for the correct training of machines. Data preparation is also involved during this stage. There is noise, irrelevant, and inconsistent information in raw data that needs to be cleaned up and standardized. Techniques used in preprocessing may include: normalization, augmentation, and resizing of images for the preparation of the data to fit the training of machine learning models. Examples of preprocessing for medical images may include: conversion of color images into grayscale images, normalization of pixel values, and segmentation of regions of interest such as tumors or lesions for individual analysis.

The sensor data, such as heart rate, skin condition, and patterns of movement, for wearable devices would have to be synchronized with the visual data for comprehensive monitoring. For instance, a camera featured on a smart watch captures facial expressions or skin changes, which are matched with physiological data such as blood pressure or oxygen levels. Suitable preprocessing of these multi-modal data sets is required in order to train machine learning models that can operate seamlessly in the real-time healthcare scenario.

Choosing Suitable Machine Learning Models

The second step involves choosing the suitable machine learning models once the data is ready. Selection of model depends on the nature of the data and the problem under consideration. In visual intelligence applications for healthcare devices, many machine learning techniques are popularly used.

a) Convolutional Neural Networks (CNNs): Due to their inherent capability to automatically extract hierarchical features from images, CNNs are the algorithm of choice for medical imaging and visual analysis. These algorithms prove to be adept pattern recognizers-whether it is to identify tumors, fractures, or abnormalities in an organ through X-rays or MRIs. It consists of layers on top of layers through which the networks progressively learn to identify edges, textures, shapes, or even more complex features in images.
b) Generative Adversarial Networks (GANs): GANs are useful for generating synthetic data with limited access to a large, labeled dataset. In the case of medical imaging, GANs can generate the realistic medical images that can be used in augmenting the training datasets, especially in rare conditions, to improve the

robustness of the model and ensure that the system generalizes well in diverse cases.

c) Reinforcement Learning (RL): Reinforcement Learning can be applied to real-time monitoring and decision-making systems that make smart healthcare devices. RL can enable devices to learn optimum actions based on the feedback received from their environment. For example, in smart wearable devices, RL might be applied continuously to change parameters such as insulin delivery in diabetic patients based on real-time data gathered by visual sensors and other biometric indicators.

Support Vector Machines (SVMs) and Random Forests: In some healthcare applications, classical ML models, such as SVMs or Random Forests, are applied for tasks, such as classification or anomaly detection. For example, SVMs can be successfully used for image or sensor data classification to recognize whether the tissue is healthy or unhealthy. Random Forests are particularly applied to decision support systems while combining the features to achieve precise predictions.

Training and Validation of the Model

Once an appropriate model is selected, the training phase follows. The labeled data sets are trained on the model, where the output that is expected to be classified or diagnosed is already provided. In this training process, a model will learn to identify the patterns present in the data by modifying its inner parameters according to a loss function, which reflects the difference between predicted and actual outcomes. Along with these issues, training healthcare models is fraught with several critical challenges such as data imbalance problems where data classes for some classes (like rare diseases) are underrepresented and overfitting, in which the model gets too specialized to the training data and fails on new data. These can be further approached with data augmentation, cross-validation, and regularization techniques. Data augmentation artificially increases the size of the dataset by applying rotations, scaling, or flipping the images-so the model is robust to variations in the data.

After this training, a model is validated using a different set of data known as validation data to ascertain that it generalizes well to examples yet unseen. Performance metrics such as accuracy, sensitivity, specificity, and area under the ROC curve (AUC) are used in judging the effectiveness of a model. In health care, these metrics do quite significantly determine how reliable the model will be when applied to real-world applications.

Model Optimization and Integration into Healthcare Devices

After training and validating a model, the next step is to optimize it for deployment on the smart healthcare devices. This may include size reduction and computational burden for the model so that it can be run on edge devices such as wearables or diagnostic tools with very limited processing power and memory. Optimization techniques, such as pruning of models (removal of less relevant parameters) and quantization (reducing the precision of numbers used within a model), make the models more efficient without losing too much accuracy. Edge computing is important in these scenarios where data processing is processed locally on the device instead of relying on cloud servers to reduce latency and improve real-time decision-making in healthcare scenarios.

Integration into healthcare devices: It involves embedding the trained and optimized model into the device's software. This requires close collaboration between data scientists, hardware engineers, and healthcare professionals to ensure seamless operation and real-time feedback. For example, in a smart wearable device, the model could analyze skin images or motion data to detect an early sign of a health issue and provide actionable insight directly to the patient or healthcare provider.

Real-time Monitoring and Continuous Learning

After integration, the system moves into the real-time deployment phase, where continuous monitoring of the patient's health and giving back feedback is carried out. In this regard, visual intelligence-powered smart healthcare devices, such as wearable monitors, real-time imaging systems, or diagnostic tools, use computer models to process visual data so that certain health issues are pinpointed in time. In addition to continually improving the system, the use of machine learning in healthcare aids in continuous learning. As more data is collected from patients in the field, a model can be retrained or fine-tuned to adapt to new patterns, improve its accuracy, and become more personalized. This has particularly been important in healthcare because the conditions of some patients can fluctuate rapidly and require models to make corresponding adjustments.

Continuous learning: Edge computing supports the continuous learning process by enabling devices to process data locally with real-time adaptations without constant communication with centralized servers. It enhances responsiveness and allows healthcare professionals to act in time based on warnings from the system whenever a potential health risk is sensed.

Ethical considerations and privacy

The final step of the implementation process involves ensuring that privacy and ethical considerations are met. The handling of sensitive patient data requires the healthcare device to work in line with the regulation of GDPR and HIPAA to ensure data privacy and security. Transparency and interpretability are also important aspects for AI models to be convinced and trusted by healthcare providers. As such, integration with XAI techniques would allow doctors a glimpse into how the system came to a particular prediction-a critical enabler of patient trust and safe practice.

Implementation of such visual intelligence through machine learning on smart healthcare devices is a challenging multi-stage process, requiring planning and proper execution in every step. Starting with the collection of data and its preprocessing, model training, optimization, and real-time deployment forms an important aspect of these healthcare devices providing the perfect accurate, reliable, and efficient solutions for health care. By tapping into machine learning and visual intelligence, healthcare devices are changing the way patient care is structured, providing for real-time monitoring capabilities, treatments tailored to a patient's needs, and next-generation diagnostic capabilities.

COLLABORATIVE STRATEGIES FOR ADOPTION

Multistakeholder engagement across clinicians, developers, policymakers, and the regulatory community should be actively involved in the adoption of visual intelligence into smart healthcare devices through machine learning. Such stakeholders take an active role to ensure technology is effectively, ethically, and maximally used to improve the care of patients in health systems. Key collaborative approaches involving training, education, and industry-specific standardization are needed for ensuring a seamless deployment of these sophisticated technologies(Aversano et al., 2024; Gao et al., 2024; Shaikh et al., 2023). Figure 4 illustrates collaborative strategies for integrating visual intelligence into smart healthcare devices.

Figure 4. Collaborative strategies for the adoption of visual intelligence in smart healthcare devices

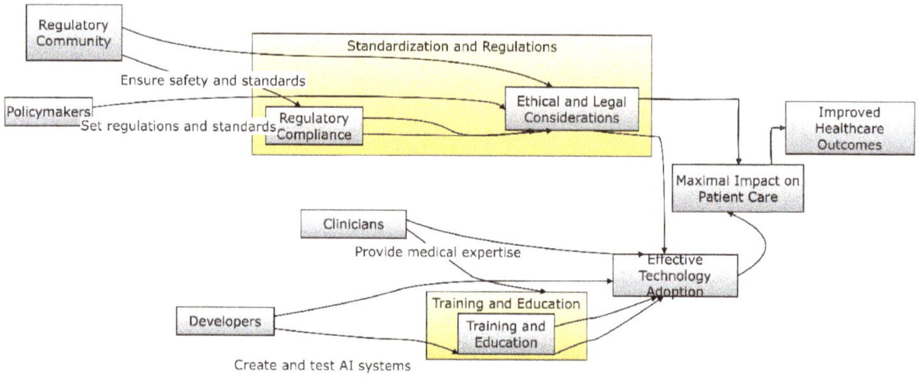

Role of Clinicians, Developers, and Policymakers

The acceptance of visual intelligence in healthcare relies on the collaborative effort between clinicians, developers, and policymakers working together to address other segments of the process in question(Gopi et al., 2024; Pitchai et al., 2024).

a) Role of Clinicians: Clinicians, from the doctor to nurses and health providers, will form the core users of a visual intelligence-enabled device. Their role will be crucial in ensuring that such devices really meet practical, clinical needs. Clinicians provide a real-world view of the need for patient care, which helps developers tailor the devices so that they can be clinically relevant, easy to use, and capable of improving patient outcomes. Their involvement in the development process ensures that these technologies align with actual workflows and patient management protocols. Additionally, clinicians must be advocates for the technology within their healthcare systems, highlighting the benefits of machine learning and visual intelligence in enhancing diagnostic capabilities, streamlining workflows, and improving patient care.
b) Developers' Role: Developers, such as data scientists, engineers, and software architects, are essential to the development and refinement of machine learning models while integrating the components into smart healthcare devices. The clinicians they work with help them understand the clinical challenge at hand; these insights are then used in the conceptualization and functionality of the device. Such collaboration ensures that developing effective, user-friendly health care systems is met with robust, scalable devices. To achieve this, the developers have to update the technology continually and utilize new medical data as well

as clinicians' feedback so that the algorithms are maximally performing and responsive to emerging needs.

c) Role of Policymakers: Policymakers and regulatory bodies have to put out frameworks that regulate the use of AI and machine learning in healthcare. They will be involving themselves highly in patient safety, data privacy, and ethical issues with the adoption process. Regulatory agencies such as the FDA in the U.S. or the European Medicines Agency (EMA) in Europe would have to develop and monitor guidelines to approve and use AI-driven healthcare technologies. In addition, policymakers need to address equity issues in accessing these technologies because the health advances don't stay confined to geographic locations or demographics. There is a need for intergovernmental collaboration among healthcare organizations and industry stakeholders to establish a regulatory regime conducive to the wide-scale adoption of safe and ethical AI in healthcare.

Training and Education on Effective Usage

For AI-powered healthcare devices to be appropriately implemented, it is important that comprehensive training and education programs be in place for all stakeholders, but most importantly for the clinicians and healthcare professionals involved. This will further ensure that not only are these AI technologies understood but also applied in clinical practice to maximize their potential for better patient outcomes.

Healthcare professionals should be adequately equipped with the knowledge and skills to utilize AI-driven devices efficiently. The training programs may include the basics of machine learning, including how AI models work and how they can aid in diagnostics as well as treatment planning. Clinicians should also be trained in interpreting the results produced by AI tools and how these results must be incorporated in the patient's care. For instance, if an AI-powered medical imaging device flags a potential issue, clinicians need to understand the confidence level of the AI's prediction and how to interpret it within the context of the patient's overall condition. Clinicians will also need to be trained in communicating AI-generated insights into understandable and trustworthy messages for patients. The secret to full adoption is not only having clinicians use the technology but ensuring that they are then able to communicate its benefits and limitations to patients and increase trust and acceptance among patients.

Educating the Developers and Data Scientists

Developers and data scientists building and deploying machine learning models for healthcare applications must be knowledgeable about both health care practices and the ethical issues surrounding patient data. This encompasses understanding medical data, which will often depend on knowledge that is specific to aspects of the human body, diseases, and treatments. The training of developers should target models that are explainable and transparent so that healthcare professionals can rely on the decisions made by AI systems. Patients must also be educated on the benefits and limitations of AI technologies. Patient education campaigns may enhance trust in AI-driven healthcare devices by illustrating how these technologies work in relation to clinical care and by de-mystifying concerns over privacy and safety. Well-informed patients are likely to accept and use AI-powered devices, and this will help improve their health outcomes.

Industry Standards and Best Practices

One of the most vital issues in the diffusion of visual intelligence for healthcare is the lack of standardized protocols and practices. But there is a lot to be done to standardize industry standards and best practices to ensure interoperability, safety, and reliability for AI-driven health care devices.

Standardization of Data: Healthcare data is highly heterogeneous within the field of machine learning and visual intelligence, coming from a variety of different sources-ranging from hospitals and clinics to wearable devices and remote monitoring tools. A uniform format and quality are crucial for information gathered through these various channels in order for machine learning models to be trained on consistent, high-quality input. Other developments include the efforts of organizations like Health Level Seven International (HL7) and the IEEE to develop standards for exchanging medical data and provide cross-device and cross-platform compatibility. Standardization will allow AI tools to seamlessly integrate into existing infrastructures of healthcare, thus improving the effectiveness of the overall system.

Best Practices Development for the AI Development and Deployment

Transparency, interpretability, and validation should be core best practices in the development of AI for healthcare. Best practices in algorithm design are aimed at developing AI models that are accurate and can explain to clinicians and patients what they are doing. This will ensure that AI-powered devices can be trusted to make life-critical decisions, such as diagnosing diseases or recommending treatment plans. Machine learning models must be validated and tested over and over in real clinical settings to make sure that these models are still accurate and relevant with new data coming(Boopathi & Khang, 2023; Durairaj et al., 2023; Pramila et al., 2023).

a) Ethics and Data Privacy Standards: Healthcare respects all ethical considerations and data privacy. Industry standards have to ensure that AI instruments follow data protection regulations such as HIPAA, GDPR, and other existing data usage laws over personal health data. Furthermore, there should be guidelines that speak to issues like biases in machine learning models to make sure that devices driven by artificial intelligence do not perpetuate healthcare disparities or harm certain patient groups. Collaboration between governments, healthcare providers, and technologists will be critical to establishing a regulatory environment that balances innovation with both patient safety and appropriate care.
b) Interoperability and Collaboration: To make visual intelligence systems work effectively in a more defined healthcare ecosystem, the standards of interoperability among devices are, therefore, as critical. Such AI devices must share data seamlessly with EHRs and other healthcare technologies in active use. The development of a standard method for data exchange and device communication ensures that AI technologies do not stand in isolation but become an integral part of patient care systems.

The success of the uptake of visual intelligence in smart healthcare devices relies on clinician and developer collaboration, policymakers, or other stakeholders' inputs. Better training, clear industry standards, and continued collaboration on healthcare organizations may maximize the developments and bring about accurate diagnostics, better patient care, and effective healthcare systems. With strong partnerships and the establishment of ethical guidelines and best practices, AI can be effectively integrated into healthcare, ultimately improving outcomes and accessibility across the globe.

CHALLENGES AND LIMITATIONS

Data Privacy and Security Issues

One of the greatest challenges with the application of visual intelligence in smart healthcare devices is data privacy and security. Healthcare data includes PII and protected health information. Unauthorized access, breaches, or misuse of this information compromise patient trust and compliance with regulations, such as HIPAA in the United States or GDPR in Europe. Often, use of AI in healthcare involves massive amounts of data. These data often include personal medical records, images, and video feeds that may be targeted through cyber threats. Robust encryption, secure data storage, and compliance with data protection laws are essential to mitigate risks(Ramudu et al., 2023; Sreedhar et al., 2024). Moreover, data security protocols and the importance of privacy maintenance are necessary for effective practices in data handling, starting from informing healthcare professionals and patients about these.

Model Interpretability and Trustworthiness

The AI models- particularly the CNNs, GANs, and reinforcement learning models-are known for their complexity and opacity. They pose problems to those trying to understand how such complex decisions are made. Hence, interpretability in AI models is important because it allows clinicians to have trust in their outputs, while more importantly, results in appropriate use of tools in healthcare settings. If the model's decisions cannot be easily explained or justified, it may lead a doctor or other health professional to have doubts or relapses into not trusting critical medical decisions being done using AI. The opacity also incurs ethical implications since it is hard to ascertain whether the tools are biased to any particular patient group in its decision-making processes. Techniques for further improvement of model transparency and XAI solutions would thus enable these aspects to be addressed, enhancing trust and acceptance among the healthcare providers.

Scalability Across Diverse Healthcare Settings

Scalability is a key consideration when deploying visual intelligence solutions across an entire spectrum of health care environments: from urban hospitals, with probably the most probable high-end resources, to the remotest, most resource-constrained rural clinics. Healthcare settings could vary in their respective levels of technology infrastructure, data management capabilities, and AI expertise. A visually intelligent system needs to be flexible and accommodate hardware and software environment differences and should be able to run on different networks. Furthermore, training data utilized to create AI models could be localized or customized in various forms to meet the needs and challenges of different healthcare settings. Effective functioning and consistent, reliable results from AI tools across a variety of settings are crucial for their acceptance and penetration into daily clinical practice. Figure 5 illustrates the challenges, emerging innovations, future trends, and ethical considerations in the adoption of visual intelligence in smart healthcare devices.

Figure 5. Challenges, emerging innovations, future trends, and ethical considerations in the adoption of visual intelligence in smart healthcare devices

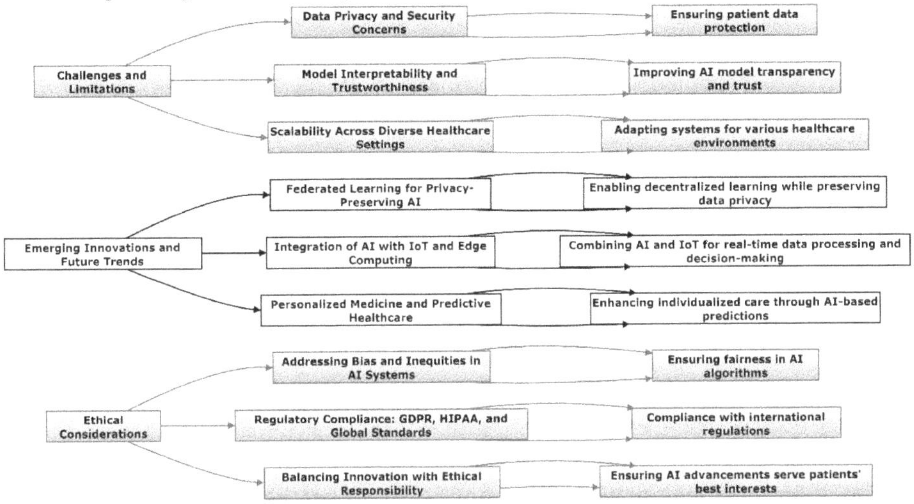

EMERGING INNOVATIONS AND FUTURE TRENDS

Federated learning for privacy-preserving AI

Federated learning is one of the recently emerging innovations that deals directly with one of the major concerns around healthcare AI: data privacy. This is because, in classic ML, data is concentrated in a particular server, thus creating many risks to the confidentiality of the patients. In contrast, federated learning allows for decentralized model training in which the data resides on local devices, such as hospitals or clinics, while only the model updates are shared across a central server. This type of approach will ensure that sensitive health data never leaves its source, thereby minimizing the probability of breaches in the data. As AI technologies for healthcare continue their development, federated learning is likely to be an increasingly important solution in the area of secure, privacy-preserving AI applications, especially in situations where sensitive patient information, such as medical images or electronic health records, is the data in question.

Integration of AI with IoT and Edge Computing

Integration of Artificial Intelligence with IoT and edge computing is among the most transformative trends in smart healthcare devices. Continuous patient data collected by IoT-enabled, for instance, wearable health monitors will be processed by AI algorithms to provide real-time insights. Edge computing enhances this process by ensuring that data is processed locally on the device or nearby to reduce latency in making a decision. This is especially useful for real-time healthcare application areas, including remote monitoring, emergency care. AI-IoT devices with edge computing would allow healthcare providers to provide a more efficient, near-real time and personalized health care even in remote or underresource areas(Karthik et al., 2023; Malathi et al., 2024; Upadhyaya et al., 2024).

Personalized Medicine and Predictive Healthcare

The future of healthcare is moving toward more personalized approaches, where treatments and care plans are tailored to the individual needs of patients. AI, particularly through machine learning, plays a pivotal role in analyzing complex datasets (genetic, clinical, and environmental) to provide personalized health insights. Predictive healthcare, powered by AI algorithms, enables early diagnosis and anticipatory care, identifying health risks before they become critical. Therefore, by integrating genetic information with lifestyle data and environmental factors, AI will thus predict disease outcomes and further offer preventative treatments or personalized treatments to that end, thereby improving patient outcomes and decreasing healthcare costs, which would keep advancing the medical world.

ETHICAL AND REGULATORY CONSIDERATIONS

Bias and Equity in AI Systems

AI systems are vulnerable to bias, which can arise from skewed training data or improper model development. In healthcare, this can lead to inequitable care, disproportionately affecting underrepresented or marginalized populations. To ensure fairness, AI models must be carefully developed and validated using diverse and representative datasets. Continuous monitoring and audits are necessary to identify and mitigate biases, ensuring AI tools do not perpetuate health disparities. Inclusivity and equity in AI design should be emphasized to create effective systems that facilitate all populations(Boopathi, 2024).

GDPR and HIPAA on global standards

The point is that any implementation of AI must comply with the strictest frameworks of regulation, such as GDPR in Europe or HIPAA in the United States, with regard to the use of personal health data. These regulations require very strict data protection, patient consent, and transparency. Global standards for AI in healthcare are in transition towards safety, privacy, and fairness. Compliance with these rules will also form a basis for regaining the confidence of patients and practitioners alike and attaining legal protection together with ethical use of AI technologies.

Balancing Innovation with Ethical Responsibility

Since this continues to innovate in healthcare, then its progress must be balanced with ethical considerations. It promises immense potential in improving patient care; therefore, developers have prioritized ethical responsibility to ensure that innovation is shaped in the best interest of humanity. Decisions regarding ethical issues in data usage and model transparency would also have to be made while safeguarding patients' rights, thus not at the expense of patients' well-being or societal trust.

CONCLUSION

The integration of visual intelligence into smart healthcare devices marks the most notable milestone in the evolution of healthcare technology. Machine learning-based systems are improving diagnostic capabilities, making patient monitoring better, and delivering care more personalized. Some applications already on the horizon include early detection of diseases through medical imaging, continuous tracking of vital signs through wearables, and remote monitoring of patients. These applications have profoundly reshaped healthcare practice to be more proactive and accessible.

Yet, the widespread use of these technologies cannot be taken lightly. Huge hurdles remain in relation to data privacy, scarce availability of good-quality datasets labeled with annotations, explainability in AI, and ensuring the robustness and reliability of visual intelligence systems across diverse populations of patients and clinical scenarios. Most importantly, ethical as well as regulatory compliance requires a balance between the safety of the patients and trust in such systems by patients while promoting technical progress.

Despite these challenges, the potential for visual intelligence to revolutionize healthcare is immense. Such emerging trends as the convergence of AI and IoT, edge computing for real-time processing, and federated learning to safeguard privacy pave the way toward next-generation smart healthcare solutions. Additionally, clinician-

AI-developer-policy-maker collaboration will be a pre-requisite in addressing these challenges and setting new standards for the safety, efficacy, and equity of healthcare technologies. Visual intelligence in a smart healthcare product has the potential to make the delivery of healthcare more effective, precise, and patient-focused. And when innovation goes on, challenges get answered, and moves toward a future where technology-driven healthcare will bring people's quality of life up.

REFERENCES

Ahmed, M., & Zubair, S. (2022). Explainable artificial intelligence in sustainable smart healthcare. In *Explainable Artificial Intelligence for Cyber Security: Next Generation Artificial Intelligence* (pp. 265–280). Springer. DOI: 10.1007/978-3-030-96630-0_12

Amin, S. U., & Hossain, M. S. (2020). Edge intelligence and Internet of Things in healthcare: A survey. *IEEE Access : Practical Innovations, Open Solutions*, *9*, 45–59. DOI: 10.1109/ACCESS.2020.3045115

Aversano, L., Iammarino, M., Mancino, I., & Montano, D. (2024). A systematic review on artificial intelligence approaches for smart health devices. *PeerJ. Computer Science*, *10*, e2232. DOI: 10.7717/peerj-cs.2232 PMID: 39650514

Baker, S., & Xiang, W. (2023). Artificial intelligence of things for smarter healthcare: A survey of advancements, challenges, and opportunities. *IEEE Communications Surveys and Tutorials*, *25*(2), 1261–1293. DOI: 10.1109/COMST.2023.3256323

Boopathi, S. (2024). Sustainable Development Using IoT and AI Techniques for Water Utilization in Agriculture. In *Sustainable Development in AI, Blockchain, and E-Governance Applications* (pp. 204–228). IGI Global. DOI: 10.4018/979-8-3693-1722-8.ch012

Boopathi, S., & Khang, A. (2023). AI-Integrated Technology for a Secure and Ethical Healthcare Ecosystem. In *AI and IoT-Based Technologies for Precision Medicine* (pp. 36–59). IGI Global. DOI: 10.4018/979-8-3693-0876-9.ch003

Dewangan, N., Vyas, P., & Mandal, S. (2022). Smart healthcare and intelligent medical systems. In *Computational Intelligence and Applications for Pandemics and Healthcare* (pp. 205–228). IGI Global. DOI: 10.4018/978-1-7998-9831-3.ch010

Durairaj, M., Jayakumar, S., Karpagavalli, V., Maheswari, B. U., & Boopathi, S. (2023). Utilization of Digital Tools in the Indian Higher Education System During Health Crises. In *Multidisciplinary Approaches to Organizational Governance During Health Crises* (pp. 1–21). IGI Global. DOI: 10.4018/978-1-7998-9213-7.ch001

Gao, X., He, P., Zhou, Y., & Qin, X. (2024). Artificial Intelligence Applications in Smart Healthcare: A Survey. *Future Internet*, *16*(9), 308. DOI: 10.3390/fi16090308

Gopi, B., Sworna Kokila, M. L., Bibin, C. V., Sasikala, D., Howard, E., & Boopathi, S. (2024). Distributed Technologies Using AI/ML Techniques for Healthcare Applications. In *Advances in Human and Social Aspects of Technology* (pp. 375–396). IGI Global. DOI: 10.4018/979-8-3693-2569-8.ch019

Jeyakumar, V., Nirmala, K., & Nithya, R. (2022). A smart virtual vision system for health monitoring. In *Biomedical Engineering Applications for People with Disabilities and the Elderly in the COVID-19 Pandemic and Beyond* (pp. 347–360). Elsevier. DOI: 10.1016/B978-0-323-85174-9.00021-2

Karthik, S., Hemalatha, R., Aruna, R., Deivakani, M., Reddy, R. V. K., & Boopathi, S. (2023). Study on Healthcare Security System-Integrated Internet of Things (IoT). In *Perspectives and Considerations on the Evolution of Smart Systems* (pp. 342–362). IGI Global.

Kharbas, V. K., Meena, Y., & Thakur, P. K. (2024). Enabling Clinical Decision-Making in Smart Healthcare through AI/ML Algorithms. *2024 15th International Conference on Computing Communication and Networking Technologies (ICCCNT)*, 1–6.

Mala, D. J. (2023). Machine learning-based intelligent assistant for smart healthcare. In *Machine Learning and Artificial Intelligence in Healthcare Systems* (pp. 265–286). CRC Press.

Malathi, J., Kusha, K., Isaac, S., Ramesh, A., Rajendiran, M., & Boopathi, S. (2024). IoT-Enabled Remote Patient Monitoring for Chronic Disease Management and Cost Savings: Transforming Healthcare. In *Advances in Explainable AI Applications for Smart Cities* (pp. 371–388). IGI Global.

Menagadevi, M., Madian, N., Thiyagarajan, D., & Rajendran, R. (2025). Smart medical devices: Making healthcare more intelligent. In *Machine Learning Models and Architectures for Biomedical Signal Processing* (pp. 487–501). Elsevier. DOI: 10.1016/B978-0-443-22158-3.00020-X

Minopoulos, G. M., Memos, V. A., Stergiou, C. L., Stergiou, K. D., Plageras, A. P., Koidou, M. P., & Psannis, K. E. (2022). Exploitation of emerging technologies and advanced networks for a smart healthcare system. *Applied Sciences (Basel, Switzerland)*, *12*(12), 5859. DOI: 10.3390/app12125859

Muhammad, G., Alshehri, F., Karray, F., El Saddik, A., Alsulaiman, M., & Falk, T. H. (2021). A comprehensive survey on multimodal medical signals fusion for smart healthcare systems. *Information Fusion*, *76*, 355–375. DOI: 10.1016/j.inffus.2021.06.007

Pitchai, R., Guru, K. V., Gandhi, J. N., Komala, C. R., Kumar, J. R. D., & Boopathi, S. (2024). Fog Computing-Integrated ML-Based Framework and Solutions for Intelligent Systems: Digital Healthcare Applications. In *Technological Advancements in Data Processing for Next Generation Intelligent Systems* (pp. 196–224). IGI Global. DOI: 10.4018/979-8-3693-0968-1.ch008

Pramila, P., Amudha, S., Saravanan, T., Sankar, S. R., Poongothai, E., & Boopathi, S. (2023). Design and Development of Robots for Medical Assistance: An Architectural Approach. In *Contemporary Applications of Data Fusion for Advanced Healthcare Informatics* (pp. 260–282). IGI Global.

Ramudu, K., Mohan, V. M., Jyothirmai, D., Prasad, D., Agrawal, R., & Boopathi, S. (2023). Machine Learning and Artificial Intelligence in Disease Prediction: Applications, Challenges, Limitations, Case Studies, and Future Directions. In *Contemporary Applications of Data Fusion for Advanced Healthcare Informatics* (pp. 297–318). IGI Global.

Ranjan, S., & Choubey, D. K. (2024). Machine Learning, Deep Learning and IoT in Smart Healthcare for Retinal Diseases Management. In *Machine Learning and IoT Applications for Health Informatics* (pp. 216–238). CRC Press. DOI: 10.1201/9781003424987-11

Sabry, F., Eltaras, T., Labda, W., Alzoubi, K., & Malluhi, Q. (2022). Machine learning for healthcare wearable devices: The big picture. *Journal of Healthcare Engineering*, *2022*(1), 4653923. DOI: 10.1155/2022/4653923 PMID: 35480146

Shaikh, T. A., Rasool, T., & Verma, P. (2023). Machine intelligence and medical cyber-physical system architectures for smart healthcare: Taxonomy, challenges, opportunities, and possible solutions. *Artificial Intelligence in Medicine*, *146*, 102692. DOI: 10.1016/j.artmed.2023.102692 PMID: 38042609

Sherwani, M. K., Aziz, A., & Calimeri, F. (2022). Role of Deep Learning for Smart Health Care. In *Computational Intelligence Techniques for Green Smart Cities* (pp. 169–186). Springer. DOI: 10.1007/978-3-030-96429-0_8

Sreedhar, P. S. S., Sujay, V., Rani, M. R., Melita, L., Reshma, S., & Boopathi, S. (2024). Impacts of 5G Machine Learning Techniques on Telemedicine and Social Media Professional Connection in Healthcare. In *Advances in Medical Technologies and Clinical Practice* (pp. 209–234). IGI Global. DOI: 10.4018/979-8-3693-1934-5.ch012

Upadhyaya, A. N., Saqib, A., Devi, J. V., Rallapalli, S., Sudha, S., & Boopathi, S. (2024). Implementation of the Internet of Things (IoT) in Remote Healthcare. In *Advances in Medical Technologies and Clinical Practice* (pp. 104–124). IGI Global. DOI: 10.4018/979-8-3693-1934-5.ch006

Venkatesh, D. A. N. (2019). Reimagining the future of healthcare industry through internet of medical things (IoMT), artificial intelligence (AI), machine learning (ML), big data, mobile apps and advanced sensors. *Artificial Intelligence (AI), Machine Learning (ML), Big Data, Mobile Apps and Advanced Sensors (October 28, 2019)*.

Yadav, S., Jayakumar, S. R. S., & Associates. (2024). Time-Efficient Diagnostics Using AI/ML Algorithms in Smart Healthcare. *2024 15th International Conference on Computing Communication and Networking Technologies (ICCCNT)*, 1–6.

Zheng, Y., Tang, N., Omar, R., Hu, Z., Duong, T., Wang, J., Wu, W., & Haick, H. (2021). Smart materials enabled with artificial intelligence for healthcare wearables. *Advanced Functional Materials*, *31*(51), 2105482. DOI: 10.1002/adfm.202105482

KEY TERMS AND DEFINITIONS

AI: The simulation of human intelligence in machines that can be designed to think and learn like humans, including machine learning, neural networks, and natural language processing, among others.

AUC (Area Under the Curve): A metric used to evaluate the performance of binary classification models, representing the area under the ROC curve; higher AUC values indicate better model performance.

CNN (Convolutional Neural Network): this is a learning algorithm broadly used in image recognition and processing, mimicking the pattern visual processing of a human brain.

COVID (Coronavirus Disease 2019) is a contagious illness caused by the SARS-CoV-2 virus: reported first in December 2019, contributing to a global pandemic.

CT (Computed Tomography): A medical imaging technology which involves the use of an X-ray to make detailed cross-sectional images of the body used primarily for the diagnosis and detection of diseases.

EHR- An electronic version of a patient's medical history: which is collected and maintained by health providers to ensure accurate and accessible data to make diagnoses, treatments, or coordinated care.

EMA (European Medicines Agency): A regulative body of the European Union which evaluates and supervises medicines and medical devices to ensure their safety, effectiveness, and quality.

FDA (Food and Drug Administration): It is a government agency of the United States that oversees as well as regulates safety and efficacy of food, drugs, medical devices, and most radiation-emitting products.

GAN (Generative Adversarial Network): Deep learning model composed of two neural networks-a generator and a discriminator, which operate against each other to produce synthetic data that mimics real data, such as images or videos.

GDPR: General Data Protection Regulation. An EU's legislation that protects and regulates an individual's human rights and rights to personal data, imposing strict rules on data collection, storage, and processing.

HIPAA (Health Insurance Portability and Accountability Act): A U.S. regulation designed to protect the privacy and security of individuals' health information, establishing standards for electronic health transactions and records.

HL (Healthcare Logistics): Managing and coordinating healthcare-related resources, including transportation, storage, and delivery of equipment and services.

IEEE- In the context of Institute of Electrical and Electronics Engineers: refers to a global professional association that manages standards in several fields such as AI, machine learning, and healthcare related areas.

ML: A subset of AI with specific emphasis on algorithms and statistical models that allow computers to learn or make decisions based on certain input without having been explicitly programmed.

MRI (Magnetic Resonance Imaging): this is the image technique in the medical sector to visualize in detail the internal structures of the body by utilizing strong magnetic fields and radio waves.

PII (Personally Identifiable Information): Information that can be used to identify an individual, such as names, addresses, social security numbers, and health information. This data should be safeguarded under both privacy regulations, such as GDPR and HIPAA.

RL: Reinforcement Learning. A subset of machine learning wherein an agent learns making decisions in an environment based on rewards and punishments it receives after executing actions.

ROC (Receiver Operating Characteristic): A graphical method for assessing the performance of a binary classifier, plotting the true positive rate against the false positive rate.

SVM (Support Vector Machine): A supervised learning algorithm in machine classification and regression to find which best separates the data from each other with a hyperplane.

XAI (Explainable Artificial Intelligence): It is the approach designed for transparent and interpretable AI, allowing humans to understand and trust the machine learning models' decision processes.

Chapter 6

Integrating Visual Intelligence With Federated Learning and IoT in Healthcare

G. K. Shwetha

Department of Computer Science and Engineering, Vidyavardhaka College of Engineering, Mysuru, India

Ashish Avasthi

https://orcid.org/0000-0003-3069-1984

Faculty of Computer Engineering, Poornima University, Jaipur, India

Manish Kumar

Department Faculty of Computer Engineering, Poornima University, Jaipur, India

Saurabh Chandra

https://orcid.org/0000-0003-4172-9968

School of Law, Bennett University, Greater Noida, India

B. S. Hari

https://orcid.org/0009-0003-1456-2709

Department of Mechanical Engineering, Kongu Engineering College, Erode, India

ABSTRACT

This chapter discusses how visual intelligence can be integrated with federated learning and IoT technologies in the healthcare segment. Health care continues to

DOI: 10.4018/979-8-3693-6094-1.ch006

rely on advanced data analytics more and more, making visual intelligence a key player in interpreting complex medical images and data. Federated learning then strengthens this by facilitating collaborative model training across decentralized devices while preserving patient privacy and data security. This enables the use of a combination of data from various sources without compromising confidential information. Multiple applications are discussed, including remote patient monitoring and diagnostic imaging, which highlight exactly how the use of these technologies can improve patient outcomes, make treatment more personalized, and streamline health care flow management. This integration leverages the strengths of visual intelligence, federated learning, and IoT to address pertinent challenges in today's healthcare environment.

INTRODUCTION

The convergence of visual intelligence, federated learning, and the Internet of Things (IoT) has been one of the most transformative paradigm shifts in health care due to the innovations they bring forth in terms of improving patient care, enhancing accuracy in diagnosis, and the overall efficiency of operations. As healthcare systems struggle with vast volumes of data coming from heterogeneous sources—including medical images and wearable devices to electronic health records—the use of advanced technologies has become essential. A part of this chapter discusses how visual intelligence can be harmonized with federated learning and IoT in order to create intelligent health solutions that not only improve the outputs of patient care but also ensure the sensitivity of information(Liu et al., 2020).

Visual intelligence is the understanding and processing of a machine towards visual information like pictures or video, and graphics. It is very significant in the medical world where making processes on diagnostic accuracy can be more automatic through image analysis. Moreover, the advanced algorithms in AI and ML are incredibly capable of processing large amounts of imaging data like X-rays, MRIs, or CT scans even more than skills of physicians. For instance, a detection system based on a computer can find outliers in an imaging study to enable a radiologist to make the appropriate choices. In the interests of visual intelligence having a growing reliance on it, big diversified datasets continue to be necessary to properly train these algorithms(Yang et al., 2021).

Federated learning thus appears to be very promising in addressing this problem of data scarcity and privacy issues perpetuated by traditional machine learning. In traditional settings, training algorithms inherently need a centralized access to data of patients, raising a lot of ethical and legal concerns. Federated learning sidesteps all these issues simply by allowing multiple health-care institutions to collaborate with each other in the joint training of models without jointly sharing sensitive data. Instead, each institution trains a local model on its data, shares updates of that model with a central server, which aggregates the updates to improve the global model. This approach maintains patient privacy and allows for robust algorithms that generalize well across different populations(Han et al., 2019). In addition, federated learning puts the power of harnessing data into the hands of institutions, making AI applications for healthcare more precise.

The Internet of Things has also advanced healthcare into new dimensions through the ability of connected devices to continuously monitor the patient. Wearable technology, smart sensors, and remote monitoring systems produce real-time data that is useful for making clinical decisions and can be used proactively for the patient. Devices which monitor even the smallest changes in vital signs, activity levels, and perhaps even emotional health give healthcare professionals information about the condition of a patient. However, the same IoT devices also present challenges, especially in terms of data management, interoperability, and security. Thus, strong frameworks are the backbone for the comprehensive realization of potential of IoT by collecting data from numerous devices, analyzing it, and utilizing it appropriately(Liu et al., 2020).

The synergy emerging from visual intelligence, federated learning, and IoT has immense possibilities for growing healthcare systems. One of the most interesting applications is in the telemedicine domain where teleconsultation and tele-diagnosis have emerged as a necessity. Telemedicine platforms will be enabled with the use of visual intelligence such that healthcare providers can use AI-driven image analysis to assess patients' conditions at a distance. For example, dermatologists may be able to analyze images of skin lesions submitted by their patients and decide whether a physical examination would be necessary. The better accessibility provided here also ensures timely intervention by the medical professional(Liu et al., 2021).

Another aspect is that the integration of IoT devices with federated learning enhances remote patient monitoring capabilities. The health metrics of patients will still be under the observation and watch of healthcare providers for potential complications, as information from wearable devices can be used to predict early. The federated learning of these sensitive data makes them private, yet more predictive models can be developed with better accuracy. Healthcare organizations can offer personalized treatment plans tailored to individual needs, which could increase patient adherence and better outcomes because of data obtained from a wide array of devices and patients(Mitra et al., 2021).

While patient care is encouraged, healthcare operations are made easier through integration. With the application of visual intelligence toward the automation of data analysis, healthcare professionals lessen the administrative burden of interpretation since data is reviewed and analyzed without presenting it to them in conventional forms of expression. This therefore gives room for more interaction with patients and less time spent on keying in data or sitting and trying to analyze them. The third point relates to an entirely new dimension that aggregated data insights can provide to the strategic decision-making of organizations at the institutional and policy level. It will lead the healthcare organizations to identify patterns and direct resources more effectively for finally improving quality care(Zhang et al., 2020).

Promise: Despite these successes, this integration is not without challenges. Healthcare needs to address a number of critical issues in order to fully realize visual intelligence, federated learning, and IoT. Data security will be of utmost concern; breaches can compromise the confidentiality of patient health information, further reducing public trust in healthcare systems. Balancing these risks against such breaches calls for more stringent measures in terms of security as well as regulatory compliance. For data to be integrated without any hassle and be able to intercommunicate smoothly, interoperability of devices and platforms must also be ensured. Standardization efforts and joint collaborative initiatives among technology providers, healthcare institutes, and regulatory bodies will be essential in pushing past these hurdles(Orlandi et al., 2023).

Another challenge is for the need of continuous learning and adaptation. Healthcare data continuously update; hence, models in place must be updated constantly for the models to remain relevant and effective. One of the great advantages of federated learning is that it can support constant model refinement by decentralized updates; however, that requires effort from participating institutions to cooperate and be transparent(Man et al., 2021).

The idea of integrating visual intelligence with federated learning and the accompanying IoT technologies might be one promising approach for delivering healthcare more effectively, accurately, and centered on patients. Different applications, case studies, and best practices followed in succeeding chapters will be discovered to cover and capitalize on these technologies in improving healthcare outcomes. With the integration of these new tools, health care systems will better be able to navigate the complexities in modern medicine and present new requirements for higher quality in care and better experiences for patients. Shaping the future of health care will, more than anything, require moving forward and embracing the integration of what best characterizes this new era(Savazzi et al., 2020).

Objectives

The chapter provides an overview of how visual intelligence, federated learning, and IoT can be merged in healthcare for the resolution of present-day challenges. It also elaborates how advanced visual analytics can be used to interpret complex medical data and ensure secure model training in a collaborative, federated learning manner, without compromising patient privacy. Lastly, it delves into studying the role of IoT to connect decentralized healthcare devices that can enhance data collection and analysis. Include targets such as the application and remote patient monitoring, diagnostic imaging, and showing how all this synergy helps in decision-making in clinics, makes treatments personalized, and facilitates optimization of health care for the sake of innovation and improvement in the outcome among patients.

Contribution and outcomes

This chapter describes the impact change will make as visual intelligence, federated learning, and IoT converge within healthcare. Advanced analytics enable complex medical data interpretation, thus facilitating the possibility of secure and decentralized training of models across systems in a manner that ensures privacy to the patients. Better patient results go with personalized treatment plus efficient health operations from monitoring of patients at a distance to applications in diagnostic imaging. This chapter highlights the point that these technologies together resolve important challenges that pave the way for innovative solutions towards improvement in clinical decision making and operational efficiency. This will be the coming together of the best practices of modern health care that would make the medical practices data-driven, patient-centric, and efficient.

BACKGROUND: VISUAL INTELLIGENCE

Visual intelligence is the technological capability that enables machines and systems to interpret, analyze, and draw conclusions from visual data such as images and video. Advanced algorithms and artificial intelligence techniques in this research area are applied mainly in the healthcare sector to push forward the diagnostics and improve patient care through computer vision and deep learning on medical images. Its scope even covers radiological images, X-rays, CT scans, MRIs, to pathology slides and video imaging data from surgical procedures or those coming from remote monitoring systems. Visual intelligence in healthcare is changing conventional approaches, leading to more accurate diagnoses and timely interventions(Bouzinis et al., 2021; Yang et al., 2022).

The most critical application of visual intelligence in medical imaging is the automated image analysis. Algorithms, trained on large datasets, may detect abnormalities, count anatomy, and assist in the decision of a radiologist to diagnose. For instance, artificial intelligence-based tools can precisely and sensitively detect the existence of a tumor in mammograms; they often are at par with, or even outperform, human specialists. Similarly, visual intelligence will take the analysis of pathological images to the next level wherein better and more accurate identification of cancerous tissues is possible by pathologists. Aside from diagnosis, this can also aid in treatment planning and monitoring by examining changes in images over time and allowing healthcare providers to track the progression of diseases and response to treatment.

Limitations of Visual Intelligence

There are several significant limitations of visual intelligence, including the fact that whereas the advantages of applying this technique are many, reliance on high-quality datasets with annotations in training models remains a challenge. Availability of such datasets can be infrequent, especially for rare conditions and does result in biases that can affect algorithms' working. Also, decisions made by AI are not very interpretable; though they may result in correct outputs, the interpretation of how and why a model has arrived at that decision is challenging-a factor that would raise many clinicians' suspicions. It also poses logistical challenges to integrate the technologies into current workflows and systems, which demands heavy investments in infrastructure and training for healthcare professionals(Zhang et al., 2022).

Hence, visual intelligence is highly promising in revolutionizing the practice of medical imagery because it has an advantage on aspects related to accuracy, efficiency, and capabilities in diagnosis. However, its issues of limitation must be addressed for practical implementation in healthcare systems. Figure 1 depicts the states and transitions involved in the federated learning process in healthcare.

Figure 1. States and transitions involved in the federated learning process in healthcare

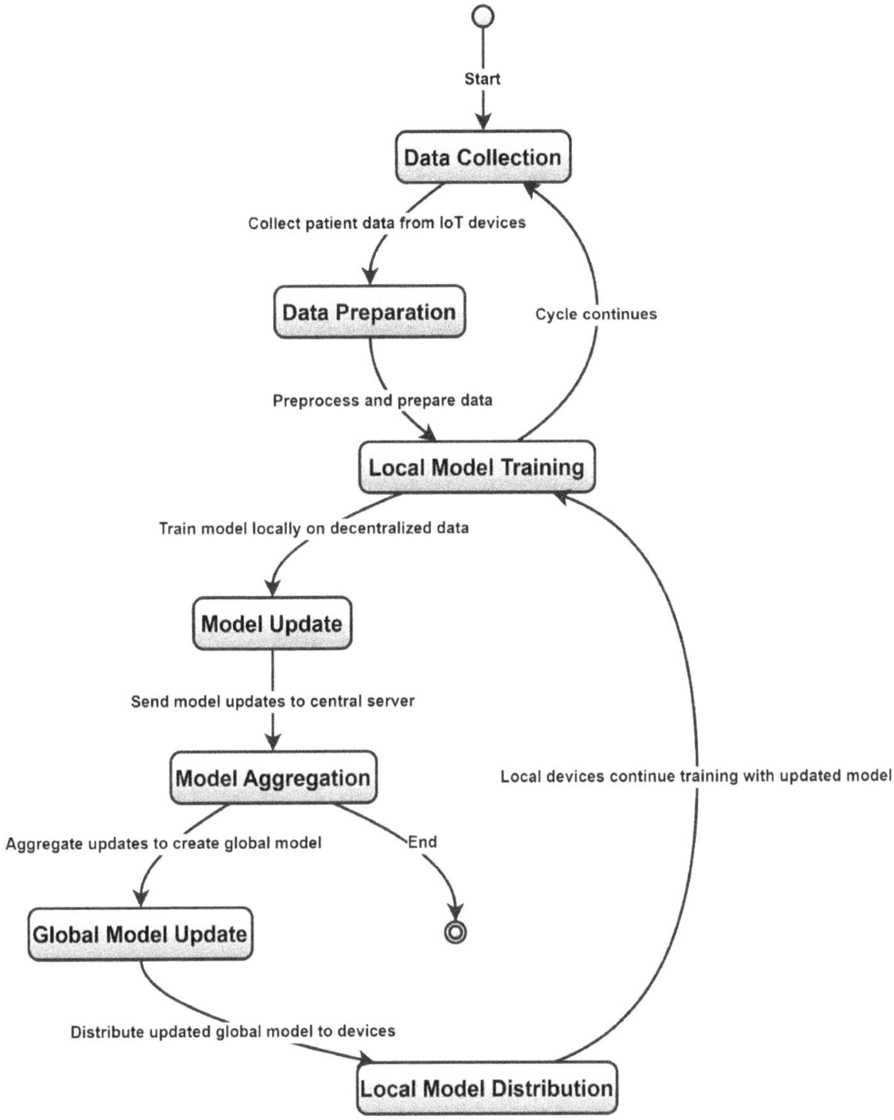

FEDERATED LEARNING IN HEALTHCARE

Federated learning is an innovative approach to machine learning that allows decentralized training of models with multiple devices or organizations while maintaining strict privacy and security of data. Traditionally, most machine learning approaches rely on the centralization of data in a single repository for training. Now, with federated learning, entities such as hospitals and clinics can jointly train a common model without sharing sensitive patient information. This approach is particularly well suited for health care applications, where protecting the confidentiality of patients and information is the utmost importance(He et al., 2021; Zhang et al., 2022). Federated learning works as if each participating local device or site trains an algorithm for itself and uploads to a central server only the updates of the model, i.e., the parameters or gradients of the model. In such a way, the central server is supposed to aggregate these updates in order to improve the model. Then, the central server is supposed to send back to each local site improved versions of the global model, in order to be further trained by local sites. The iterative process continues until the model reaches satisfactory performance. Maintaining data locally in federated learning resolves associated risks of sharing data, thereby addressing very critical concerns based on patient privacy and the regulation that is HIPAA in the United States and GDPR in Europe.

The main advantage of federated learning in healthcare is that it supports privacy and security in data. Compared to traditional scenarios of machine learning, sensitive health information has been transferred to centralized servers, and this raises intense concerns about unauthorized access and data breaches. Federated learning, as designed, ensures that patients' data never leaves the local device or institution and therefore exposes the least sensitive possible information. This approach not only provides confidentiality regarding the identity of patients but also generates trust among patients and healthcare providers since patients are liable to share their health data if they are sure that it is safe. Furthermore, federated learning supports institutions in fulfilling the requirements of legal and ethical principles related to patient data while benefiting from collaborative research and model development. It allows researchers to build more general and robust models trained with different populations of patients, bringing the AI-applications' performance in healthcare--like diagnostic algorithms and predictive analytics--closer to the highly accurate and practical benchmark that is 95% or higher accuracy.

Some case studies demonstrate that federated learning works well in healthcare. Here, the goal was to build a deep learning model for the prediction of patient outcomes on the basis of EHR data among a group of collaborating healthcare institutions. Each participating institution trained a local model on the data it itself maintained in its EHR system and transmitted only the updates of the model to a central server. The aggregated model had much better predictive accuracy than models trained on individual datasets, which convincingly demonstrated that, in federated learning, the power of distributed sources of data could be taken advantage of in a fully patient privacy-preserving manner. Yet another interesting case was the application of federated learning to medical imaging. Researchers collaborated with several hospitals to propose a federated model for detecting diabetic retinopathy from retinal fundus images. The researchers received high diagnostic accuracy by training the model on decentralized datasets without transferring sensitive image data and kept it under the regulations related to data protection. This is one of the cases of how federated learning helps collaborate institutions maintain patient privacy while improving the performance of AI models.

Apart from those discussed above, federated learning is also being experimented toward real-time patient monitoring and decision support systems. In one pilot study, the researchers developed a federated learning framework which they used to develop predictive models for identifying at-risk patients for sepsis through continuous vital sign monitoring. The study aimed at creating a general model using data from different hospitals that would predict sepsis effectively in various patients. Results Superior performance of federated model over its peers trained on single-site data have exposed the potential of enhancing patient outcomes. Furthermore, COVID-19 and other health crises have well underlined the critical need for responses that are time-sensitive; thus, federated learning has been applied to enable collaborative research toward developing models for the detection of viruses and prognosis of patients without compromising data privacy. A federated learning framework has been proven to be a tool necessary to handle urgent healthcare challenges by letting researchers from different parts of the world share their insights and learnings while keeping data local.

Although there are several benefits of implementing federated learning within healthcare, there are also challenges due to the technical complexities of ensuring the smooth functioning of federated systems across different computation resources and changing network conditions within institutions. In reality, consistency of model performance across multiple sites may be difficult when data regarding quality, volume, or, most importantly, patient demographics is fundamentally different. Developing robust frameworks and protocols that easily create seamless collaboration while maintaining the reliability and effectiveness of the federated learning approach will be important to solve these issues(Ramudu et al., 2023; Sreedhar et al., 2024; Ugandar et al., 2023).

Another challenge is the development of standardized protocols and frameworks for sharing data, training models, and evaluation. There is a general need in establishing common guidelines to facilitate the meaningful interaction among participating institutions in federated learning. Thus, efforts toward the standardization of methodologies for federated learning in healthcare are crucial to overcome these barriers and facilitate its further adoption.

Federated learning is that transformative approach to machine learning in the health sector, bringing decentralized collaboration with prioritized safety on data secrecy and privacy. This kind of approach addresses crucial challenges in the health landscape because it enables multiple institutions to be involved in model development without having to share sensitive patient data. The advantages of this kind of approach are exemplified through case studies which demonstrate how it can improve predictive accuracy and enhance patient outcomes. However, for federated learning to realize its full potential, much more work is needed to deal with the remaining technical challenges, standardize protocols, and foster a culture of collaboration among healthcare organizations. As the health care sector continues to evolve, federated learning promises to be an exciting frontier for innovative solutions capable of successfully tapping into the power of data while at the same time providing patient data protection and regulatory compliance.

THE ROLE OF IOT IN HEALTHCARE

The IoT is a transformative force in healthcare as it drives improvements that bring benefits to the care of patients, improve the operational efficiency of operations, and introduce innovation in medical practice. The IoT refers to the network of interconnected devices that are usually equipped with sensors, software, and communication capabilities for collecting and exchanging data over the internet. From the wrist-worn devices that monitor the vital signs of the patient to a complex system integrating medical equipment, environmental sensors, and patient data management systems, the IoT technologies used within the health care sector can widely differ. IoT enables healthcare providers to make decisions more informatively, respond faster to the needs of the patient, and respond progressively to improve the delivery of care through its real-time capabilities of data collection and analysis(Bouzinis et al., 2021; Mohammed et al., 2020; Pei et al., 2022). The Internet of Things (IoT) is playing a pivotal role in healthcare, enhancing patient care, operational efficiency, and innovation as figure 2.

Figure 2. Role of IoT in healthcare: impact on patient care, operational efficiency, and innovation

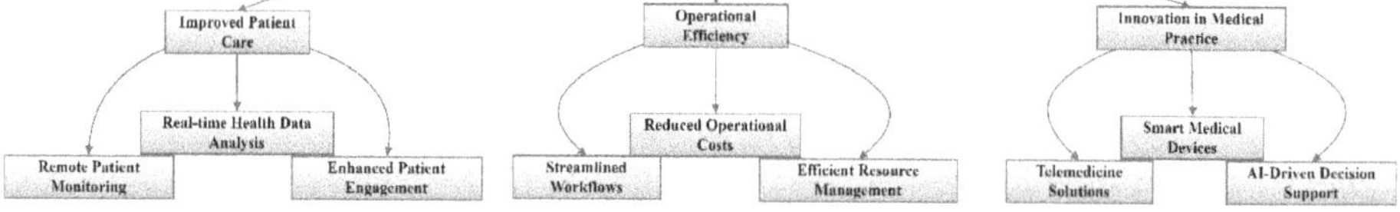

There exist a range of IoT technologies that are now being used in healthcare, which include wearable devices, remote patient monitoring systems, smart hospital equipment, and connected health applications. Wearable devices encompass all the tools and devices embedded with sensors that monitor physiological parameters, heart rate, blood pressure, and activity level. Such devices can easily send reports to healthcare providers in real time, making it possible for continuous monitoring and timely intervention. Another important area of application of IoT in health systems is the one related to remote patient monitoring systems, which allows health care providers to view the health parameters outside traditional clinical settings, thus saving frequent hospital visits and establishing proactive management of chronic conditions. Smart Hospital Equipment(Upadhyaya et al., 2024; Venkateswaran et al., 2023), Such as Connected Beds, Infusion Pumps Improves Workflow Efficiency and Enhances Patient Safety with Real-time Tracking of Medical Devices and their Performance. Over and above this, IoT applications in telehealth facilitate virtual consultations, which patients can attend from the comfort of their homes while ensuring providers have a registry of health information(Sreedhar et al., 2024).

The applications for IoT in patient monitoring and management are virtually limitless and transformative. Some of the major benefits include improved chronic disease management. IoT devices such as blood glucose monitors can be a relief for patients with conditions like diabetes, hypertension, or heart disease as it keeps the patient's health in check. A CGM, for instance, can monitor the real time level of a patient's blood sugar and alert him to potential issues before they manifest. This allows the patient to make better decisions to control his or her health, which facilitates adherence to treatment plans and lowers hospitalizations. In addition, IoT-based blood pressure and heart rate monitoring equipment facilitate remote monitoring by healthcare professionals on cardiovascular health in patients, thereby leading to timely interventions that help minimize risks associated with unmanaged conditions.

IoT can also significantly contribute to post-operative care and rehabilitation. Connected devices after surgery allow patients to track the rate of their recovery, so that healthcare teams have the critical information about their healing journey. By generating a higher clinician's index of suspicion and warning the clinician about potential complications, remote monitoring systems will ensure that the patient receives timely follow-up care. IoT devices in rehabilitation enable the creation of customized exercise programs for the patients by keeping track of the performance as well as progress of the patients. The data about adherence to treatment by a patient helps healthcare providers to intelligently alter the treatment plan and, hence optimizes the outcome of recovery(Upadhyaya et al., 2024).

However, various challenges present it from large-scale applications across the healthcare domain. Data security and privacy is the key concern. While the IoT devices are gathering huge amounts of sensitive patient information, data breach and cyberattacks bring the biggest worries with them for healthcare organizations. This would ensure that the right security measures were in place, such as encryption, secure authentication, and regular software updates, to protect the patient's data. There is also the problem of compliance with legislations, such as in the United States with the Health Insurance Portability and Accountability Act (HIPAA). The health care provider has to ensure that its IoT systems meet adequate data protection standards to prevent legal implications and foster trust between the patients and the health care providers.

Interoperability is yet another significant challenge facing IoT integration in health care. The effective accomplishment of an exchange of data among different technologies requires the accommodation of an array of devices and systems produced in large numbers globally. Many IoT devices operate on proprietary platforms that cannot easily interface with existing electronic health record systems and other healthcare technologies. Interoperability also calls for standardization of data formats and communication protocols that will enable access, location, and application of patient data by various healthcare providers.

Healthcare organizations also need a skilled workforce to process and interpret the IoT data. Although IoT technology can produce a vast volume of data, it presents opportunities for insights to improve patients' care, and health care organizations usually lack the capability to analyze and make practical use of this data effectively. The potential of such systems must be leveraged through creating a skillful workforce in data analytics and IoT technologies. Health professionals must be educated so they understand and then interpret the data that IoT creates, giving them the basis for enhanced decision-making with respect to care and outcomes(Upadhyaya et al., 2024). Another very important factor in considering the use of IoT technology in healthcare is the cost:. IoT solutions frequently involve a tremendous investment in equipment, infrastructures, and training upfront. Therefore, even though the long-term payoffs of IoT, such as lower hospital readmissions and better patient outcomes, are likely to make the payback suitable, health care organizations are unlikely to invest into new technology without earning its ROI. Other than this, cost-effective development of IoT solutions and proving their value through robust evidence and multiple case studies shall form the backbone of encouraging its widespread use(Malathi et al., 2024; Upadhyaya et al., 2024; Venkateswaran et al., 2023).

Healthcare IoT has a transformative role with the potential to revolutionize patient monitoring and management. It has the potential to link a plethora of connected devices and technologies in order to enhance the quality of care for patients, better outlay outcomes, and streamline operations. However, to realize the full potential of IoT, healthcare organizations must address challenges faced within these areas: data security, interoperability, workforce training, and cost. The landscape of health care is changing, requiring IoT technologies to support the delivery of patient-centered care within a rapidly changing environment. Overcoming these challenges and investment in innovative solutions will enable healthcare providers to tap into the potential of IoT towards improving health outcomes, making operations more efficient, and assisting them in adopting a more proactive approach in all their patient care endeavors.

SYNERGY OF VISUAL INTELLIGENCE, FEDERATED LEARNING, AND IOT

The integration of visual intelligence, federated learning, and IoT is positioned to transform the landscape in healthcare, especially with respect to enhancing telemedicine, improving patient monitoring while farther away from healthcare providers, and streamlining healthcare operations. These technologies offer innovative solutions that promote efficiency, improve patient outcomes, and maintain data privacy and security(Mehta et al., 2023; Michieli & Ozay, 2021; Pei et al., 2022; Zhang et al., 2024). The figure 3 illustrates the integration of visual intelligence, federated learning, and IoT in a synergistic manner.

Figure 3. Synergy of visual intelligence, federated learning, and IOT

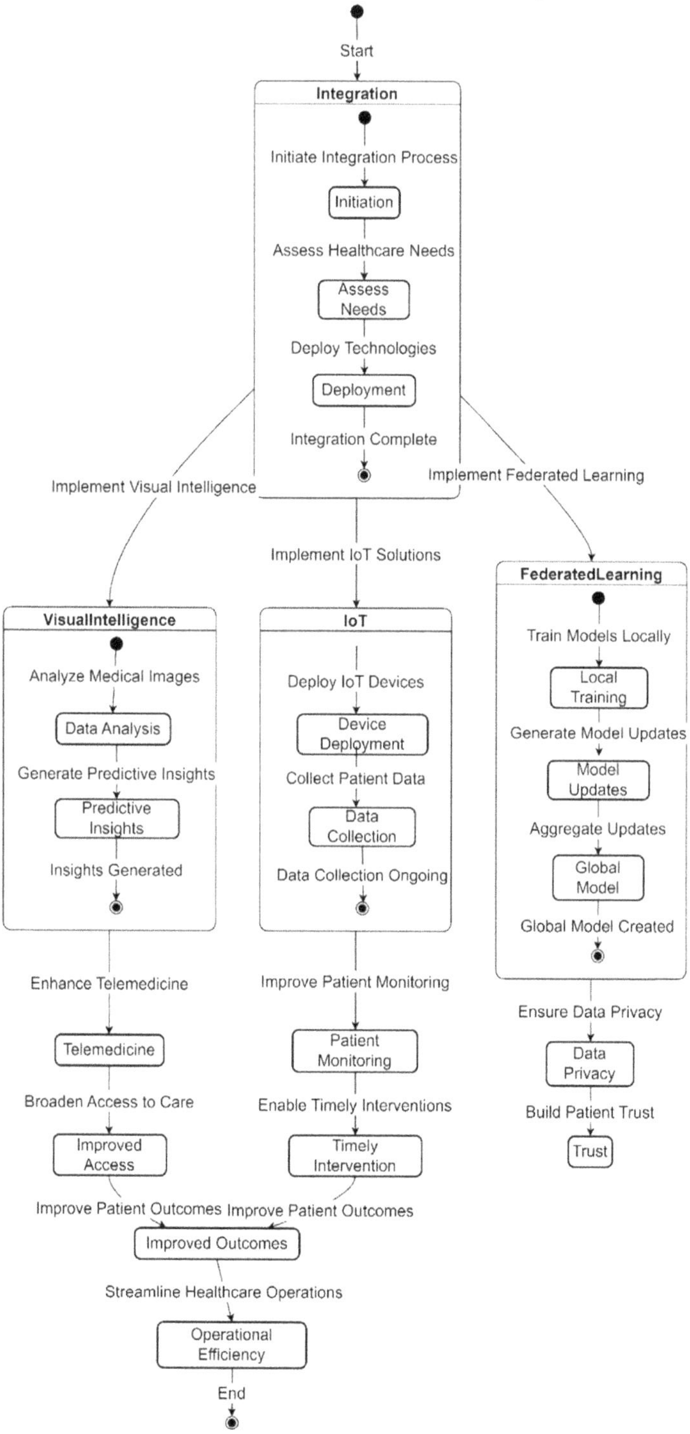

Improving Telemedicine through Visual Intelligence

Telemedicine has grown at a tremendous rate in the recent past, more so after the COVID-19 pandemic; such a pandemic forced people to look for solutions for remote health care. Visual intelligence can be described as system ability to understand and analyze visual data, hence very key in improving telemedicine services. Advanced imaging technologies, such as the algorithms of machine learning and AI, enable healthcare providers to study medical images in real time-this would include X-rays, MRIs, and CT scans through virtual consultations(Agrawal et al., 2023; Reddy et al., 2023).

Telemedicine can be practiced more accurately for diagnosis and recommendation of treatment through visual intelligence. For instance, using AI-based imaging sources, clinicians will be able to identify anomalies even one would miss, thus always ensuring that second and third opinions are precise, though they may be miles away. This capability is highly beneficial in access-constrained areas where general practitioners can deliver expert-level consultation backed by intelligent visual analysis. This would be because it can enhance patients' telemedicine experience through clearer communication by diverse objects in view with accompanying annotations such as images and 3D models to better illustrate their conditions and treatment options.

The federated learning approach in telemedicine allows for the continuous improvement of visual intelligence algorithms but preserves the patients' privacy. The federated approach enhances diagnostic tools by enabling multiple healthcare institutions to collaborate and train AI models using their own data without sharing sensitive information, enhancing accuracy and robustness. It ensures that the visual intelligence of various systems has the chance to benefit from diverse datasets to improve its performance in cross-patients and respective medical conditions. This means that telemedicine is going to be an even more powerful and trustworthy answer for care delivery, which eventually drives toward better patient outcomes and satisfaction.

Remote Patient Monitoring and Predictive Analytics

RPM is one more the key application of IoT in healthcare. This offers a chance to healthcare providers to keep patient vital signs along with health metrics under real-time monitoring so that proactive intervention can be performed and the number of visits to the hospital can be minimized. The integration of visual intelligence in RPM systems aids in the understanding of the health condition of patients. For instance, by cameras mounted on wearable devices, skin lesion or any other physical symptoms can be captured for further analysis and interpretation by the algorithms within the visual intelligence, which would emphasize any problem identified(-Boopathi, 2023; Malathi et al., 2024).

Predictive analytics, together with the synergy realized between IoT, Visual intelligence, and Federated learning, may significantly enhance the functions of RPM capabilities. Using the multimodal historical and real-time data from multiple sources, including wearable devices, electronic health records, and imaging studies, healthcare professionals are able to create predictive models that would identify patients who might deteriorate into a critical condition. Such examples include an algorithm using machine learning to predict the probability of readmission to the hospital of a chronically ill patient, depending on their vital signs and histories. Such predictions enable physicians, therefore, to intervene before the onset of complications and improve patient outcomes.

In addition to the above, federated learning bolsters the predictions analytics capabilities of RPM by enabling organizations to pool knowledge safely and without compromising the privacy of patients. Federated learning enables the development of more generalized and accurate algorithms for predicting patient risks by training models on data collected from multiple institutions without sharing sensitive patient information. Therefore, healthcare providers can understand more about patient risks, and interventions could be led towards meaningful care delivery.

Aggregating Healthcare Operations

Integrating visual intelligence, federated learning, and IoT is the wave that streamlines healthcare operations to improve healthcare efficiency and cut costs. Visual intelligence can further enhance all workflows of operational efficiency by automating some of the tasks, for example, image analysis and data entry in order to free health care professionals to engage more fully in direct patient care. For example, AI algorithms may sort through medical images, thus raising a flag on abnormalities for review by radiologists. Visual intelligence can be used to track medical supplies and equipment through images, thereby enabling ideal stock levels within a healthcare facility(Pitchai et al., 2024; Sreedhar et al., 2024).

Moreover, Internet of Things devices can optimize patient flow and resource utilization efficiencies within healthcare settings. In this context, real-time monitoring of the flow of patients, bed occupancy, and utilization of medical equipment can further enhance healthcare operational performance management and resource utilization efficiencies. Through generated data from devices, healthcare providers can identify bottlenecks in patient care and devise targeted interventions to enhance throughput and reduce waiting times.

Federated learning is also paramount in the process of streamlining operations because it enables healthcare organizations to learn from the experiences of their peers while maintaining data security. Hospitals can, for instance share best practice practices in the management of patients and attaining operational efficiency based on aggregated insights drawn from the data while at the same time maintaining confidentiality of information regarding patients. This sets a stage for a culture of continuous improvement and innovation within the health sector. In addition, federated learning, visual intelligence, and IoT can enhance better communication between healthcare providers and facilitate them to communicate and collaborate together. Creating shared platforms that integrate visual data, real-time monitoring information, and predictive analytics will enable the healthcare teams to collaborate with each other for decision making concerning patient care. Thus, improved communication tools can ensure coordination among interdisciplinary teams that generally enhances the outcome of a patient .

Synergistic relationship of visual intelligence, federated learning, and IoT in healthcare has been envisioned to change the frontiers of better improvement in telemedicine, enhancements in remote patient monitoring, and smoothing of operations. With data analytics and the use of advanced imaging technologies, federated learning will ensure more accurate diagnoses and recommendations for further treatment, thereby keeping patient data confidential and fully secure. Predictive analytics, through remote patient monitoring, improves the effectiveness and enables proactive interventions for better outcomes on the patients' side. Further, streamlined healthcare operations will only bring efficiency and lower costs to both providers and patients. Together, the advancement of these technologies will unmistakably catapult a healthcare system into a more efficient, effective, and patient-centered process. The potential for innovation in healthcare is immense and embracing this synergy will be the key to meeting all the challenges of modern delivery in healthcare.

CHALLENGES AND CONSIDERATIONS

The confluence of visual intelligence, federated learning, and IoT in healthcare offers promising opportunities but presents many challenges and considerations in its proper implementation to assure effectiveness with the highest benefit. Among these are data security and privacy concerns, issues of interoperability and standardization, and the necessity of continuous learning or adaptation of models(He et al., 2021; Michieli & Ozay, 2021; Mohammed et al., 2020). The integration of visual intelligence presents numerous challenges and considerations, as illustrated in Figure 4.

Figure 4. Challenges and considerations associated with the integration of visual intelligence

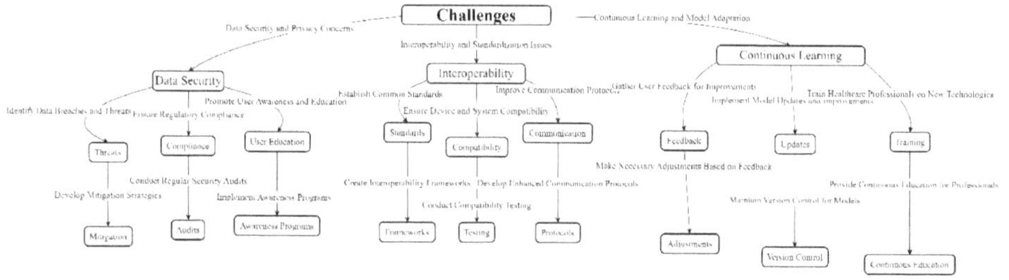

Data Security and Privacy Concerns

But one of the biggest challenges in health technology is data security and patient confidentiality. Most of the collected data by the IoT devices, visual intelligence systems, and federated learning that sent around the world is private information of patients. This sensitive information can be vulnerable to cyber attacks and breaches when not protected adequately, having disastrous consequences for both patients and healthcare organizations.

This federated learning can include some enhancements to mitigate privacy concerns through the development of machine learning models without sensitive data centralization. However, data still resides at its source but its model updates shared among the participating entities. There is still a risk, as in the case of model inversion attacks, for malicious actors to infer sensitive patient information from parameters of the model developed. Therefore, strong encryption protocols, secure authentication mechanisms, and periodic audits must provide patient data protection.

Healthcare providers also have to meet numerous regulatory requirements. Other leading examples include the Health Insurance Portability and Accountability Act of the United States of America and the General Data Protection Regulation of Europe. It can be extremely comprehensive and labor-intensive when dealing with these requirements while bringing in new technologies within a health system. Staff trainings as well as system updates are much needed to always ensure that one does not violate the rules at hand.

Interoperability and Standardization Challenges

The third significant integration challenge in the visual intelligence, federated learning, and IoT paradigm is the lack of interoperability and standardization in the healthcare systems and devices. Health care providers often use a different kind of technology, wherein many of these technologies run on different platforms and formats. This fragmentation can hinder seamless communication among devices or systems while limiting the effectiveness of integrated solutions in healthcare. The optimum realization of benefits from visual intelligence and IoT in healthcare could be achieved with the development of standardized protocols for data formats, communication, and device compatibility. This would smoothen interoperability among dissimilar systems, thereby allowing for enhanced data analysis for proper patient care. Absence of standardization can make it difficult for the healthcare organization to introduce new technologies in their system, which can create inefficiency and may result in suboptimal patient outcomes. In addition, multi-level collaborations among healthcare providers, technology vendors, regulatory bodies, and policymakers are required in order to ensure interoperability. Crucial for facilitating health care innovation, collaborative frameworks with a shared vision for handling the challenges discussed are in need of being set up to properly deal with these challenges.

Continuous Learning and Model Adaptation

Healthcare is dynamic by nature, and models of machine learning must constantly learn and adapt to new data towards visual intelligence and predictive analytics. Updating is usually necessary so that the accuracy as well as the efficacy of such models are maintained. Model retraining proves to be resource-intensive and also quite complex in federated learning environments where the data are decentralized. Such a challenge would demand development of significant strategies for continuous learning from real-time data coming from IoT devices on the part of healthcare organizations while ensuring preservation of patient privacy. Such an implementation could probably come about by using adaptive learning algorithms, perhaps incrementally updating models without that demanding the use of substantial computational resources or creating significant data transfers.

Healthcare providers have to incorporate user input and clinical knowledge into developing and refining and updating machine learning continuously. Involving healthcare experts in the design and assessment of these systems assures that the machines learn things that can work in real-time; thus, they improvise their utility. Hence, although much promise exists in incorporating visual intelligence, federated learning, and IoT in healthcare, issues pertaining to problems of data security and privacy, interoperability, and continuous learning must be addressed. Healthcare organizations can help take positive action towards improved patient care and outcomes while also respecting regulatory standards and maintaining patient privacy by planning in-depth strategies and encouraging cooperation from all interested parties.

FUTURE DIRECTIONS AND INNOVATIONS

Due to the fast pace of change in technologies, the healthcare landscape is constantly changing. With increasing integration of visual intelligence, artificial intelligence, and the Internet of Things, comes a host of emerging future directions and innovations that influence trends in visual intelligence and AI development, the potential impact of 5G and edge computing, and implications on healthcare policy and practice(Mehta et al., 2023; Michieli & Ozay, 2021; Mohammed et al., 2020; Pei et al., 2022). The figure 5 depicts the future directions and innovations in healthcare.

Figure 5. Future directions and innovations in healthcare

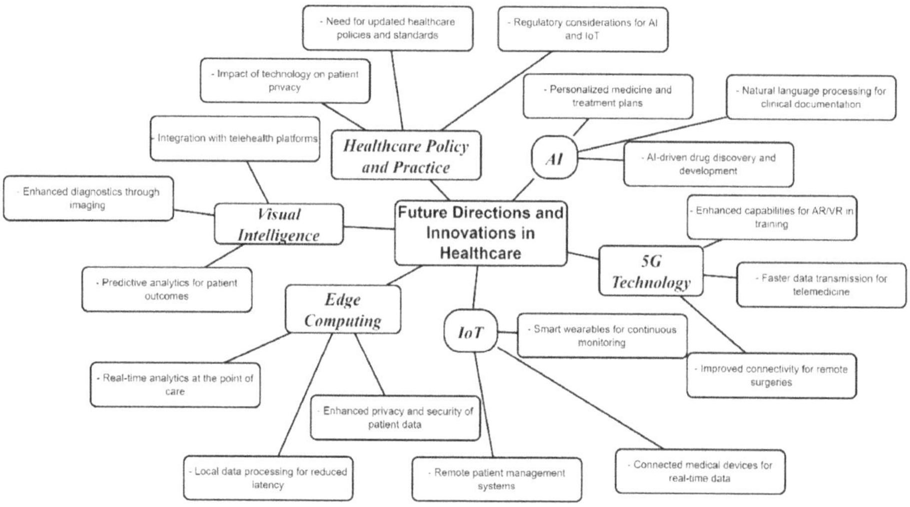

Future Directions of Visual Intelligence and AI

Perhaps one of the most promising trends in visual intelligence is its increasing application in medical imaging. Deep learning algorithms, especially convolutional neural networks, have been able to bring about great success in image classification, segmentation, and anomaly detection. In terms of being more complex, future breakthroughs and innovations might allow for models that could be brought up while analyzing tricky visual data in real-time to have actionable insights at the point of care. Advances in explainable AI will make these systems more transparent so that the rationale for conclusions reached can be understood, thus fostering the trust needed between providers and end-users to apply these technologies.

A new trend being explored currently includes multimodal data analysis, where visual data come together with patient data types such as genomics, EHRs, and wearable sensor data. Such an approach would result in individualized, effective treatment plans through finding correlations and patterns that would not have been there when analyzing data in isolation. The ability to tap into diverse datasets will be key towards the development of robust AI systems that can be fashioned around a patient's individual needs and preferences.

Impact of 5G and Edge Computing

The rollout of 5G networks and edge computing will undoubtedly transform the health care industry to push toward faster data transmission, improved connectivity, and reduced latency. It could also possibly enable a real-time exchange of large volumes of data between IoT devices for real applications in remote patient monitoring. For instance, high-resolution medical images may be transmitted instantly, and specialists can comment on a case without delay from any remote location. This capacity is crucial in emergency situations, whereby timely interventions make all the difference in the outcome for patients. dge computing is complementary to 5G, as it is closer to the source of data processing and reduces the need for a lot of data to be transmitted to centralized cloud servers(Molakatala et al., 2024; Sreedhar et al., 2024). This is particularly important for applications requiring real-time analysis that no one wants to wait for-visual intelligence system in surgery or diagnostics. By processing at the edge, healthcare organizations can ensure quick vital decisions, thus safeguarding safety with better patient care and operational efficiency.

5G and edge computing will also be applied to very innovative applications of AR and VR in health care, the applications whereby training of surgeons can occur remotely, consultancy via remote means, and patient education. Healthcare will enable trying real-life situations in a controlled environment with the help of AR and VR. The more immersive experiences that these technologies may generate will lead to more engagement in learning among medical professionals and between patients and their providers.

Implications for Health Care Policy and Practice

The technologies will have profound implications on health care policy and practice. Of these, important policy and practice imperatives at the apex are needed to engage frameworks for allowing the uses of AI and visual intelligence in clinical settings with safety, effectiveness, and ethics considerations. Some examples are requirements for directions in data privacy, security, and consent use when handling sensitive information within patient files. Policymakers would need to extend incentives to healthcare organizations to encourage acceptance of these technologies, rewards for innovation along with access for all. Technology evolves with such a velocity that the healthcare personnel must be forever trained and updated. For visual intelligence and AI to be further integrated into clinical practice, more will depend on providers' developing expertise regarding knowledge and skills about how to apply the tools appropriately. It may happen in the form of providing training programs and other resources that guide clinicians to better understand and interpret insights formed through AI(Ramudu et al., 2023; Satav et al., 2023).

Furthermore, there should be incentives from the health care organizations to promote the development of interdisciplinary teams comprising data scientists, clinicians, and IT specialists to encourage collaboration during the implementation of these technologies. It is in this setting that a healthcare provider has the opportunity to nurture innovation and lifelong learning, hence being better able to deal with the fast-paced environment and provide quality patient-centered care. Therefore, the future of healthcare would be bright with ongoing trends in visual intelligence, AI, and advanced connectivity revolutionizing the industry. By embracing such innovations and solving the related challenges, healthcare organizations will be able to improve patient outcomes, enhance operation efficiency, and create a more efficacious and equitable healthcare system. And most importantly, forward and satisfying collaboration among stakeholders and thoughtful policymaking combined with continuous education will be required to unlock the full potential of these transformative technologies.

CASE STUDIES

In the last few years, healthcare systems in different parts of the world have been facing two challenges with respect to patient increase volumes: quality care. To address such challenges, a regional healthcare organization in the United States recently designed a novel remote patient monitoring program based on the integration of visual intelligence through the implementation of federated learning and IoT technology. This report describes the combined approach and elaborates how it effectively enhanced the outcomes for patients and operational effectiveness while ensuring data security(Mehta et al., 2023; Orlandi et al., 2023; Zhang et al., 2024).

Implementation

The healthcare organization had set out to monitor the chronic patients who needed constant monitoring and interventions, especially heart disease and diabetes. IoT devices like wearables-based heart rate monitors and glucose sensors would fetch critical health information regularly from the patients' homes for the organization. Real-time information relayed by these devices could be visualized on a central platform through sophisticated algorithms of visual intelligence. It translated the data produced by various devices into insights. For instance, imaging instruments, which are AI-powered, had scrutinized visual inputs from telemedicine visits to enable healthcare workers to evaluate patients' conditions based on remote consultations. By using a convolutional neural network, it could detect unusual patterns in the parameters like irregular beating of the heart or fluctuations of blood glucose and pass on warning to healthcare teams on time.

The organization chose a federated learning model for the enhancement of data privacy and security. It was from the local healthcare facilities that the AI algorithms learned the decentralized patient data, containing the sensitive information within them. Instead of uploading raw data to a central server, providers train models in their facilities locally and exchange only the updates of these models with the central system. Thus, patient data remains secure in conformity with regulations like HIPAA.

Outcomes

The integration of visual intelligence, federated learning, and IoT technologies eventually led to the enhancement in the efficiency of operations regarding patient care. After six months of starting the telemonitoring program, the organization achieved a 30% reduction in hospital readmission rates for patients suffering from chronic conditions. The health providers were eventually in a position to intervene based on real-time responses as the patients showed certain warning trends; for example, as heart rates increase or blood sugar levels deviate. Patients found care very convenient to be monitored remotely; it was commented upon to be more satisfying. There were responses from their team of health care within a short period. The visual tools of intelligence made possible to give understandable insights regarding the health metrics for patients thus empowering them to take active roles in managing the conditions. The federated model significantly reduced the risk of data breaches. The organization improved its cybersecurity posture with the minimization of data transfer and keeping sensitive information on local facilities. The success in that model boosted the level of patient's confidence to collaborate with the remote monitoring program.

Challenges and Concerns

Despite the positive outcomes, challenges were noted during the implementation of this integrated approach in the healthcare organization. Ensuring interoperability between different devices and health information systems was essential to successfully implementing this program. The organization coordinated with the various technology vendors in relation to standardizing data formats and communication protocols to make integration much smoother. Another issue is that the healthcare professionals must be regularly trained. The clinicians are supposed to learn how to read appropriately the insights generated by AI and use a monitoring system effectively. Training programs and workshops were designed for the staff on a routine basis to equip them with the relevant skills.

This case study, therefore, clearly brings out the transformative potential of visual intelligence, federated learning, and IoT technologies in healthcare. Based on improved patient monitoring and engagement regarding data privacy, this regional health organization experienced better outcomes and operational efficiency. As the new scenario unfolds further in the healthcare landscape, the integrated approaches will be significantly more decisive to achieve high-quality personalized care to the patients.

CONCLUSION

In conclusion, visual intelligence, federated learning, and IoT integration for health therefore relate paradigm changes in the delivery and management of patient care. This chapter outlined how these technologies can transform aspects of diagnosis accuracy, remote monitoring, and the privacy of the data. Visual intelligence enables healthcare providers to gain actionable insights from the massive medical data, while federated learning tackles the perceived concerns over privacy in relation to model training where no sensitive information from patients will be shared. The Internet of Things technologies advance these aspects further by continuously monitoring patients in a real-time manner that leads to timely intervention and better results.

While these innovations hold great promise, several challenges exist for data security, interoperability, and model adaptation for updates. Resolving these will take a collective effort from stakeholders, regulatory guidelines and continuous education of healthcare providers. Embracing these innovations will be key in empowering patient engagement in health care, making operations easier, and creating a more efficient and equitable system in health care. Ultimately, the integration of visual intelligence, federated learning, and IoT technologies herald a new future in

REFERENCES

Agrawal, A. V., Pitchai, R., Senthamaraikannan, C., Balaji, N. A., Sajithra, S., & Boopathi, S. (2023). Digital Education System During the COVID-19 Pandemic. In *Using Assistive Technology for Inclusive Learning in K-12 Classrooms* (pp. 104–126). IGI Global. DOI: 10.4018/978-1-6684-6424-3.ch005

Boopathi, S. (2023). Internet of Things-Integrated Remote Patient Monitoring System: Healthcare Application. In *Dynamics of Swarm Intelligence Health Analysis for the Next Generation* (pp. 137–161). IGI Global. DOI: 10.4018/978-1-6684-6894-4.ch008

Bouzinis, P. S., Diamantoulakis, P. D., & Karagiannidis, G. K. (2021). Wireless Federated Learning (WFL) for 6G Networks[4]Part I: Research Challenges and Future Trends. *IEEE Communications Letters*, *26*(1), 3–7. DOI: 10.1109/LCOMM.2021.3121071

Han, X., Yu, H., & Gu, H. (2019). Visual inspection with federated learning. *Image Analysis and Recognition: 16th International Conference, ICIAR 2019, Waterloo, ON, Canada, August 27–29, 2019. Proceedings*, *16*(Part II), 52–64.

He, C., Shah, A. D., Tang, Z., Sivashunmugam, D. F. N., Bhogaraju, K., Shimpi, M., Shen, L., Chu, X., Soltanolkotabi, M., & Avestimehr, S. (2021). Fedcv: A federated learning framework for diverse computer vision tasks. *arXiv Preprint arXiv:2111.11066*.

Liu, F., Wu, X., Ge, S., Fan, W., & Zou, Y. (2020). Federated learning for vision-and-language grounding problems. *Proceedings of the AAAI Conference on Artificial Intelligence*, *34*(07), 11572–11579. DOI: 10.1609/aaai.v34i07.6824

Liu, W., Lin, H., Wang, X., Hu, J., Kaddoum, G., Piran, M. J., & Alamri, A. (2021). D2MIF: A malicious model detection mechanism for federated learning empowered artificial intelligence of things. *IEEE Internet of Things Journal*.

Liu, Y., Huang, A., Luo, Y., Huang, H., Liu, Y., Chen, Y., Feng, L., Chen, T., Yu, H., & Yang, Q. (2020). Fedvision: An online visual object detection platform powered by federated learning. *Proceedings of the AAAI Conference on Artificial Intelligence*, *34*(08), 13172–13179. DOI: 10.1609/aaai.v34i08.7021

Malathi, J., Kusha, K., Isaac, S., Ramesh, A., Rajendiran, M., & Boopathi, S. (2024). IoT-Enabled Remote Patient Monitoring for Chronic Disease Management and Cost Savings: Transforming Healthcare. In *Advances in Explainable AI Applications for Smart Cities* (pp. 371–388). IGI Global.

Man, D., Zeng, F., Yang, W., Yu, M., Lv, J., & Wang, Y. (2021). Intelligent Intrusion Detection Based on Federated Learning for Edge-Assisted Internet of Things. *Security and Communication Networks*, *2021*(1), 9361348. DOI: 10.1155/2021/9361348

Mehta, S., Kukreja, V., & Gupta, A. (2023). Revolutionizing Maize Disease Management with Federated Learning CNNs: A Decentralized and Privacy-Sensitive Approach. *2023 4th International Conference for Emerging Technology (INCET)*, 1–6.

Michieli, U., & Ozay, M. (2021). Prototype guided federated learning of visual feature representations. *arXiv Preprint arXiv:2105.08982*.

Mitra, A., Ngoko, Y., & Trystram, D. (2021). Impact of federated learning on smart buildings. *2021 International Conference on Artificial Intelligence and Smart Systems (ICAIS)*, 93–99. DOI: 10.1109/ICAIS50930.2021.9395938

Mohammed, I., Tabatabai, S., Al-Fuqaha, A., El Bouanani, F., Qadir, J., Qolomany, B., & Guizani, M. (2020). Budgeted online selection of candidate IoT clients to participate in federated learning. *IEEE Internet of Things Journal*, *8*(7), 5938–5952. DOI: 10.1109/JIOT.2020.3036157

Molakatala, N., Kumar, D. A., Patil, U., Mhatre, P. J., Sambathkumar, M., & Boopathi, S. (2024). Integrating 5G and IoT Technologies in Developing Smart City Communication Networks. In *Blockchain-Based Solutions for Accessibility in Smart Cities* (pp. 147–170). IGI Global. DOI: 10.4018/979-8-3693-3402-7.ch006

Orlandi, F. C., Dos Anjos, J. C., Leithardt, V. R., Santana, J. F. D. P., & Geyer, C. F. (2023). Entropy to mitigate non-IID data problem on federated learning for the edge intelligence environment. *IEEE Access : Practical Innovations, Open Solutions*, *11*, 78845–78857. DOI: 10.1109/ACCESS.2023.3298704

Pei, X., Deng, X., Tian, S., Zhang, L., & Xue, K. (2022). A knowledge transfer-based semi-supervised federated learning for IoT malware detection. *IEEE Transactions on Dependable and Secure Computing*, *20*(3), 2127–2143. DOI: 10.1109/TDSC.2022.3173664

Pitchai, R., Guru, K. V., Gandhi, J. N., Komala, C. R., Kumar, J. R. D., & Boopathi, S. (2024). Fog Computing-Integrated ML-Based Framework and Solutions for Intelligent Systems: Digital Healthcare Applications. In *Technological Advancements in Data Processing for Next Generation Intelligent Systems* (pp. 196–224). IGI Global. DOI: 10.4018/979-8-3693-0968-1.ch008

Ramudu, K., Mohan, V. M., Jyothirmai, D., Prasad, D., Agrawal, R., & Boopathi, S. (2023). Machine Learning and Artificial Intelligence in Disease Prediction: Applications, Challenges, Limitations, Case Studies, and Future Directions. In *Contemporary Applications of Data Fusion for Advanced Healthcare Informatics* (pp. 297–318). IGI Global.

Reddy, M. A., Gaurav, A., Ushasukhanya, S., Rao, V. C. S., Bhattacharya, S., & Boopathi, S. (2023). Bio-Medical Wastes Handling Strategies During the COVID-19 Pandemic. In *Multidisciplinary Approaches to Organizational Governance During Health Crises* (pp. 90–111). IGI Global. DOI: 10.4018/978-1-7998-9213-7.ch006

Satav, S. D., Hasan, D. S., Pitchai, R., Mohanaprakash, T., Sultanuddin, S., & Boopathi, S. (2023). Next generation of internet of things (ngiot) in healthcare systems. In *Sustainable Science and Intelligent Technologies for Societal Development* (pp. 307–330). IGI Global.

Savazzi, S., Nicoli, M., & Rampa, V. (2020). Federated learning with cooperating devices: A consensus approach for massive IoT networks. *IEEE Internet of Things Journal*, *7*(5), 4641–4654. DOI: 10.1109/JIOT.2020.2964162

Sreedhar, P. S. S., Sujay, V., Rani, M. R., Melita, L., Reshma, S., & Boopathi, S. (2024). Impacts of 5G Machine Learning Techniques on Telemedicine and Social Media Professional Connection in Healthcare. In *Advances in Medical Technologies and Clinical Practice* (pp. 209–234). IGI Global. DOI: 10.4018/979-8-3693-1934-5.ch012

Ugandar, R., Rahamathunnisa, U., Sajithra, S., Christiana, M. B. V., Palai, B. K., & Boopathi, S. (2023). Hospital Waste Management Using Internet of Things and Deep Learning: Enhanced Efficiency and Sustainability. In *Applications of Synthetic Biology in Health, Energy, and Environment* (pp. 317–343). IGI Global.

Upadhyaya, A. N., Saqib, A., Devi, J. V., Rallapalli, S., Sudha, S., & Boopathi, S. (2024). Implementation of the Internet of Things (IoT) in Remote Healthcare. In *Advances in Medical Technologies and Clinical Practice* (pp. 104–124). IGI Global. DOI: 10.4018/979-8-3693-1934-5.ch006

Venkateswaran, N., Kumar, S. S., Diwakar, G., Gnanasangeetha, D., & Boopathi, S. (2023). Synthetic Biology for Waste Water to Energy Conversion: IoT and AI Approaches. *Applications of Synthetic Biology in Health. Energy & Environment*, 360–384.

Yang, H., Lam, K.-Y., Xiao, L., Xiong, Z., Hu, H., Niyato, D., & Vincent Poor, H. (2022). Lead federated neuromorphic learning for wireless edge artificial intelligence. *Nature Communications*, *13*(1), 4269. DOI: 10.1038/s41467-022-32020-w PMID: 35879326

Yang, H., Yuan, J., Li, C., Zhao, G., Sun, Z., Yao, Q., Bao, B., Vasilakos, A. V., & Zhang, J. (2021). BrainIoT: Brain-like productive services provisioning with federated learning in industrial IoT. *IEEE Internet of Things Journal*, *9*(3), 2014–2024. DOI: 10.1109/JIOT.2021.3089334

Zhang, R., Mao, J., Wang, H., Li, B., Cheng, X., & Yang, L. (2024). A survey on federated learning in intelligent transportation systems. *IEEE Transactions on Intelligent Vehicles*, 1–17. DOI: 10.1109/TIV.2024.3446319

Zhang, X., Hu, M., Xia, J., Wei, T., Chen, M., & Hu, S. (2020). Efficient federated learning for cloud-based AIoT applications. *IEEE Transactions on Computer-Aided Design of Integrated Circuits and Systems*, *40*(11), 2211–2223. DOI: 10.1109/TCAD.2020.3046665

Zhang, Z., Ma, S., Yang, Z., Xiong, Z., Kang, J., Wu, Y., Zhang, K., & Niyato, D. (2022). Robust semisupervised federated learning for images automatic recognition in Internet of Drones. *IEEE Internet of Things Journal*, *10*(7), 5733–5746. DOI: 10.1109/JIOT.2022.3151945

KEY TERMS

AI refers to the simulation of human intelligence through machines to enable them to perform tasks like solving problems: making decisions, and processing natural language.

ML can be described as a subcategory of AI: where systems can learn and improve automatically from experience without explicit programming using algorithms to analyze data and make predictions or decisions.

MRI (Magnetic Resonance Imaging): This is a medical imaging technique that is based on the use of magnetic fields and radio waves to create clear images of the organs and tissues within the body.

CT (Computed Tomography): A type of medical imaging that uses X-rays to create highly detailed cross-sectional images of the body.

HIPAA (Health Insurance Portability and Accountability Act): US legislation that creates standards for the protection of medical records and personal health information is safeguarded with appropriate standards set in place for privacy and security.

GDPR (General Data Protection Regulation): EU regulation regarding rules for the protection of personal data and privacy for individuals in the EU as well as exporting data outside the European Union.

Electronic Health Record: A digital version of any patient's existing paper chart that can be electronically accessed and shared with other healthcare providers responsible for the patient's healthcare needs, including medical history, diagnosis, treatments, and other relevant information.

Coronavirus Disease (COVID): A more infectious viral disease caused by a new coronavirus, SARS-CoV-2, which was declared a worldwide pandemic in 2020.

CGM: Continuous Glucose Monitoring - the continuous real-time glucose levels are monitored continuously through a sensor implanted under the skin, and this is widely used by people with diabetes in the management of their conditions.

ROI: Return on Investment - it describes the efficiency or profitability of an investment that has been made through net return is divided by the initial cost of investment.

Internet of Things is a collection of connected devices in communication and data sharing with the internet to develop intelligent applications in health care: transportation, and automating homes.

PM essentially addresses the application of technology toward the remote monitoring of patient health: whereby the health care providers can monitor remotely the state and condition of the patient.

AR: Technology that adds a layer to what people see, with visual, as well as auditory information, on top of actual reality.

VR: Computer-generated environment that one could use to immerse oneself in a potentially three-dimensional space to entertain, train, or educate.

IT: Information Technology refers to computers, storage, networking, and other physical devices, of which the basic function is to process, store, and communicate electronic data within an organization, including support of business operations and personal activities.

Chapter 7
IoT-Enhanced Additive Manufacturing and Federated Learning for Smart Healthcare Systems

Shaik Mahamad Shakeer
https://orcid.org/0000-0002-4809-2229
School of Computer Science and Engineering, Vellore Institute of Technology (VIT), Vellore, India

M. Rajasekhara Babu
https://orcid.org/0009-0008-4621-0034
School of Computer Science and Engineering, Vellore Institute of Technology (VIT), Vellore, India

ABSTRACT

This chapter explores the privacy-utility trade-offs in IoT-enhanced additive manufacturing and federated learning systems within smart healthcare. IoT-driven additive manufacturing transforms healthcare by enabling customized medical devices and implants, while federated learning facilitates collaborative, decentralized AI model training without compromising raw data privacy. However, balancing privacy protection and system utility remains challenging, as stringent privacy measures often hinder data richness and model accuracy. The chapter explores strategies like differential privacy, homomorphic encryption, and secure multi-party computation to mitigate risks and ensure robust privacy, while evaluating the impact of regulatory frameworks. This chapter discusses the importance of balancing privacy and utility in personalized healthcare, promoting sustainable and secure IoT-augmented systems in clinical settings through case studies and comparative analysis.

DOI: 10.4018/979-8-3693-6094-1.ch007

INTRODUCTION

Rapid advancements in technology over the last couple of years have opened up new health care scenarios through the horizon, where combining the technologies of IoT (Internet of Things), additive manufacturing, and AI-driven methodologies, such as federated learning, change the age-old paradigms. Innovations are revolutionizing medical device design, healthcare system management, and patient care. It has opened up new avenues for having very high-grade customized medical devices, implants, and prosthetics for individual patients. The federated learning approach in artificial intelligence decentralizes the actual learning process, avoiding centralization of sensitive patient data and thus offering the way forward to critical privacy concerns. Together, they form a promising revolution for smart systems in healthcare but raise a significant problem: privacy-utility trade-off(Okokpujie & Tartibu, 2024).

This chapter explores the heart of the trade-off: the subtle balance to be struck between very strict data privacy standards and high utility and performance of IoT-enhanced systems. Health is a data-intensive industry, and patient information's sensitivity makes privacy an essential issue. With all these grave consequences, a breach can lead to the loss of money, reputation, and patient trust. On the other hand, this information, especially if it is abundant and accurate, forms the core on which the utility of health care depends. Richer data leads to better accuracy and precision of AI models because it enables superior diagnostics, predictive analytics, and treatment personalization. This delicate interplay forms the basis of the discussion in this chapter(Bhuvaneshwari et al., 2024).

IoT-advanced additive manufacturing has started changing healthcare dramatically. It enable the production of patient-specific medical devices using real-time data from IoT sensors. For example, a patient's anatomical structure can be exactly replicated through 3D printed implants and prosthetics, promoting more comfort, functionality, and optimal outcomes. Additionally, IoT integration permits the continuous monitoring of device performance and patient recovery for the critical insights that would benefit healthcare providers. However, the devices prone to reliance in collecting and transmitting sensitive health information offer areas of vulnerability from unauthorized access and misuse. Such issues necessitate robust data privacy measures and secure communication protocols to prevent security incidents, yet they often compromise system efficiency and real-time functionality(Babu et al., 2024).

The other development is federated learning, which has come up to address some of the privacy issues with centralized data collection. It provides decentralized model training and lets several entities develop AI models together, without sharing raw data such as hospitals, clinics, and research institutions. This approach not only preserves data privacy but also complies with stringent regulatory frameworks such as the

General Data Protection Regulation (GDPR) and the Health Insurance Portability and Accountability Act (HIPAA). However, federated learning is not without its limitations. Communication overhead, model accuracy, and system scalability are some of the technical challenges that arise, further complicating the privacy-utility equation(Serral et al., 2024).

The privacy-utility trade-off is, therefore, a technical, but also a regulatory and ethical problem. Laws and regulations for protecting the patient's data often impose various restrictions that may block the development and implementation of advanced technologies. In fact, while GDPR and HIPAA enforce data protection practices, they also present compliance difficulties for organizations seeking to implement data-driven solutions. In addition to these issues, considerations of ethics, including informed consent, ownership over data, and equitable use of AI models further complicate matters. Privacy and utility would go hand in hand by requiring a solution that integrates technical innovation with policy reform, stakeholder collaboration, and public engagement(Premavathi et al., 2024).

To deal with these issues, this chapter identifies several different techniques for privacy preservation and assesses them in the context of IoT-enhanced additive manufacturing and federated learning systems. Methods that look most promising include differential privacy, secure multi-party computation, and homomorphic encryption. They ensure sensitive data can only be allowed for meaningful analysis and high system utility. For instance, differential privacy introduces controlled noise into datasets and is useful when deriving meaningful insights without exposing individual data points. Similarly, secure multi-party computation enables multiple parties to jointly compute functions over their data without revealing it to each other, fostering collaboration without compromising confidentiality(Kaur, 2024). Homomorphic encryption takes data protection a step further by allowing computations to be performed on encrypted data, ensuring that sensitive information remains secure even during processing.

The chapter also examines the role of regulatory frameworks in shaping the adoption of these technologies. While respecting rules like GDPR and HIPAA are of course necessary, regulatory compliance should not strangle innovation. The balance between the requirements of regulation and the incentives for innovation requires a forward-looking approach to the design of policy: it must innovate in a way that does not compromise public trust. For example, regulatory sandboxes whereby innovators test new technologies in controlled environments may represent a solution in finding a middle ground between compliance and innovation(Raman & Mitra, 2023a).

Case studies comprise a significant component of this chapter, reflecting real-world applications of IoT-enhanced additive manufacturing and federated learning in health care. The case studies delineate the practical challenges and benefits related to maintaining privacy-utility equilibrium. For instance, one case explores how an international hospital network could use IoT-enabled devices to create customized implants in patients while utilizing federated learning for predictive analytics. This strategy dramatically enhanced patient outcome statistics but presented difficult problems in terms of data security and interoperability. Another case study looks at federated learning models implementing differential privacy for research into rare disease, demonstrating how privacy-preserving technologies can enable sensitive-but-useful scientific findings(Shchepkina et al., 2024).

Conclusively, this chapter presents a comprehensive understanding of the inherent trade-offs between privacy utility in IoT-enhanced additive manufacturing and federated learning for smart healthcare systems. By analyzing the technical, regulatory, and ethical dimensions of such trade-offs, the present chapter tries to provide actionable insight for researchers, practitioners, and policymakers into innovative solutions which can help develop secure, efficient, and patient-centered healthcare systems(Vanitha et al., 2023). As we move toward a future in which technology will play an increasingly central role in healthcare, addressing these trade-offs will be crucial to realizing the full potential of IoT and AI in transforming medical science and improving global health outcomes.

Contrubution

This chapter contributes to the understanding of privacy utility in IoT-enhanced additive manufacturing and federated learning in smart healthcare systems. The study addresses advanced methodologies such as differential privacy, secure computation, and encryption to preserve the data without losing its utility. This study has passed through the regulatory frameworks, for instance, GDPR and HIPAA, to weigh upon their impact on innovation along with the compliance achieved within the health care domain. The chapter provides actionability through detailed case studies for achieving robust privacy as well as operational efficiency. It thereby offers strategies for developing customized, secure, and efficient healthcare solutions powered by the technologies of IoT and federated learning.

Objectives

This chapter shall aim to:

a) Explore privacy utility trade-offs in IoT-enhanced additive manufacturing and federated learning for smart healthcare systems.
b) Examine methodologies with differential privacy, secure computation, and encryption so that data security does not compromise system utility.

c) Analyse regulatory frameworks such as GDPR and HIPAA from a perspective of their effect on innovation with compliance with the healthcare sector.
d) Insights through case studies to achieve robust balance between privacy and operational efficiency.
e) Help develop deeper insights into strategies that can enable personalized, secure, and efficient healthcare systems through IoT and federated learning technologies.

IOT-ENHANCED ADDITIVE MANUFACTURING IN HEALTHCARE

Additive manufacturing, often referred to as 3D printing, has become a revolutionary technology in healthcare, opening unprecedented opportunities for designing and developing personalized medical devices and implants. When combined with IoT, the true potential of additive manufacturing can be realized, namely, real-time data exchange, intelligent automation, and customization. This section discusses the crucial role IoT-enriched additive manufacturing plays in the creation of customized medical solutions and detailed experimental approaches that bring this integration into reality. Figure 1 shows the design to final assembly process, with IoT integration occurring after 3D printing for performance monitoring and patient data collection(Hassan et al., 2021; Raman & Mitra, 2023b).

Figure 1. Process of IoT-enhanced Additive Manufacturing in Healthcare

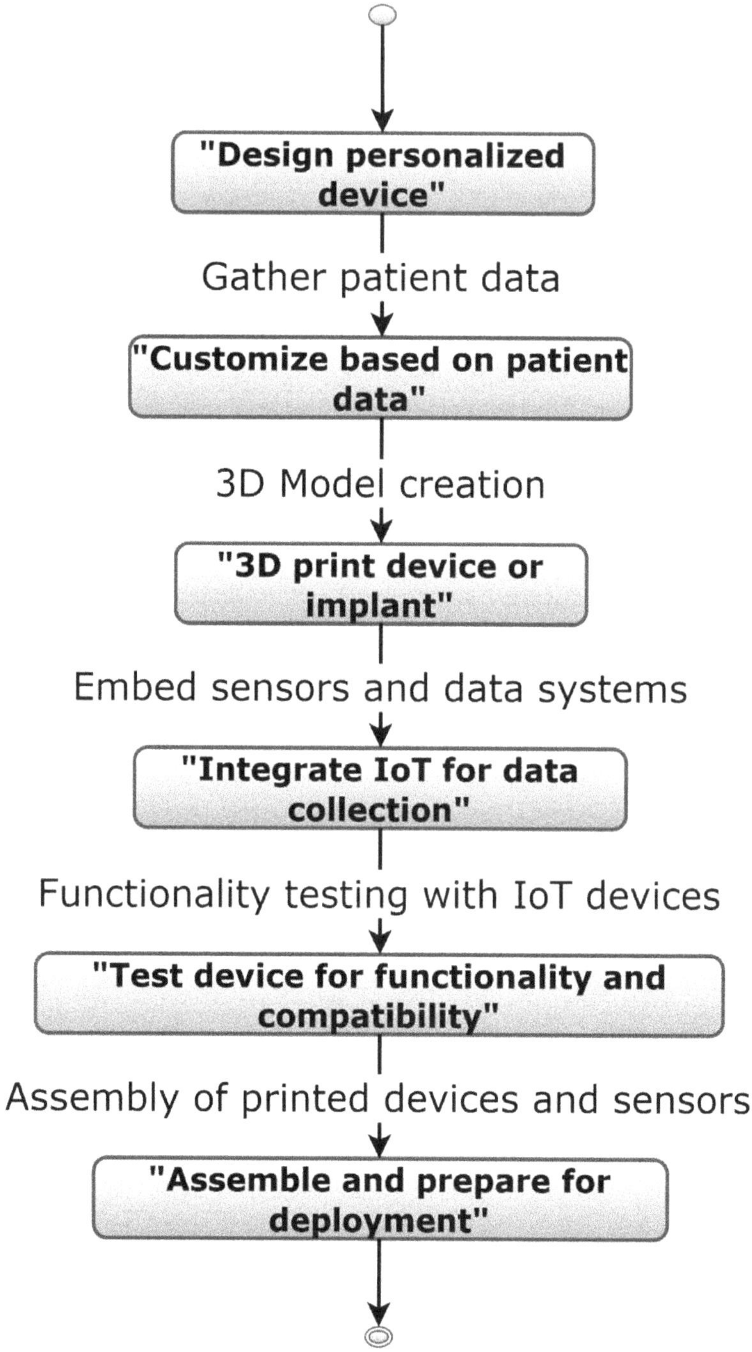

Role in Personalized Medical Devices and Implants

Improving patient outcomes and satisfaction are crucial drivers for personalization in health care. Among the technologies stimulating this trend is IoT-enhanced additive manufacturing. It has the huge advantage of promoting the development of particularly patient-specific devices and implants tailored to specific anatomical and physiological requirements(Anderson & Smith, 2024; Huang et al., 2024).

Accuracy and Customization: IoT-enabled sensors capture specific patient information through imaging scans and physiological parameters and then process this data using advanced algorithms. The patient-specific data are the basis for designing an implant and a medical device that accounts for the unique anatomy of each patient. For instance, through 3D printing, prosthetics and orthopedic implants can be obtained with precise dimensions and materials that enhance effectiveness and comfort.

Real-Time Monitoring and Feedback: IoT devices embedded within medical implants allow for continuous monitoring of patient health and device performance. For instance, sensors in orthopedic implants can track load distribution and healing progress, transmitting real-time data to healthcare providers. This dynamic feedback loop ensures timely interventions and enhances patient safety.

Efficiency in Production: Long processes and huge wastage of materials in traditional manufacturing methods for medical devices are often the case. IoT-enhanced additive manufacturing contributes to streamlined production through digital designs and exact material deposition. This not only reduces lead times but also provides opportunities for cost and environmental impact reduction, in turn making personalized health care accessible.

Regulatory compliance and traceability: The integration of IoT ensures that every step involved in the manufacturing process is recorded, thereby improving traceability and ensuring all regulatory standards are met, such as FDA and ISO certifications. This transparency is therefore of paramount importance for quality assurance of manufactured medical devices.

Applications for intricate cases: IoT-enabled additive manufacturing is very valuable in the treatment of complex medical conditions. It has already been applied for creating cranial implants for skull-injured patients and airway splints for children with congenital breathing problems. In such applications, this technology is used to be lifesaving.

Experimental Procedure

Experimental incorporation of IoT and additive manufacturing in healthcare involves a multi-step process including data acquisition, design optimization, production, and validation(Anderson & Smith, 2024; Huang et al., 2024). Below is an overview of the general procedures usually involved in such an experimental approach:

Patient-Specific Data Collection: Advanced imaging technologies including MRI, CT scans, and 3D ultrasound record accurate anatomical data. IoT sensors monitor the real-time physiological parameters, for example, heart rate or pressure distribution.

Data Integration: The acquired data is processed on IoT platforms with AI algorithms to formulate an exhaustive patient profile.

Design Optimization

Modeling Software: CAD computer-aided design software is used to develop a digital 3D model of the device or implant.

Simulation and Testing: IoT-enabled tools that simulate the real world, such as stress, loads, and temperature changes, maximize the design for performance and durability.

Additive Manufacturing Process

Material: Biocompatible material such as medical-grade titanium or polymers for the particular application and patient needs.

3D Printing Process: The additive manufacturing machine produces the device layer-by-layer as the digital model guides it. It checks on parameters such as temperature, material deposition, and the alignment of each layer in real time to ensure precision.

Post-Process and Quality Assurance

After Process: Sterilization, polishing, and others are applied to prepare the device for medical usage.

Quality Control: IoT systems track a high degree of metrics during their production, which can be carefully checked for quality ensuring that the device meets all medical and regulatory standards.

Clinical Validation

The device is tested strenuously in simulated environments to test its functionality and robustness.

In-Vivo Trials: With the device getting regulatory approval, the device is implanted in patients and controlled conditions. The IoT devices continuously track its performance after implantation and send back data for further refinement.

Feedback Loop and Iterative Improvements

Feedback from IoT systems is used in continuous areas of improvement, not only in the designed device but also in manufacturing processes. This series of iterative improvement approaches will continue to enhance the quality of products and patient outcomes.

IoT-advanced additive manufacturing, as this field continues to improve, will likely find new application avenues in healthcare. AI-driven design automation, smart materials that heal themselves, and blockchain for safeguarding data are emerging trends. Collaborative teamwork between technologists, healthcare providers, and regulatory bodies will be a critical input toward addressing scalability-related issues, data security concerns, and ethical questions. IoT-enhanced additive manufacturing will allow for the production of highly customized, intelligent medical devices that can revolutionize patient care by being more precise, efficient, and responsive. This integration addresses current problems in health care but also presents opportunities for innovative solutions to balance the needs of patients with the pursuit of technological advancement.

FEDERATED LEARNING FOR SMART HEALTHCARE SYSTEMS

Federated learning (FL) is considered the technological and innovative approach to be adopted in AI, especially in healthcare, as it overcomes the main challenges in data privacy, security, and efficiency. As such, this decentralized training of AI models offers more-than-one possibility of collaboration among numerous healthcare institutions to develop robust AI models without a need to share sensitive patient data. This chapter discusses the federated learning principles, as well as the benefits for smart healthcare systems, keeping in mind the fact that data privacy is also a critical element in collaborative learning processes. Figure 2 demonstrates how federated learning facilitates efficient, privacy-preserving machine learning in healthcare.

Figure 2. Federated Learning for Smart Healthcare Systems

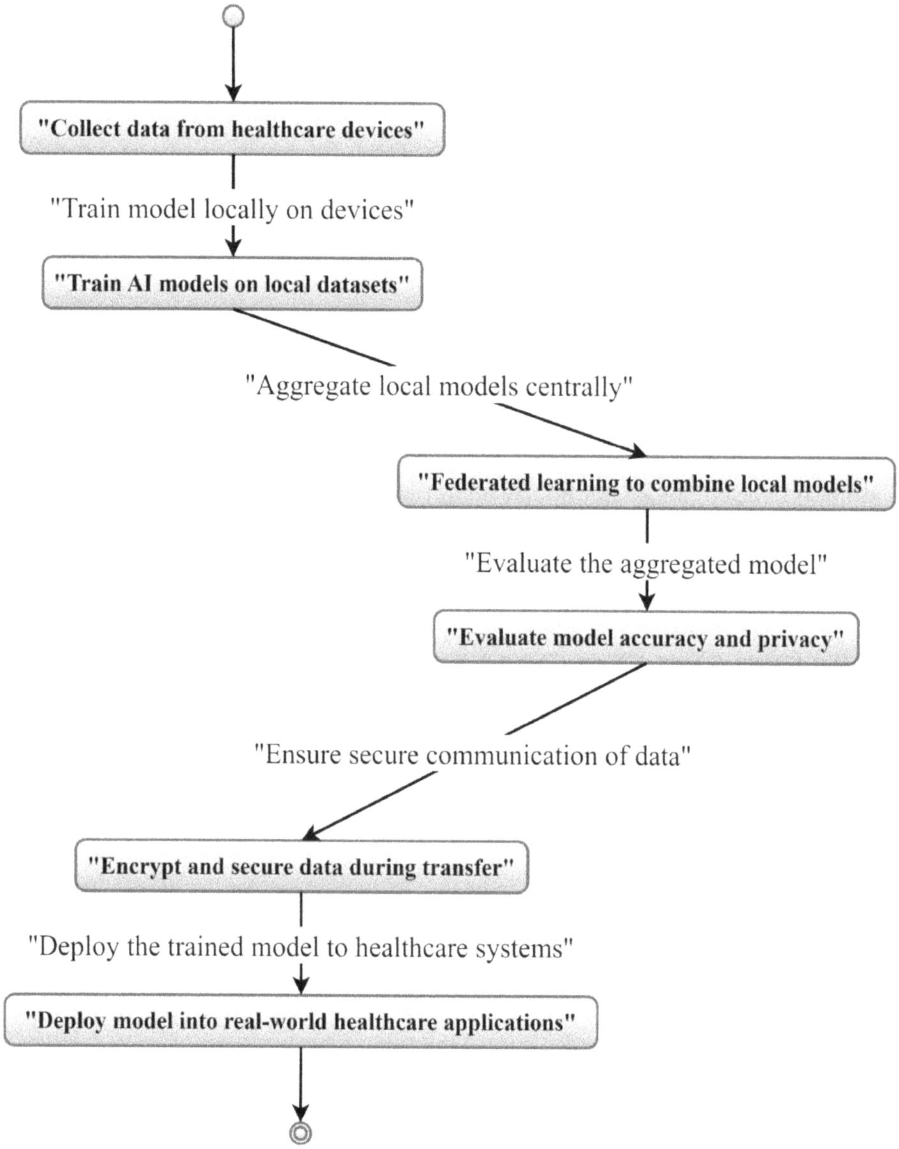

Decentralized AI Model Training: Principles and Benefits

The main concept behind federated learning is the principle of decentralized model training. Traditional machine learning approaches usually need centralization of data from various sources in one point location, say in the cloud server, for their analysis and model development. Obviously, it raises big concerns about privacy, mainly in healthcare, given the sensitivity of patient data, with HIPAA and GDPR setting major strictures in its governing regulations. Federated learning, on the other hand, enables institutions to train AI models locally, directly on their data, and share only model updates, such as gradients or weights, and not the raw data itself(Minnema et al., 2018; Morrison et al., 2018a).

Principles of Federated Learning

Local Model Training: This is an instance of federated learning, wherein each participant in the health-care institution, such as hospitals, clinics, or research centres, trains a local model using its own datasets. This training is done at the local level without moving the data from their source, thus maintaining control and security at every site.

Model Aggregation: Once the local models are trained, they will be forwarded to a central server, where an aggregation process takes place. An aggregation process at the central server aggregates updates at the model weights or gradients received from all participating nodes and combines them into a global model. This global model is then rediffused back to the participating institutions, where further local training may continue.

Iterative Process: The training process is iterative, with repeated cycles of local model training and global model aggregation. Each iteration enables the global model to learn through the assimilation of varied datasets, producing a robust AI model that learns to generalize across wide health-care contexts.

Benefits of Federated Learning in Health Care

Data Privacy and Security: The most important advantage of federated learning in healthcare would be the guarantee of patient data privacy. As raw patient data is never leaving the local institution, chances to be penetrated or accessed illegitimately are minimized. This especially matters when information is highly confidential and touches on secrecy, such as medical records, imaging data, and genetic information(Akhtar, 2024; Salmi, 2021).

Compliance with Regulations: The approach of federated learning is well-suited to the stringent regulations set forth by laws such as HIPAA in the United States and GDPR within the European Union, which mandate strict controls over the handling and sharing of healthcare data. It ensures that patient data remains on local servers, and only aggregated model updates are shared, thus facilitating compliance with such legal frameworks while still enabling meaningful data-driven research in the domain.

Enhanced AI Models: Federated learning enables the development of AI models trained on various datasets emanating from different healthcare institutes. This diversity enhances the model's ability to generalize to handle a wide range of patient conditions, demographics, and medical practices. The resulting model tends to be more accurate and reliable when deployed in real healthcare environments.

Low Cost and Resource Intensity: Federated learning reduces the need for centralizing large volumes of data, which can be expensive in terms of storage, transmission, and processing. By allowing local institutions to train models and share only essential updates, federated learning helps optimize resources and reduces the overhead costs of data transfer and centralized data storage.

Scalability and Flexibility: Federated learning is naturally scalable. It can easily be applied in all kinds of health systems sizes, ranging from small clinics to large hospital networks. New members of the federated learning network can easily join to contribute to the development of the model without sending sensitive data across different institutions' boundaries.

Facilitating Collaborative Research: Federated learning allows multiple institutions to collaborate, making it easier for researchers to develop powerful models without the inconveniences of data-sharing barriers. Collaboration between multiple institutions would lead towards a more varied and innovative healthcare solution by integrating insights from different patient populations and medical practices into AI models.

Ensuring Data Privacy in Collaborative Learning

Federated learning does provide many inherent benefits with regard to privacy by design; however, guaranteeing robust data privacy remains an essential challenge, particularly in healthcare. With medical data being highly sensitive, additional protection must be incorporated into the federated learning process in order to ensure patient data security as well as preserving the integrity of the collaborative learning environment(Han et al., 2022; Hashemi et al., 2022).

Differential Privacy: Differential privacy is one of the most widely used techniques in federated learning to ensure that individual data points remain private. It involves adding controlled noise to the data or the model updates, making it difficult to identify any individual's information. By using differential privacy, federated learning systems can prevent sensitive patient information from being inferred, even if the model updates are accessed by malicious actors. The noise, calibrated appropriately, minimizes its influence on the average performance of the model but keeps the output private.

Homomorphic Encryption: As it has come to pass, with homomorphic encryption, computations can directly be performed on the encrypted data without decryption, so the model updates can be secured in federated learning. A central server aggregates encrypted model updates and, instead, decrypts the final global model. This ensures individual data points as well as intermediate updates remain secure throughout the process. It is truly computationally intensive in terms of usage but has this really great layer of security over data privacy.

Secure Multi-Party Computation (SMPC): SMPC is a cryptographic protocol that allows a group of parties to perform a joint computation on their individual data without revealing any data to other parties. In federated learning, SMPC can be used for securely aggregating model updates from different participants. A local model update is computed by each institution in privacy and then combined together securely without revealing raw data or intermediate results to other parties. SMPC preserves privacy by making sure that the data is kept private throughout the learning process.

FedAvg: Federated averaging is another technique used in federated learning; it aggregates the model parameters across many participating devices while minimizing the exposure of sensitive data. It works by simply averaging the updates received from each local model then integrating them into the global model. By design, this approach also limits how much data needs to be shared and reduces the exposure of sensitive patient information.

Data Anonymization and Secure Communication: Addressing: Apart from cryptographic methods, federated learning systems often integrate data anonymization techniques to prevent personally identifiable information being related to specific data points. Anonymization in general removes or alters the identifiable information, such as names, addresses, and contact details, before this is used to train any model. Secure communication protocols, including encrypted communication channels, are also necessary to prevent interception of model updates or other sensitive information during transmission.

Regulatory and Ethical Considerations: There is a need to have regulatory and ethical considerations of collaborative learning as federated learning continues to gain grounds in healthcare. Ethical federated learning practice much be ensured through clear transparency over how the data is used, and informed consent maintained with the patient. Health care organizations must, therefore, keep abreast of the federated learning systems to ensure that they meet the thresholds set for data privacy and protection rules.

Federated learning presents a very promising solution to the issues of data privacy in healthcare AI. Decentralized training and aggregation in federated learning allow healthcare institutions to collaborate on building powerful models without the need to compromise patient privacy. Sensitive medical data remains protected at all stages of the learning process with the incorporation of privacy-preserving techniques such as differential privacy, homomorphic encryption, and secure multi-party computation. As healthcare organizations continue embracing AI and data-driven innovations, federated learning represents a critical tool for creating intelligent, privacy-preserving, and scalable healthcare systems.

INTEGRATION OF IOT-ENHANCED ADDITIVE MANUFACTURING AND FEDERATED LEARNING FOR SMART HEALTHCARE SYSTEMS

Internet of Things (IoT)-augmented additive manufacturing and federated learning (FL) integration within smart healthcare systems is transforming the way patient care is designed, medical devices customized, and the analysis of medical data. The technologies enable personalized on-demand health care solutions while addressing typical challenges related to data privacy and patient-specific device requirements, as well as distributed learning in health care environments. Some of the key implementations of these technologies in health care are described below(Han et al., 2022; Hashemi et al., 2022; Wang et al., 2021). The IoT-enhanced additive manufacturing and federated learning system in smart healthcare illustrates a sequence of data flow and interactions as shown in Figure 3.

Figure 3. IoT-enhanced additive manufacturing and federated learning system in smart healthcare

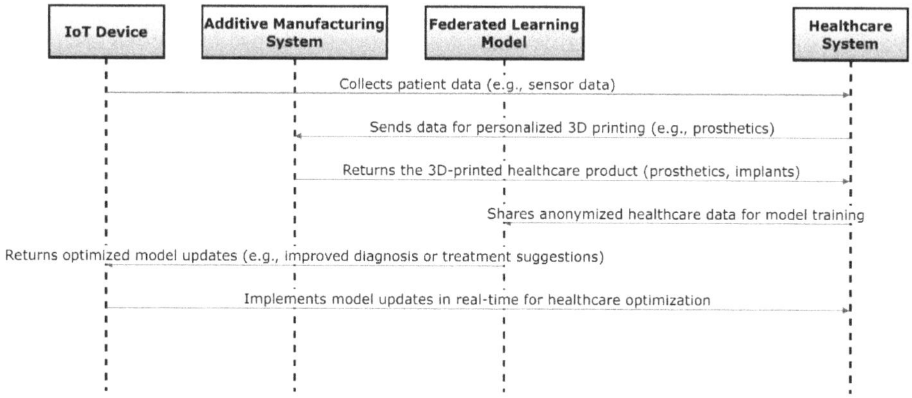

IoT-Enriched Additive Manufacturing for Intelligent Health Systems Personalized Medical Devices and Implants

Some of the most important applications of IoT-enhanced additive manufacturing in the healthcare sector include the development of individualized medical devices and implants. For example, additive manufacturing, or 3D printing, enables the manufacturing of patient-specific devices, such as prosthetics, implants, and orthotic supports, with exact anatomy matching the patient. IoT plays a vital role in this process by incorporating sensors in the devices that collect real-time data on their performance and the patient's condition(Guduri et al., 2023; Tripathy et al., 2024). For instance, IoT-based implants may monitor the biomarkers such as pressure, temperature, or pH levels within the body. The results may then be communicated to the healthcare providers, thus continuously monitoring the device function(Gaur et al., 2023). In addition, the data can be used to make decisions concerning the required adjustments or replacements so that better patient outcomes can be realized.

Real-Time Feedback and Remote Monitoring: Additive manufacturing, along with IoT devices, also enables the creation of "smart" medical implants that can monitor patients in real-time. For example, smart orthopedic implants may have sensors that observe any stress, strain, and patient movement. This information will inform the assessment of the healing process, determine any complications, and assist in interference before the problems become life-threatening. On another hand, IoT technology makes it possible for healthcare providers to monitor these implants from a distance, thus reducing the frequent visits to hospitals and improving care given to patients. The remote monitoring capacity is highly preferred in long-term recovery because patients may need consistent tracking for a long time.

Supply Chain Optimization: In addition to patient care, IoT-enhanced additive manufacturing can revolutionize healthcare supply chains. 3D printing can be used to create medical devices locally, reducing dependency on traditional supply chains and minimizing the time required to produce and distribute devices. IoT sensors track inventory levels, monitor usage, and ensure that devices are available when needed, reducing waste and stockouts.

Federated Learning for Smart Healthcare Systems

Decentralized AI Model Training: Federated learning (FL) is a promising new approach in the training of AI models wherein it enables decentralized and cooperative training of deep learning models on distributed patient data without needing to transfer those data into centralized repositories. Such decentralization is very important in preserving patient privacy, especially in conjunction with norms like HIPAA or GDPR. In FL, for example, local institutions like hospitals or clinics train models locally on their datasets. The model parameters or updates are communicated to a central server rather than the raw data, thus allowing for the building of robust AI models without violating confidentiality of patient data. A typical application of FL in healthcare may involve developing diagnostic models that predict the onset of diseases such as cancer or cardiovascular conditions. Such models can be trained on data from different hospitals and research institutes without patients' records having to be shared across institutions. In fact, using decentralized algorithms protects sensitive information while allowing an AI model to generalize well across different populations by including diverse data sets(Gopi et al., 2024; Kushwah et al., 2024; Pitchai et al., 2024).

Collaborative Decision-Making and Personalized Healthcare: FL is also used for collaborative decision-making over personalized healthcare. For example, several healthcare providers might share their datasets of patient reactions to treatments. A federated learning model could then process this data to yield personalized recommendations for treatments based on a rich collective of clinical experiences. Since the data never leaves its source, patient privacy can be maintained, but even so, healthcare providers can make use of a rich, collective knowledge base. For instance, the application of federated learning comes in precision medicine. Precision medicine is aimed at tailoring treatments to individual patients on the basis of their genetic, environmental, and lifestyle factors. Models trained across different institutions will actually create personalized health models that supply more accurate predictions for each patient without exposing the private health data.

Real-Time Predictions and Patient Monitoring: Federated learning facilitates real-time predictions through harnessing the IoT structure in healthcare. For example, patients connected through wearable devices can seamlessly stream health data—heart rate, blood sugar levels, physical activity—into a central FL system. Such data streams can then be analyzed by learning models built across many hospitals and used to raise timely alerts about potential health issues. If there are early signs of a heart attack or diabetic episode, the system can alert both the patient and the healthcare provider to intervene in time(Boopathi, 2023; Malathi et al., 2024).

Based on this, federated learning can help monitor the effectiveness of treatment plans and predict the possibility of complications coming from historical data aggregated from multiple institutions. This loop of constant feedback will lead to better patient management and less risk of preventable events, therefore improving general health outcomes.

IoT and federated learning in integrated smart health systems

The combination of IoT-enhanced additive manufacturing and federated learning establishes an infrastructure that is strong in the creation of smart healthcare systems. The latter can then gather rich, real-time data of patient health through IoT devices and additive manufacturing that enables customized medical devices and implants for production. Federated learning can then use the data to improve healthcare decision making and prompt development of specific treatment plans without compromising patient data confidentiality(Morrison et al., 2018b, 2018a; Riazi et al., 2018).

For instance, in a patient who has undergone surgery, IoT-enabled implants will be continuously sending data regarding healing through transmitting the amount of strain put on the implant or body parts. This information could possibly be used through federated learning models trained from data collected from multiple hospitals to predict when the implant might need adjustment or when complications might arise. This would allow healthcare professionals to make data-driven decisions and intervene before the situation becomes critical, improving patient outcomes. A key benefit of federated learning in this context is that it ensures privacy by design. Since patient data never leaves the local institution's servers, and only model parameters are shared, the risk of a data breach is significantly reduced. It is especially critical in healthcare, as breaches may lead to more severe consequences for individuals and the organization itself. Federated learning contributes towards helping healthcare institutions comply with regulatory requirements by ensuring patient privacy and improving the utility of healthcare data, while still advancing AI capability(Malathi et al., 2024; Upadhyaya et al., 2024).

Healthcare data are generated in many formats, due to differences in quality and granularity. Data heterogeneity in federated learning must be dealt with and should thereby extend the effectiveness of AI models across various sources. Both IoT devices and federated learning require solid infrastructure to handle the largest amounts of real-time data. Healthcare providers need to invest in scalable solutions to handle the computing load and ensure seamless, real-time data transmission. Data privacy laws and regulations, such as HIPAA or GDPR, are applicable while these technologies are implemented. The healthcare systems would need to implement tight safeguards and audit mechanisms to comply with them. With continued advancement in technology, these challenges will be mitigated in all likelihood, thus integrating IoT-enhanced additive manufacturing and federated learning more smoothly in the healthcare sector.

Enabled by technologies like IoT-enhanced additive manufacturing and federated learning, new settings of smart healthcare systems will be developed. These systems will allow specific patient care, enhance medical devices, promote data privacy, and improve the utilisation of medical AI models for areas of delivering real-time insights, support individual treatment, and advance medical innovation respecting privacy.

PRIVACY-UTILITY TRADE-OFFS: KEY CONSIDERATIONS

Probably, the most important issue in implementing AI and machine learning is to balance data privacy with model utility in healthcare systems. The privacy-utility trade-off is indeed a big challenge in designing solutions that rely on large datasets, such as electronic health records (EHRs), medical imaging, or patient health monitoring. Optimal trade-off will be achieved by understanding the implications of preserving privacy while maintaining the utility of AI models used in decision-making, diagnosis, and patient care(Abdulhameed et al., 2019; Zhong et al., 2018). In this scenario, two key considerations—data sensitivity and the balance between model performance and privacy—will shape how AI systems for healthcare continue to be effective but still protect the patient's information. The concept of privacy-utility trade-offs in healthcare systems is illustrated in Figure 4.

Figure 4. Concept of privacy-utility trade-offs in healthcare systems

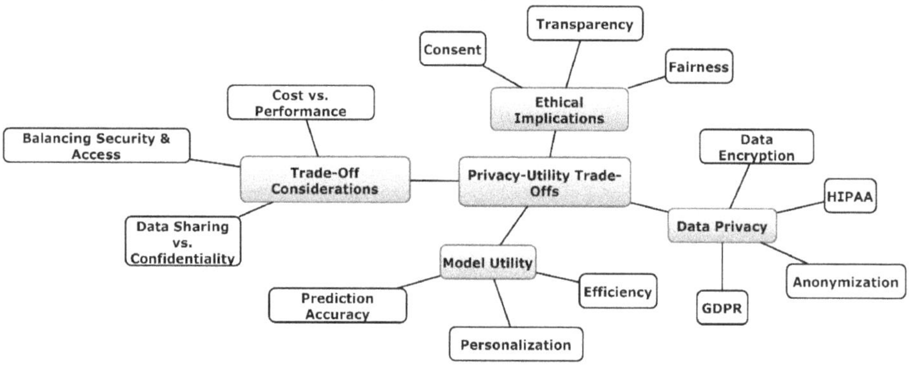

The most significant issue with health care data management is its sensitivity. Healthcare data is one of the most sensitive types of personal information because medical records, genetic data, and even the health conditions of individuals are highly confidential. Unlike general data, which can be anonymized or pseudonymized without much harm to its utility, health data demands a far greater degree of protection because it indirectly relates to an individual's well-being.

Healthcare data comes in a number of forms that can be considered sensitive. These may include: medical diagnoses, treatment, genetic data, and mental health records. For example, diseases or disorders of HIV, mental health disorders, or genetic predispositions all often hold a certain stigma within society. More recently, patient data is being shared at greater detail levels via devices such as wearable health devices. In addition to these regulations - in the United States, for example, the Health Insurance Portability and Accountability Act, or HIPAA; in Europe, the

General Data Protection Regulation - these data types are also highly sensitive so that stringent safeguarding against data breaches, unauthorized access, or misuse is in order.

Re-identification risks exist even when health data is appropriately anonymized. Advanced analytics techniques can potentially link anonymized data with external information, thus revealing a patient's identity. The potential for re-identification is particularly high when datasets contain rich and granular information, such as genetic data, which is unique to each individual. Hence, the healthcare system needs to be vigilant about data aggregation levels and should further make sure that de-identification or encryption methods are implemented at all stages of data usage and model training to avoid breaches of privacy.

The ethical considerations regarding the privacy of healthcare data add another dimension to this trade-off. Patients need to feel assured of how their personal information is being handled and assured about what's going to be done with their data, especially where models and algorithms from AI are involved in making decisions. It is through the transparent informed consent process that this kind of trust may be developed, together with assurances that patients would know about any arrangements to share data. Furthermore, AI models should respect patient autonomy and avoid perpetuating biases that may harm specific groups of people based on their health conditions, demographics, or socioeconomic status.

Balancing Model Performance with Privacy

One of the central challenges in the privacy-utility trade-off is in balancing the protection of patient data with the possible compromise of the performance and accuracy of AI models. AI models for healthcare diagnosis, prognosis, and treatment recommendations rely on large, high-quality datasets to optimize their performance; therefore, including mechanisms of privacy-preserving such as data anonymization, encryption, and differential privacy can lead to a degraded quality of the models and the reduction of their ability to be predictive(Boopathi et al., 2023; Palaniappan et al., 2023).

Impact of Privacy-Preserving Techniques on Model Accuracy: While privacy-preserving techniques are indeed indispensable to protect patient information, they do interfere with the quality of AI models. As an example, differential privacy introduces noise into the data or model updates for purposes of non-re-identification, which can decrease the model's accuracy due to distorted patterns in the data. Similarly, methods like data anonymization or cryptographic techniques such as homomorphic encryption may incur computational complexity, so that the training time becomes longer or less accurate outputs from the model(Sonia et al., 2024).

The more significant the privacy guarantees, the more the model performance is likely to degrade.

Fine-Tuning the Privacy-Utility Trade-Off: Finding an appropriate balance requires dialing in the privacy mechanisms applied to the data. Another important factor is the privacy budget. It refers to the amount of noise added into the data, or to updates into the model. For example, in differential privacy, the noise level is traded off against that in which the model is capable of learning over it. A lower privacy budget leads to more noise and a greater loss in accuracy. Conversely, more than a budget leads to less noise and preserves model accuracy with larger risk to privacy. Therefore, health care systems are to decide at what point they allow the privacy lost not to compromise the utility of the model. This is a delicate balance that must be periodically readjusted both for privacy standards as they evolve and for healthcare organizations as their AI models improve.

Federated Learning as a Solution: The promise of balancing privacy with utility lies in federated learning. Here, a decentralized approach allows healthcare institutions to train models on their local data without sharing raw data. This enables the model to benefit from data distributed across several institutions without compromising the privacy of individual data by only sharing and aggregating updates, such as weights or gradients, at a central server. Federated learning can maintain model utility by allowing for more accurate training of models on diverse datasets while keeping sensitive patient data, for example, inside its origin. In addition, federated learning can use privacy-preserving techniques like differential privacy or secure multi-party computation to further enhance data security during the collaborative learning process.

Differential Privacy and Utility Trade-Off: Differential privacy is one of the most popular techniques used for individual privacy protection for model training. However, model accuracy comes with trade-offs. Noise added can interfere with the fine-tuned patterns discovered by the model, leading to a less precise prediction. The level of noise needs to be calibrated accordingly so that privacy protection is addressed without compromising on the desired model performance. Research in this direction led to techniques such that differential privacy can be applied with little or no loss of accuracy, thereby enabling healthcare systems to build robust models that do not compromise on privacy.

Interpretability in Privacy-Preserving Models: In addition to privacy and model accuracy, the interpretability of AI models is important in healthcare settings. Clinicians and healthcare providers need to understand and have trust in the predictions and recommendations made by AI systems. Therefore, privacy-preserving techniques should not only safeguard patient data but also ensure that the final model remains interpretable and explainable. These further builds credibility with health professionals and ensures that AI-based decisions are transparent and defensible.

The trade-off between privacy and utility is fundamental in the design of AI models applied in healthcare. As AI becomes ubiquitous in healthcare systems for the betterment of patient care, personalized medicine, and clinical decision-making, there is a need to find a balance between the protection of confidential patient information and the utility of the AI model. While privacy-preserving techniques like differential privacy, federated learning, and secure multi-party computation provide important protection to data, they often compromise model accuracy or increase computational complexity. Healthcare organizations will have to consider these trade-offs and tailor approaches so that privacy requirements are well met but do not compromise the effectiveness of AI systems. By continually refining these strategies and investing in innovative privacy-preserving technologies, healthcare systems can unlock the complete potential of AI while keeping patient data safe and secure.

CASE STUDIES AND PRACTICAL APPLICATIONS

The confluence of IoT-driven additive manufacturing and federated learning in healthcare is changing the paradigms of medical device production and predictive analytics in healthcare. These technologies provide innovative solutions for better patient outcomes, enhance operational efficiency, and ensure data privacy(Boopathi & Kumar, 2024; Senthil et al., 2023). Two case studies describing their practical application are as follows.

Case Study: Customized Orthopedic Implants for Personalized Healthcare

Probably, the most influential application of IoT-driven additive manufacturing comes in the form of personalized orthopedic implants. For example, a leading orthopedic company recently designed a customized knee implant for a patient by using 3D printing technology. The first step was collecting detailed CT scans of the patient's knee; subsequently, these scans were sent to create a 3D model of the entire joint. It was then integrated with IoT-enabled software to evaluate the biomechanics and joint movement patterns of the patient.

Customized Implant with IoT Sensors for Monitoring: The customized implant had an embedded IoT sensor, which tracked the performance of the implant after surgery in real-time. The pressure, temperature, and strain inside the knee were tracked by the sensors and were important information used by healthcare professionals.: After the implantation, it was possible to track the patient's recovery remotely through a smartphone app connected to the implant. The implanted device was updating the healthcare provider about the condition of the patient constantly, ensuring an immediate response in case of any problems(Boopathi & Khang, 2023; Upadhyaya et al., 2024; Venkateswaran et al., 2023).

the customized implant significantly eased the comfort of a patient as well as facilitated mobility. Moreover, the integration of IoT allowed for continuous monitoring that would allow identification of any complications at an early stage and hence decreased hospital visits and improved recovery as a whole. This case shows how IoT-driven additive manufacturing can not only create personalized medical devices but also enhance their functionality by real-time monitoring, thus ensuring better health outcomes for patients.

Case Study: Early Detection of Heart Disease Using Federated Learning

In predictive healthcare analytics, federated learning has proved to be of immense value in training AI models without sensitive data on a patient. There is one interesting application: early heart disease detection. A federation of hospitals created a federated learning model that predicts the risk of heart disease for a patient based on multiple criteria ranging from age to medical history to lifestyle and lab results.

Implementation:

Every hospital trained its own model on local patient data, including historical health records and diagnostic results. Instead of collecting sensitive data in a central server, only the model updates, meaning trained parameters, were shared; thus, it ensured preservation of privacy and more fittingly followed HIPAA and GDPR guidelines.

Federated learning aggregates model updates coming from various institutions to produce a capable AI model that generalizes well across divergent patient populations, with no infringement of the privacy of individual patient data. The trained federated model could predict the probability of a patient developing heart disease with high accuracy. It was very useful in picking up patients at an advanced risk who may not have presented any overt signs of the disease. The system also made corresponding suggestions for lifestyle or early intervention that could decrease the chances of heart attacks or strokes.

CHALLENGES AND FUTURE DIRECTIONS

In fact, the integration of IoT-enhanced additive manufacturing and federated learning in healthcare systems offers great transformative potential but poses significant technical and ethical challenges that cover both layers-applications development, deployment, and scalability in real-world healthcare scenarios. Overcoming these challenges will help ensure that these innovations are implemented appropriately and responsibly(Boopathi & Kumar, 2024; Palaniappan et al., 2023; Senthil et al., 2023). Figure 5 presents the challenges and future directions in integrating IoT-enhanced additive manufacturing and federated learning in healthcare systems.

Figure 5. Challenges and future direction

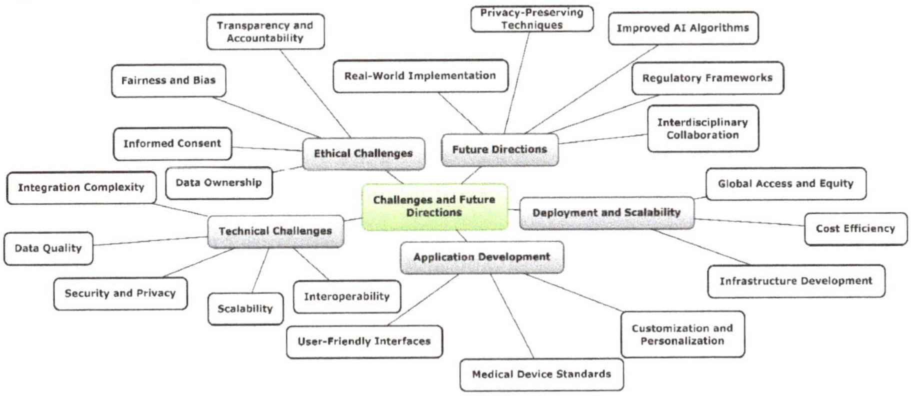

Technical Challenges

Data Interoperability and Integration: One of the most problematic technical challenges is achieving seamless interoperability in data exchange between various healthcare systems. For example, millions of data values are transferred from IoT devices, including those from sensors within personalized implants. Nonetheless, such a large amount of data is often produced from fragmented sources with different formats, standards, and protocols, which causes interference in integration with healthcare IT infrastructures. Robust integration frameworks are essential for potential standardization, sharing, and analytics of the same data across the different platforms and systems for the effective usage of the full potential of IoT and federated learning.

Scalability: Any large volume of data to be handled regarding IoT is required to be scalable, as federated learning also demands the growing number of healthcare providers and patients. In the case of federated learning, efficient model update aggregation from participating institutions without delay is very necessary. In the case of medical devices made IoT-enabled, real-time data streaming and analysis need to be processed in a manner not overloading the system's resources. Scalable solutions for big data management and compute to the required level to make them successful can be key.

Security and Integrity of Data: Federated learning ensures that the data itself never crosses the boundaries of the local device, yet model updates aggregated between healthcare institutions are susceptible to cyber threats. All forms and means of ensuring model update security, the transmission channels, and the storage system have to be protected against unauthorized access. The same goes for IoT devices: particularly for ones used in personalized medical implants, which may be vulnerable to hacking and alterations in the data. All data—both from local devices and aggregation models of learning—need to be secure and tamper-proof. Earning user confidence is therefore one of the greatest challenges.

Device Reliability and Accuracy: In additive manufacturing, 3D-printed medical devices, such as implants, have to make sure that they meet the standards of safety and performance required. IoT-enhanced implants have to be highly reliable with correct sensor readings avoiding wrong diagnoses or treatment plans. Additionally, there is a need for continuous monitoring and testing of the devices to ensure that they work optimally over time. The problem of course is the quality control on a varied range of customized devices without sacrificing on safety.

Ethical Challenges

Data Privacy and Consent: One of the key ethical challenges facing both IoT and federated learning is patient data privacy. In IoT-enhanced devices, the constant collection of sensitive health information creates questions about who has access to that data and how that data is used. Federated learning systems also minimize data sharing but do involve aggregation of model updates, potentially leaking private insights about individual patients. The ethical challenge here is to ensure that the data of the patients used is done so with informed consent and within data protection regulations, and clearly, boundaries around how the health data of the patients are being used(Malathi et al., 2024; Upadhyaya et al., 2024).

Bias in AI Models: In federated learning, model updates are aggregated from various institutions that may serve diverse patient populations. Thus, if the data used to train the model contain underrepresented groups, this may lead to biased predictions and inequalities in healthcare. The issue is more delicate when the disparities exist across different demographics like race, ethnicity, and socio-economic status. There is, therefore an ongoing challenge of how to ensure federated-learning-trained AI models are both fair and inclusive but not at the expense of perpetuating biases already present.

Accountability and Liability: With the growing reliance on IoT devices and AI-driven systems for diagnosis, treatment, and monitoring, determining who is accountable in the case of a malfunction or incorrect prediction becomes increasingly complex. If a personalized medical device fails or a predictive model generates a wrong diagnosis, who is responsible? Is it the manufacturer of the device, the healthcare provider using it, or the developers of the AI model? These questions raise critical ethical issues related to liability and accountability in healthcare systems leveraging these advanced technologies.

Future Trends in Privacy-Preserving Technologies

Some promising trends and advancements in privacy-preserving technologies are ahead and may solve the potential challenges and enhance the capabilities of IoT-driven additive manufacturing and federated learning in healthcare(Boopathi et al., 2023; Mohanty et al., 2023):

Federated Learning with Differential Privacy: A natural response to worries about data privacy, federated learning systems are being infused with differential privacy techniques. This technique makes it infeasible for individual data points to be distinguishable even if the model update is leaked out. Differential privacy, which introduces noise in a controlled form to the model updates, could give much stronger guarantees that sensitive information is confidential while still enabling the model to learn efficiently from the data.

Blockchain for better security and transparency: Due to its reliability in securing IoT data and federated learning systems, blockchain technology is becoming increasingly popular. Blockchain may make immutable records of all updates of the model and the data transactions happening, thus ensuring transparency and accountability in the healthcare system. Moreover, it can be used with smart contracts for automating the management of data access and consent so that data privacy is maintained throughout the process(Sundaramoorthy et al., 2024; Tagesse et al., 2024).

Edge Computing for Real-Time Data Processing: The emergence of edge computing is anticipated to greatly boost the performance and privacy of IoT-driven healthcare systems. Edge computing processes information locally on IoT devices or at adjacent edge servers, eliminating the risks of data transmission instead of uploading it to cloud-based platforms in a centralized manner. This trend assures the privacy and security of medical data while allowing real-time analysis and decision-making processes(Das et al., 2024; Maguluri et al., 2023).

Advanced AI techniques for enhancing anonymization and encryption of data might gain momentum in the coming years for privacy-preserving technologies. AI algorithms could be specifically designed to anonymize the data while preserving its utility and bring new techniques to safeguard patient information with desired patterns preservation yet assure privacy without harming the performance of healthcare models.

CONCLUSION

The convergence of IoT-enhanced additive manufacturing and federated learning is revolutionizing healthcare delivery with the promise of personalized treatments and increased process efficiency. The inherent tension between privacy and utility, however, poses significant challenges. While such sensitive patient data needs to be protected so that trust is maintained, regulations are followed, and security risks are mitigated, robust data availability is essential for the optimization of AI models, predictive accuracy enhancement, and innovation in smart healthcare systems. A chapter through which we went ahead to discuss privacy-preserving techniques with differential privacy and homomorphic encryption in balancing data-protection with performance in the system. Case studies demonstrated the actual impact of these methods, showing promise for the retention of privacy as well as high-utility application supports in personalized medicine and decentralized diagnostics.

Regulatory frameworks like GDPR and HIPAA were also analyzed, underscoring their dual role in fostering data security and imposing constraints on technological progress. Navigating these frameworks requires stakeholders to adopt innovative privacy strategies while maintaining compliance. Moreover, interdisciplinary collaboration among technologists, healthcare providers, and policymakers is vital to harmonize privacy concerns with clinical utility.

This insight aims to guide the design of secure, efficient and scalable systems, which fully leverage the collective capabilities of IoT and federated learning. In addition to addressing the privacy-utility tradeoff, this chapter makes a contribution toward fulfilling the promise of sustainable and secure smart healthcare ecosystems that seek to build patient trust and promote data-driven innovation. The way forward should include refinement of privacy techniques, harmonization of regulation around the world, and facilitation of equitable access to such disruptive technologies.

REFERENCES

Abdulhameed, O., Al-Ahmari, A., Ameen, W., & Mian, S. H. (2019). Additive manufacturing: Challenges, trends, and applications. *Advances in Mechanical Engineering, 11*(2), 1687814018822880. DOI: 10.1177/1687814018822880

Akhtar, Z. (2024). Exploring Biomedical Engineering (BME): Advances within Accelerated Computing and Regenerative Medicine for a Computational and Medical Science Perspective Exploration Analysis. *J Emerg Med OA, 2*(1), 01–23.

Anderson, J., & Smith, R. (2024). *Heart Health Guardian: An IoT-Enhanced Cardiovascular Disease Prediction and Recommendation Platform.* EasyChair.

Babu, C. S., Felixa, S., Vidya, A., Singh, D. J., & Associates. (2024). IoT-Enhanced Haptic Feedback: Revolutionizing Healthcare Wellbeing in AR and VR. In *Modern Technology in Healthcare and Medical Education: Blockchain, IoT, AR, and VR* (pp. 186–215). IGI Global.

Bhuvaneshwari, V., Sadaieswaran, R., Malathi, P., Legapriyadharshini, N., Thirumalaikumari, T., & Raja, S. (2024). IoT-Enhanced Innovations in Drug Delivery Systems for Targeted Therapy in Autoimmune Disorders. *2024 10th International Conference on Advanced Computing and Communication Systems (ICACCS), 1*, 1275–1281.

Boopathi, S. (2023). Internet of Things-Integrated Remote Patient Monitoring System: Healthcare Application. In *Dynamics of Swarm Intelligence Health Analysis for the Next Generation* (pp. 137–161). IGI Global. DOI: 10.4018/978-1-6684-6894-4.ch008

Boopathi, S., & Khang, A. (2023). AI-Integrated Technology for a Secure and Ethical Healthcare Ecosystem. In *AI and IoT-Based Technologies for Precision Medicine* (pp. 36–59). IGI Global. DOI: 10.4018/979-8-3693-0876-9.ch003

Boopathi, S., & Khare, R. KG, J. C., Muni, T. V., & Khare, S. (2023). Additive Manufacturing Developments in the Medical Engineering Field. In *Development, Properties, and Industrial Applications of 3D Printed Polymer Composites* (pp. 86–106). IGI Global.

Boopathi, S., & Kumar, P. (2024). Advanced bioprinting processes using additive manufacturing technologies: Revolutionizing tissue engineering. *3D Printing Technologies: Digital Manufacturing, Artificial Intelligence, Industry 4.0*, 95.

Das, S., Lekhya, G., Shreya, K., Shekinah, K. L., Babu, K. K., & Boopathi, S. (2024). Fostering Sustainability Education Through Cross-Disciplinary Collaborations and Research Partnerships: Interdisciplinary Synergy. In *Facilitating Global Collaboration and Knowledge Sharing in Higher Education With Generative AI* (pp. 60–88). IGI Global.

Gaur, R., Prakash, S., Prasad, L. N., Kumar, S., Abhishek, K., & Guduri, M. (2023). A secure and efficient scheme based on unlinkability and anonymous traceable protocol for cloud-assisted IoT environment. *Journal of Circuits, Systems, and Computers*, *32*(18), 2350316. DOI: 10.1142/S0218126623503164

Gopi, B., Sworna Kokila, M. L., Bibin, C. V., Sasikala, D., Howard, E., & Boopathi, S. (2024). Distributed Technologies Using AI/ML Techniques for Healthcare Applications. In *Advances in Human and Social Aspects of Technology* (pp. 375–396). IGI Global. DOI: 10.4018/979-8-3693-2569-8.ch019

Guduri, M., Chakraborty, C., Maheswari, U., & Margala, M. (2023). Blockchain-based federated learning technique for privacy preservation and security of smart electronic health records. *IEEE Transactions on Consumer Electronics*, *70*(1), 2608–2617. DOI: 10.1109/TCE.2023.3315415

Han, D., Ren, X., Luo, C., Zhang, Y., Zhang, X. Y., Zhang, X. G., Jiang, W., Hao, J., & Xie, Y. M. (2022). Experimental and computational investigations of novel 3D printed square tubular lattice metamaterials with negative Poisson's ratio. *Additive Manufacturing*, *55*, 102789. DOI: 10.1016/j.addma.2022.102789

Hashemi, S. M., Parvizi, S., Baghbanijavid, H., Tan, A. T., Nematollahi, M., Ramazani, A., Fang, N. X., & Elahinia, M. (2022). Computational modelling of process–structure–property–performance relationships in metal additive manufacturing: A review. *International Materials Reviews*, *67*(1), 1–46. DOI: 10.1080/09506608.2020.1868889

Hassan, A., Prasad, D., Khurana, M., Lilhore, U. K., & Simaiya, S. (2021). Integration of internet of things (IoT) in health care industry: An overview of benefits, challenges, and applications. *Data Science and Innovations for Intelligent Systems*, 165–180.

Huang, Y., Wang, Y., Li, X., Chen, H., Si, Y., Zhang, Y., Zhou, H., Yang, Y., Li, M., Xie, Y., & Associates. (2024). CMS-Robot: A Cloud Medical Service Robot Merging SLAM and IoT for Enhanced Healthcare Delivery. *2024 IEEE 19th Conference on Industrial Electronics and Applications (ICIEA)*, 1–6.

Kaur, J. (2024). Urban Oasis: Harnessing IoT for Green Healthcare in Smart City Landscape. In *Technologies for Sustainable Healthcare Development* (pp. 325–348). IGI Global.

Kushwah, J. S., Gupta, M., Shrivastava, S., Saxena, N., Saini, R., & Boopathi, S. (2024). Psychological Impacts, Prevention Strategies, and Intervention Approaches Across Age Groups: Unmasking Cyberbullying. In *Change Dynamics in Healthcare, Technological Innovations, and Complex Scenarios* (pp. 89–109). IGI Global.

Maguluri, L. P., Arularasan, A., & Boopathi, S. (2023). Assessing Security Concerns for AI-Based Drones in Smart Cities. In *Effective AI, Blockchain, and E-Governance Applications for Knowledge Discovery and Management* (pp. 27–47). IGI Global. DOI: 10.4018/978-1-6684-9151-5.ch002

Malathi, J., Kusha, K., Isaac, S., Ramesh, A., Rajendiran, M., & Boopathi, S. (2024). IoT-Enabled Remote Patient Monitoring for Chronic Disease Management and Cost Savings: Transforming Healthcare. In *Advances in Explainable AI Applications for Smart Cities* (pp. 371–388). IGI Global.

Minnema, J., van Eijnatten, M., Kouw, W., Diblen, F., Mendrik, A., & Wolff, J. (2018). CT image segmentation of bone for medical additive manufacturing using a convolutional neural network. *Computers in Biology and Medicine*, *103*, 130–139. DOI: 10.1016/j.compbiomed.2018.10.012 PMID: 30366309

Mohanty, A., Jothi, B., Jeyasudha, J., Ranjit, P., Isaac, J. S., & Boopathi, S. (2023). Additive Manufacturing Using Robotic Programming. In *AI-Enabled Social Robotics in Human Care Services* (pp. 259–282). IGI Global. DOI: 10.4018/978-1-6684-8171-4.ch010

Morrison, T. M., Pathmanathan, P., Adwan, M., & Margerrison, E. (2018a). Advancing regulatory science with computational modeling for medical devices at the FDA's Office of Science and Engineering Laboratories. *Frontiers in Medicine*, *5*, 241. DOI: 10.3389/fmed.2018.00241 PMID: 30356350

Morrison, T. M., Pathmanathan, P., Adwan, M., & Margerrison, E. (2018b). Advancing regulatory science with computational modeling for medical devices at the FDA's Office of Science and Engineering Laboratories. *Frontiers in Medicine*, *5*, 241. DOI: 10.3389/fmed.2018.00241 PMID: 30356350

Okokpujie, I. P., & Tartibu, L. K. (2024). Study of the economic viability of internet of things (IoTs) in additive and advanced manufacturing: A comprehensive review. *Progress in Additive Manufacturing*, 1–20.

Palaniappan, M., Tirlangi, S., Mohamed, M. J. S., Moorthy, R. S., Valeti, S. V., & Boopathi, S. (2023). Fused Deposition Modelling of Polylactic Acid (PLA)-Based Polymer Composites: A Case Study. In *Development, Properties, and Industrial Applications of 3D Printed Polymer Composites* (pp. 66–85). IGI Global.

Pitchai, R., Guru, K. V., Gandhi, J. N., Komala, C. R., Kumar, J. R. D., & Boopathi, S. (2024). Fog Computing-Integrated ML-Based Framework and Solutions for Intelligent Systems: Digital Healthcare Applications. In *Technological Advancements in Data Processing for Next Generation Intelligent Systems* (pp. 196–224). IGI Global. DOI: 10.4018/979-8-3693-0968-1.ch008

Premavathi, T., Shekhar, A., Raj, A., Mohan, K., Palaniappan, D., & Shukla, M. (2024). The Utilization of Internet of Things (IoT) in the Field of Robotics Process Automation. In *Applications of New Technology in Operations and Supply Chain Management* (pp. 337–359). IGI Global. DOI: 10.4018/979-8-3693-1578-1.ch018

Raman, R., & Mitra, A. (2023a). IoT-Enhanced Workplace Safety for Real-Time Monitoring and Hazard Detection for Occupational Health. *2023 International Conference on Artificial Intelligence for Innovations in Healthcare Industries (ICAIIHI), 1*, 1–5. DOI: 10.1109/ICAIIHI57871.2023.10489803

Raman, R., & Mitra, A. (2023b). IoT-Enhanced Workplace Safety for Real-Time Monitoring and Hazard Detection for Occupational Health. *2023 International Conference on Artificial Intelligence for Innovations in Healthcare Industries (ICAIIHI), 1*, 1–5. DOI: 10.1109/ICAIIHI57871.2023.10489803

Riazi, M. S., Weinert, C., Tkachenko, O., Songhori, E. M., Schneider, T., & Koushanfar, F. (2018). Chameleon: A hybrid secure computation framework for machine learning applications. *Proceedings of the 2018 on Asia Conference on Computer and Communications Security*, 707–721. DOI: 10.1145/3196494.3196522

Salmi, M. (2021). Additive manufacturing processes in medical applications. *Materials (Basel), 14*(1), 191. DOI: 10.3390/ma14010191 PMID: 33401601

Senthil, T., Puviyarasan, M., Babu, S. R., Surakasi, R., Sampath, B., & Associates. (2023). Industrial Robot-Integrated Fused Deposition Modelling for the 3D Printing Process. In *Development, Properties, and Industrial Applications of 3D Printed Polymer Composites* (pp. 188–210). IGI Global.

Serral, E., Torres, V., & Valderas, P. (2024). Modeling IoT-enhanced business processes. In *Handbook on Business Process Management and Digital Transformation* (pp. 363–386). Edward Elgar Publishing. DOI: 10.4337/9781802206098.00025

Shchepkina, N., Negi, G. S., Bhalla, L., Nangia, R., Jyoti, J., & Surekha, P. (2024). IoT-Enhanced Public Safety in Smart Environments: A Comparative Analysis Using the Public Safety IoT Test. *BIO Web of Conferences, 86*, 01100.

Sonia, R., Gupta, N., Manikandan, K., Hemalatha, R., Kumar, M. J., & Boopathi, S. (2024). Strengthening Security, Privacy, and Trust in Artificial Intelligence Drones for Smart Cities. In *Analyzing and Mitigating Security Risks in Cloud Computing* (pp. 214–242). IGI Global. DOI: 10.4018/979-8-3693-3249-8.ch011

Sundaramoorthy, K., Singh, A., Sumathy, G., Maheshwari, A., Arunarani, A., & Boopathi, S. (2024). A Study on AI and Blockchain-Powered Smart Parking Models for Urban Mobility. In *Handbook of Research on AI and ML for Intelligent Machines and Systems* (pp. 223–250). IGI Global.

Tagesse, T., Arulkumar, S., Mahalingam, S., Subbarao Tadepalli, N. V. R., Munjal, N., & Boopathi, S. (2024). Analyzing Fuel Cell Vehicles in India via the PESTLE Framework and Intelligent Battery Management Systems (BMS): Blockchain in E-Mobility. In *Advances in Mechatronics and Mechanical Engineering* (pp. 107–129). IGI Global. DOI: 10.4018/979-8-3693-5247-2.ch007

Tripathy, S. S., Guduri, M., Chakraborty, C., Bebortta, S., Pani, S. K., & Mukhopadhyay, S. (2024). An adaptive explainable AI framework for securing consumer electronics-based IoT applications in fog-cloud infrastructure. *IEEE Transactions on Consumer Electronics.*

Upadhyaya, A. N., Saqib, A., Devi, J. V., Rallapalli, S., Sudha, S., & Boopathi, S. (2024). Implementation of the Internet of Things (IoT) in Remote Healthcare. In *Advances in Medical Technologies and Clinical Practice* (pp. 104–124). IGI Global. DOI: 10.4018/979-8-3693-1934-5.ch006

Vanitha, N. S., Karthikeyan, A., Ramani, R., Meenakshi, T., & Sujatha, S. (2023). IoT Enhanced Induction Motor Drive in Electric Vehicle Propulsion Using Field Oriented Control. *2023 7th International Conference on Electronics, Communication and Aerospace Technology (ICECA)*, 288–292.

Venkateswaran, N., Kumar, S. S., Diwakar, G., Gnanasangeetha, D., & Boopathi, S. (2023). Synthetic Biology for Waste Water to Energy Conversion: IoT and AI Approaches. *Applications of Synthetic Biology in Health. Energy & Environment*, 360–384.

Wang, D. D., Qian, Z., Vukicevic, M., Engelhardt, S., Kheradvar, A., Zhang, C., Little, S. H., Verjans, J., Comaniciu, D., O'Neill, W. W., & Vannan, M. A. (2021). 3D printing, computational modeling, and artificial intelligence for structural heart disease. *JACC: Cardiovascular Imaging*, *14*(1), 41–60. DOI: 10.1016/j.jcmg.2019.12.022 PMID: 32861647

Zhong, L., Zhang, J.-M., Su, B., Tan, R. S., Allen, J. C., & Kassab, G. S. (2018). Application of patient-specific computational fluid dynamics in coronary and intracardiac flow simulations: Challenges and opportunities. *Frontiers in Physiology*, *9*, 742. DOI: 10.3389/fphys.2018.00742 PMID: 29997520

KEY TERMS AND DEFINITIONS

Artificial Intelligence: The simulation of human intelligence in machines that can perform tasks such as learning, problem-solving, and decision-making.

General Data Protection Regulation: A regulation by the European Union that governs the protection of personal data and privacy for individuals.

Health Insurance Portability and Accountability Act: The U.S. legislation that provides data privacy and security provisions to safeguard medical information.

FDA (Food and Drug Administration): This is the agency of the U.S. government charged with responsibility for food, drugs, and medical devices.

ISO (International Organization for Standardization): ISO is an international body that develops and publishes international standards.

MRI (Magnetic Resonance Imaging): This is a medical imaging technique that uses magnetic fields and radio waves to create detailed images of organs and tissues.

CT (Computed Tomography): A form of imaging that employs X-rays and computer processing to draw cross-sectional images of the body.

CAD (Computer-Aided Design): Software program used for creating precision drawings or models, often utilized in manufacturing as well as architecture.

FL (Federated Learning): A form of machine learning that trains algorithms on decentralized devices while keeping data localized for privacy.

EHR (Electronic Health Record): An electronic version of a patient's medical history, kept by healthcare providers.

HIV (Human Immunodeficiency Virus): A virus that attacks the immune system, leading to AIDS if untreated.

IT: It refers to the use of computers, networks, and software for storing, processing, and transmitting information.

Chapter 8
Study on Challenges and Future Prospects of Glomerulus-on-a-Chip: A Pathway for Future Kidney on Chip Technology

Bhagyashree Saud
National Institute of Technology Silchar, India

Koushik Guha
https://orcid.org/0000-0002-5046-2786
National Institute of Technology Silchar, India

Pratim Sengupta
https://orcid.org/0000-0003-0515-5485
Nephrocare India Ltd, Kolkata, India

Sergei Selishchev
National Research University of Electronic Technology (MIET), Moscow, Russia

K. Srinivasa Rao
KL University, Vaddeswaram, India

ABSTRACT

Glomerulus-On-a-Chip (GoC) is an innovative in vitro organ model which is a recent advancement in the field of microfluidic-based organ-on-a-chip research. GoC is basically used to study glomerulopathy, test drug nephrotoxicity and to imitate the functions of filtering membrane in the glomerulus. As part of the glomerulus-on-a-chip, a microfluidic device is used to co-culture podocytes and endothelial cells and

DOI: 10.4018/979-8-3693-6094-1.ch008

physical stimulation is used to enhance cell function so that a functional filtration barrier can be constructed. The "glomerulus-on-a chip" technology in conjunction with the cell culture technology could potentially eliminate the need for animal testing by offering an alternate organ model. This review paper provides an overview of the characteristics of the current "glomerulus-on-a-chip systems", with an emphasis on challenges involved in selective permeability verification tests. Finally, we discuss the possible future approaches that should be created to address those issues and enable further "glomerulus-on-a-chip" technology progress.

1 INTRODUCTION

An international issue has emerged with kidney diseases in recent years. Around 10-15% of the world population reportedly have been affected by kidney diseases. People affected with severe kidney diseases are incurring significant costs for dialysis care of between $35,000 and $100,000 every year. Taking minimal sodium level diet to adopting organ protection techniques have greatly improved the therapy of kidney illness over the past two decades. However, management and therapy for glomerular disorders have not seen much progress in the recent years.

Consequently, there is a need for the exploration of efficient and proactive therapies to enhance the prognosis of glomerulopathy patients. Damage to the "glomerular capillary wall" is directly associated with a disease called proteinuria which leads to loss of protein from the body through urine. This surrogate objective is crucial from a therapeutic standpoint. Consequently, it is essential to assess the filtration barrier's function of selective permeability when researching glomerular illness (Zhou et al., 2016). Traditional methods in the disciplines of nephrology and non-clinical drug discovery research are restricted to two-dimensional cell culture systems and animal trials (Wang et al., 2017). "The two-dimensional cell culture technique was applied to study the different changes in the mathematical equations of genes and proteins in response to chemicals and culture conditions" (Musah et al., 2017). Although co-culturing podocytes and endothelial cells was attempted to create glomerular filtration barriers it was not possible to replicate the physiological and physical environment for the cells (Petrosyan et al., 2019). Contrarily, experiments on animals are employed to examine the functions of particular genes, the effectiveness of chemicals in the treatment of sickness, and drug testing. Costly and time-consuming, animal research involves a high risk of uncontrolled effects on many organ systems. The emergence and development of cell culture methods with pluripotent stem cells is witnessed in past decade in case of kidney organoid and "organ-on-a-chip (OoC) technology" (Petrosyan et al., 2019). These methods of culture are superior to 2D cell culture systems because they can express tissue-specific characteristics generally. However, it was unable to effectively examine "the size and charge selective" permeable function of the "filtration barrier" in the "glomerulus due to absence of glomerular endothelial cell (GEnC) infiltration below the podocytes" (Iampietro et al., 2020).The formation of GoCs, which can replicate the "filtration barrier" in the "glomerular capillary wall" has been the subject of research. It is attempted to "co-culture endothelial cells and podocytes" in various ways. These cells are either grown on a porous membrane with holes on both sides or on a extracellular matrix (ECM)-containing gel wall that permits medium perfusion in a three-dimensional micro environment to replicate the flow of fluids across the "glomerular filtration barrier". Researchers also tried to simulate the effects of actual physical stimulations, including stretching the cell base. In order to examine the "selective permeability" of the "glomerular filtration barrier", GoCs are perfused with a solution containing "fluorescently labelled molecules" of different molecular sizes (Zhou et al., 2016)(Wang et al., 2017)(Musah et al., 2017)(Petrosyan et al., 2019)(Iampietro et al., 2020)(Xie et al., 2020)(Roye et al., 2021). Furthermore, research on GoC is further extended by integration of human "stem cell derived podocytes and endothelial cells" from patients with hereditary diseases (Musah et al., 2017)(Petrosyan et al., 2019) (Roye et al., 2021).This review discusses the challenges that are associated with implementing GoC technology, assessing the glomerular permeability and in the end discusses the future scopes for further advancement in this field.

The paper is organized as follows: Section 2 illustrates selective permeability of glomerular filtration barrier, section 3 describes the types of GoCs, Section 4 describes permeability assessment ways, and section 5 and 6 discusses the future scope and conclusion respectively.

2 SELECTIVE PERMEABILITY OF GLOMERULAR FILTRATION BARRIER

The nephron is the basic filtration unit of kidney. There are millions of nephrons inside a kidney that continuously work together to purify our blood. The first stage of urine generation occurs in the glomerulus, making it a crucial component of the nephron. The mass of capillaries that make up glomerular tissue are grouped in a ball-like form (Figure 1)."Glomerular endothelial cells (GEnC), glomerular basement membrane (GBM), and the podocyte layer make up the three levels of the glomerular capillary wall" (Roye & Musah, 2022)('t Hart et al., 2023).

Figure 1. Structure of nephron and human glomerulus

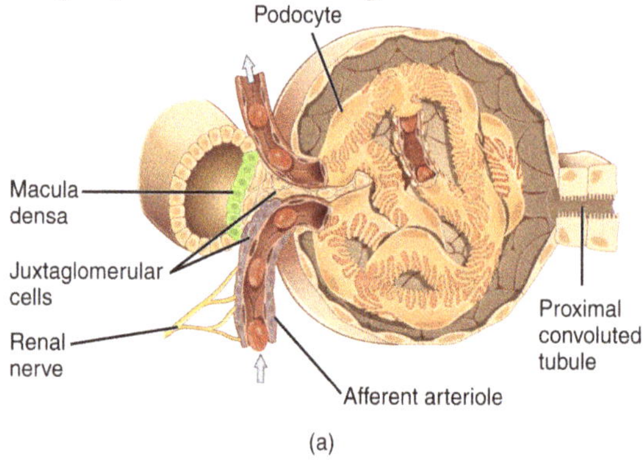

Source- Adapted from (Wikimedia Commons, n.d.) and licensed under CC BY 3.0.

Figure 2. Structure of glomerular filtration barrier

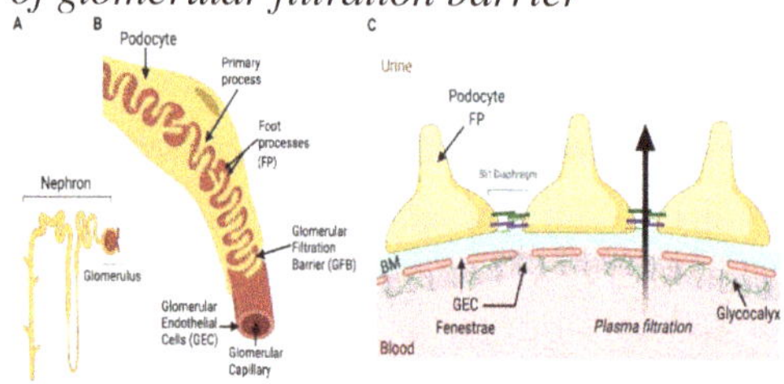

Source- Adapted from (Ebefors et al., 2021) and licensed under CC BY 4.0.

The structure of "glomerular filtration barrier" is illustrated in Figure 2. The GEnCs have numerous fenestrations with a diameter of about 100 nm, and they add a thin layer of cytoplasm lining to the vessel walls (Satchell & Braet, 2009). In humans, the GBM is a stiff layer of extracellular matrix that has a thickness of around 300 nm and resembles a gel (Miner, 1999). The podocyte cell layer is the third layer that covers the glomerular capillaries with many primary and secondary foot processes extending from the cell body (Figure 2 (a)). Slit diaphragms, which contain a number of membrane proteins, are situated between the foot processes. Each of these three layers together form the glomerulus "filtration barrier" that performs selective filtration of blood (Wang et al., 2017). "The effective glomerular filtration pressure acting through the filtration barrier is around 20 mmHg" (Benzing & Salant, 2021). "The sieving coefficient of molecules" that pass past the "filtration barrier" is impacted by this filtration pressure (Benzing & Salant, 2021). The filtration pressure also takes part in regulating the glomerular filtration rate in our body (Figure 1). The Selective permeability of these layers refers to passage of tiny molecules like "water and electrolytes" across the barrier, whereas bigger molecules such as "albumin" and other big proteins are prevented (Benzing & Salant, 2021).

3 GLOMERULUS-ON-A-CHIP

In OoCs in the "μTAS field," the microfluidic device technology is utilised. The process uses "photolithography and soft lithography to create microscale pillar formations, channels, and micropores" in micro-electromechanical systems (MEMS) (Kim et al., 2008). These chips are mostly made of "Polydimethylsiloxane (PDMS)", a form of "silicone rubber", due to their biocompatibility, clarity, and ease of handling (Kim et al., 2008). Alginate hollow fibres are employed as cell culture platforms (Xie et al., 2020) and resins are currently being used to prevent sorption of drugs in PDMS (Petrosyan et al., 2019)(Iampietro et al., 2020). By encouraging cell functions, researchers are trying to improve filtration barriers in GoC. The challenge in GoC research is growing glomerular cells, particularly podocyte cells, under the appropriate cell culture conditions. Thereby, this study area is moving comparatively more slowly than other organ models that have been created thus far.

3.1 Microfluidics based Glomerulus-on-a-Chip Devices

It is important to study how the selective permeability was evaluated and how the filtering barrier was replicated in the current GoC technology. The different reported microfluidic devices in GoC are explained below.

Two-Channel Porous Membrane Device

Figure 3. A) Glomerulus-on-A-chip (GoC) of two-layered with a porous membrane device Polygonal line folds for flow channels were moulded onto top and bottom polydimethylsiloxane plates. The porous membrane was placed between the top and bottom plates. B) The device's detailed structure and manipulation C) Co-culture in GoC D) Environment physiology in GoC.

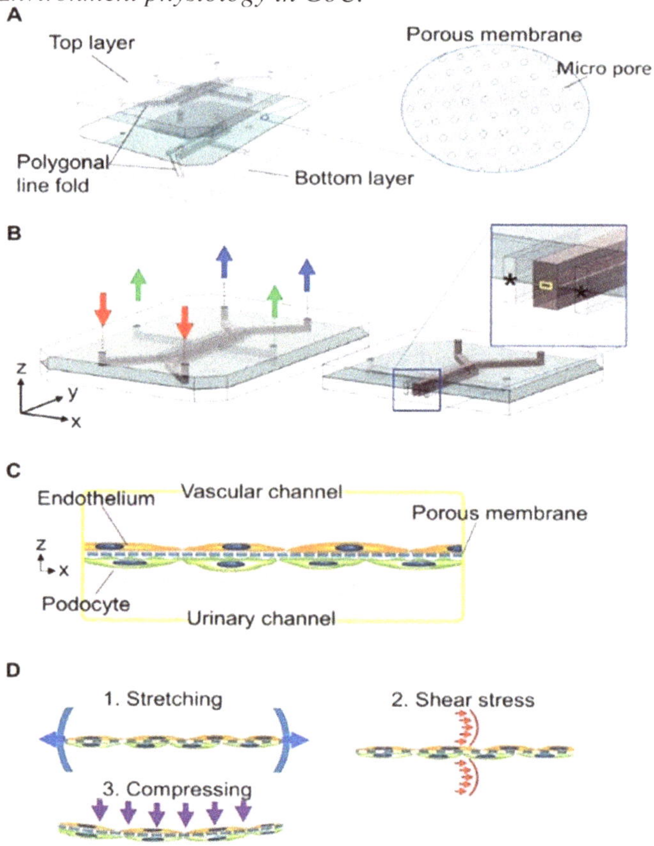

Source- (Doi et al., 2022)

A "porous membrane" is sandwiched between two layers of "vertically aligned microfluidic channels" in this form of GoC (Figure 3 A). The device's detailed structure and manipulation is shown in figure 3 B while co-culture in GoC and environment physiology in GoC are shown in figure 3 C and 3 D respectively. The foundation for the cultivated cells is provided by this "porous membrane". To replicate the "glomerular filtration barrier", "podocytes and endothelial cells" are cultivated on both sides of the "porous membrane". The materials used for porous membranes are generally PDMS, "polycarbonate (PC), or polyethylene terephthalate" (Quirós-Solano et al., 2018). The device employed by Musah et al and Roye et al uses intermittent negative pressure in microchannels that allows the "porous membrane" to mimic "vascular pulsation" by stretching (Figure 3 D1) (Musah et al., 2017) (Roye et al., 2021).

Central Gel Channel Device. This device contains a "central ECM gel" with a thickness in the range of several hundred micrometres, which serves as a "scaffold for cultured cells". There are two perfusion channels on both sides of the central gel channel in the XY direction (Figure 4 A). Pillar-like guides are placed to hold the gel in place between two channels. This shape enables the grown cells to adhere to the gel scaffold after being seeded through the perfusion channel (Wang et al., 2017) (Petrosyan et al., 2019). Place the isolated glomeruli between the pillars (Figure 4 B1) or podocytes and then endothelial cells can be seeded into one perfusion channel to mimic the "glomerular filtration barrier" in the device (Figure 4 B2).

Figure 4. A) Bilateral flow glomerulus-on-A-chip with central gel channels; A1) Detailed structure of the device showing micropillars and vascular, scaffold (gel), and urinary channel; A2)phase guides at both side edges of the scaffold channel. B)Cell culture at the gel-media interface; B1) Seeded isolated glomeruli were stuck between the micropillars; B2) seeding podocytes and glomerular endothelial cells in the small box area shown in A2.

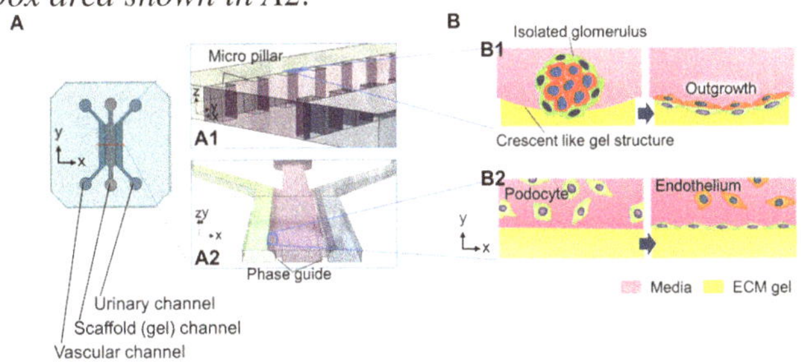

Source- (Doi et al., 2022)

Hollow Alginate Fiber Device. A microfluidic device with a sheath construction and a calcium ion solution can create hollow alginate fibres, which are frequently employed in cell fibre applications (Ikeda et al., 2017) (Figure 5 A1, A2). Xie et al have modified a hollow alginate fiber fragment with a knot in the center made of multiple micro-convex surfaces to mimic a glomerular topography. Placed in the chamber, the hollow alginate fiber's ends are joined to the inlet and outflow chambers (Figure 5 B1). In order to replicate the glomerular filtration barrier, endothelial cells are seeded from the inlet into the "hollow alginate fibre" and "podocytes" are applied to the surface of the fibre using a hanging drop approach. This device shows better recreation of the glomerular topography more than the other GoC devices (Figure 5 B2). The device requires continuous addition of 5 mM CaCl2 to the cell culture medium to maintain the "alginate cross linking".

Figure 5. A) Glomerulus-on-A chip with hollow alginate fibers. B) Leakage test using alginate hollow fiber.

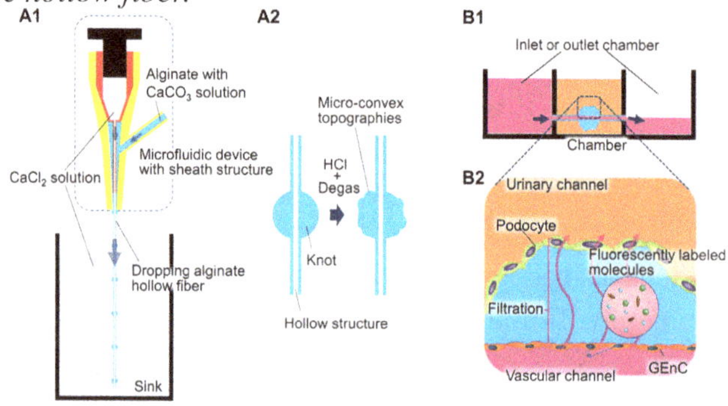

Large Scale Fluidic Device. This device is comparatively larger than the other reported devices of GoC. A "porous membrane" of around 20 mm diameter is placed in the middle of a cylindrical chamber mostly made of resin. The membrane is removable and is tightly sandwiched between the upper and lower channels. Peristaltic pumps power the medium perfusion tubes that connect the top and lower cylinders. Compared to other microfluidic devices, this one's enormous scale makes operation easier (Iampietro et al., 2020).

A tabular representation of the summarized reported work on GoC is presented in the following table.

Table 1. Summarized Works on GOC

Authors	Material used in device	Scaffold used	Structure of Device	Molecules used for assessment of barrier integrity
Zhou et al(2016)	"PDMS" (Zhou et al., 2016), "Polycarbonate Porous membrane" (Zhou et al., 2016)	Cultrex Basement Membrane Extract	Two layered channel with porous membrane (Zhou et al., 2016)	"Fluorescently labelled inulin, albumin, and IgG" (Zhou et al., 2016)
Wang et al (2017)	PDMS (Polydimethylsiloxane)	Matrigel	"Bilateral flow with central gel channels"	"IgG, Albumin"
Musah et al (2018)	"PDMS Porous membrane"	Laminin-511	"Two-layered channel with porous membrane"	"Inulin, albumin"
Petrosyan et al (2019)	"Glass Proprietary polymers"	"Cultrex 3-D Culture Matrix Rat Collagen I"	"Bilateral flow with central gel channels"	Albumin
Iampietro et al (2020)	"Silicone, ABS, cover glass, PET porous membrane"	None	"Upper and lower Cylindrical chambers separated by a porous membrane"	Albumin
Xie et al (2020)	"RGD conjugate Alginate"	None	"Hollow fiber with micro-concave topography knot"	"Fluorescently labeled inulin, Ficolls, and BSA" [6]
Roye et al (2021)	"PDMS, PDMS Porous membrane"	Laminin-511	"Two-layered with porous membrane"	Albumin
Roye et al (2022)	"PDMS"	PDMS	Two channel microfluidic chip	Inulin and Albumin
Daan C et al (2023)	Polycarbonate membrane	PDMS	membrane with a semi-permeable surface divides two parallel microfluidic channels	"Fluorescently labelled dextran"

4 SELECTIVE PERMEABILITY ASSESSMENT IN GLOMERULUS-ON- A-CHIP

In order to assess the filtration barrier's maturity and selective permeability function in GoC, researchers performed permeability testing and molecular biological evaluations. Molecules including "inulin (5 kDa), albumin (70 kDa), and IgG (150 kDa)" are used in the "permeability" experiments (Zhou et al., 2016)(Wang et al., 2017)(Musah et al., 2017)(Petrosyan et al., 2019)(Iampietro et al., 2020) (Roye et al., 2021). These molecules are "fluorescently labelled" for analyzing the filtering barrier's capacity to selectively filter lumen fluid concerning molecular weight through microscope derived image (Figure 6). Similar to this, in other situations, "fluorescently-labeled Ficoll and dextran" of different molecular sizes are also utilized (Xie et al., 2020). In essence, the approach involves infusing the medium with "fluorescently labelled molecules" only through "vascular channels" (Zhou et al., 2016)(Wang et al., 2017)(Musah et al., 2017)(Petrosyan et al., 2019)(Iampietro et al., 2020) (Roye et al., 2021). The clearance of each fluorescently labelled molecule, which is determined by its concentration in the "vascular and urinary channels", is used to evaluate the filtration barrier's effectiveness (Musah et al., 2017) (Roye et al., 2021). Some disease model of GoC are also worked upon to study function of filtration barrier in those conditions and to understand effects of various drugs on the barrier functionality. Various diseased models use transplantation of derived podocytes from people with the inherited condition Alport syndrome and infusing cytotoxic drug-containing medium to study the effects (Wang et al., 2017) (Musah et al., 2017)(Petrosyan et al., 2019)(Iampietro et al., 2020)(Xie et al., 2020)(Roye et al., 2021).

5 CHALLENGES ASSOCIATED WITH GLOMERULUS-ON- A-CHIP TECHNOLOGY

The filtration barrier's maturity, which is mostly related to the cell source and culture conditions of the podocytes, is the main biological challenge confronting the current GoC. Their development has not yet been compared in vivo to that of human adults, despite the fact that the human podocytes generated from the stem cells discussed in this article have shown some advantages over immortalized podocytes. Podocyte cell sources are primarily challenging because of the incompatibility between podocyte maturation and cell number. Furthermore, there is opportunity for enhancing the culture conditions for the podocytes in the GoCs, as the interdigitated foot processes and the slit diaphragm created between the foot processes have not been observed to be reproduced in the GoCs (Doi et al., 2022).

6 FUTURE SCOPE

The primary issue that is faced by the present GoC technology is to build a perfectly mimicking glomerulus filtration barrier. Although the human podocytes produced from stem cells have several advantages over the immortalised podocytes, it is still unclear how these human podocytes mature. Also, the function of the cultured podocytes needs to be compared with human podocytes residing in-vivo (Musah et al., 2017)(Petrosyan et al., 2019). Yoshimura et al.'s cell culture method for generating "podocyte aggregates from nephron progenitor cells showed great podocyte induction efficiency and production of maturation markers in vitro at a protein level comparable to that of adult human glomeruli" (Yoshimura et al., 2019). In order for the podocytes in the GoCs to fully mimic the functions of the "glomerular filtration barrier", the culture conditions can therefore be improved. Another way for mimicking glomerular filtration barrier could be using non-cell-based techniques. A microfluidic device without using complex cell culture technique can be attempted to develop so that it can serve as an integral part of artificial kidney.

We at NMDC NIT, Silchar have been working on designing a non-cell based microfluidic device for replicating glomerular filtration barrier. FEM simulation tool COMSOL 6.1 is used to design the model. The simulated structure for our model is shown in figure 6.

Figure 6. a) 2D view of microfluidic structure for size dependent glomerular filtration; b) 2D view of velocity simulation; c) 3D view of velocity simulation

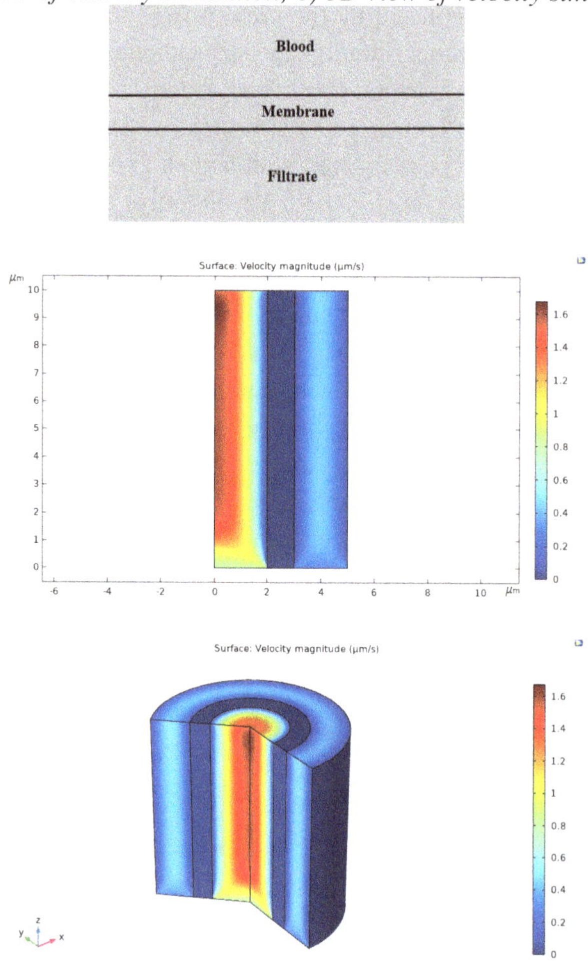

Figure 6 (a) represents 2D view of cylindrical microfluidic structure. Figure 6(b) and (c) represents 2D and 3D velocity profile of fluid passing through the two channels respectively. The microfluidic channel is made of two cylindrical channels separated by a membrane. The inner channel carries blood and the outer channel carries filtered blood. The membrane separating the two channels acts as a dialysis membrane. Velocity in outer channel is low as compared to the inner channel which indicates that a very little fraction of filtrate is formed at a particular time from the blood. Further work needs to be done in optimizing the channel and more analysis needs to be carried out to reach required filtration rate. Besides charge dependent filtration factor also needs to be incorporated in the design.

7 CONCLUSION

The microfluidic devices discussed in the review needs to clarify the structural design and come up with comparative analysis on the cell culture techniques. It needs to be made clear whether podocytes and endothelial cells should be cultivated in close proximity or separated by a porous membrane. The device should replicate the difference in pressure across the filtering barrier, which is roughly 20 mmHg inside human glomerulus, to help with filtration (Benzing & Salant, 2021). These issues stem from the physical stimulus which can be attempted to reproduce through the device. The chemical exchange and crosstalk between the cells to promote the filtration barrier's maturity and assessment of permeability of different molecules of varying size and charge needs to be incorporated in the device. Interdisciplinary collaborations with mathematicians would help develop new mathematical models which in turn will explain the variance between the results from in vivo and in vitro data. Engineers, cell biologists, physicians, pharmacologists, and mathematicians are currently working collaboratively to develop practical GoC applications that could help cut down on the expense of animal testing and drug development. By offering both preventive and therapeutic uses, this will benefit individuals with ESRD and uncommon genetic illnesses.

ACKNOWLEDGEMENT

The authors would like to express their gratitude to NMDC (National MEMS Design Centre) at NIT Silchar for providing the essential financial support to complete the study.

REFERENCES

Benzing, T., & Salant, D. (2021). Insights into glomerular filtration and albuminuria. *The New England Journal of Medicine*, *384*(15), 1437–1446. DOI: 10.1056/NEJMra1808786 PMID: 33852781

Doi, K., Kimura, H., Matsunaga, Y. T., Fujii, T., & Nangaku, M. (2022). Glomerulus-on-a-chip: Current insights and future potential towards recapitulating selectively permeable filtration systems. *International Journal of Nephrology and Renovascular Disease*, *15*, 85–101. DOI: 10.2147/IJNRD.S344725 PMID: 35299832

Ebefors, K., Lassén, E., Anandakrishnan, N., Azeloglu, E. U., & Daehn, I. S. (2021). Modeling the glomerular filtration barrier and intercellular crosstalk. *Frontiers in Physiology*, *12*, 689083. DOI: 10.3389/fphys.2021.689083 PMID: 34149462

Iampietro, C., Bellucci, L., Arcolino, F. O., Arigoni, M., Alessandri, L., Gomez, Y., Papadimitriou, E., Calogero, R. A., Cocchi, E., Van Den Heuvel, L., Levtchenko, E., & Bussolati, B. (2020). Molecular and functional characterization of urine-derived podocytes from patients with Alport syndrome. *The Journal of Pathology*, *252*(1), 88–100. DOI: 10.1002/path.5496 PMID: 32652570

Ikeda, K., Nagata, S., Okitsu, T., & Takeuchi, S. (2017). Cell fiber-based three-dimensional culture system for highly efficient expansion of human induced pluripotent stem cells. *Scientific Reports*, *7*(1), 2850. DOI: 10.1038/s41598-017-03246-2 PMID: 28588295

Kim, P., Kwon, K. W., Park, M. C., Lee, S. H., Kim, S. M., & Suh, K. Y. (2008). Soft lithography for microfluidics: a review.

Miner, J. H. (1999). Renal basement membrane components. *Kidney International*, *56*(6), 2016–2024. DOI: 10.1046/j.1523-1755.1999.00785.x PMID: 10594777

Musah, S., Mammoto, A., Ferrante, T. C., Jeanty, S. S., Hirano-Kobayashi, M., Mammoto, T., ... & Ingber, D. E. (2017). Mature induced-pluripotent-stem-cell-derived human podocytes reconstitute kidney glomerular-capillary-wall function on a chip. *Nature biomedical engineering, 1*(5), 0069.

Petrosyan, A., Cravedi, P., Villani, V., Angeletti, A., Manrique, J., Renieri, A., De Filippo, R. E., Perin, L., & Da Sacco, S. (2019). A glomerulus-on-a-chip to recapitulate the human glomerular filtration barrier. *Nature Communications*, *10*(1), 3656. DOI: 10.1038/s41467-019-11577-z PMID: 31409793

Quirós-Solano, W. F., Gaio, N., Stassen, O. M. J. A., Arik, Y. B., Silvestri, C., Van Engeland, N. C. A., Van der Meer, A., Passier, R., Sahlgren, C. M., Bouten, C. V. C., van den Berg, A., Dekker, R., & Sarro, P. M. (2018). Microfabricated tuneable and transferable porous PDMS membranes for Organs-on-Chips. *Scientific Reports*, *8*(1), 13524. DOI: 10.1038/s41598-018-31912-6 PMID: 30202042

Roye, Y., Bhattacharya, R., Mou, X., Zhou, Y., Burt, M. A., & Musah, S. (2021). A personalized glomerulus chip engineered from stem cell-derived epithelium and vascular endothelium. *Micromachines*, *12*(8), 967. DOI: 10.3390/mi12080967 PMID: 34442589

Roye, Y., & Musah, S. (2022). Isogenic kidney glomerulus chip engineered from human induced pluripotent stem cells. *Journal of Visualized Experiments*, *189*, e63821. PMID: 36408985

Satchell, S. C., & Braet, F. (2009). Glomerular endothelial cell fenestrations: An integral component of the glomerular filtration barrier. *American Journal of Physiology. Renal Physiology*, *296*(5), F947–F956. DOI: 10.1152/ajprenal.90601.2008 PMID: 19129259

'tHart, D. C., Yildiz, D., Palacio-Castañeda, V., Li, L., Gumuscu, B., Brock, R., Verdurmen, W. P. R., van der Vlag, J., & Nijenhuis, T. (2023). Co-culture of glomerular endothelial cells and podocytes in a custom-designed glomerulus-on-a-chip model improves the filtration barrier integrity and affects the glomerular cell phenotype. *Biosensors (Basel)*, *13*(3), 339. DOI: 10.3390/bios13030339 PMID: 36979551

Wang, L., Tao, T., Su, W., Yu, H., Yu, Y., & Qin, J. (2017). A disease model of diabetic nephropathy in a glomerulus-on-a-chip microdevice. *Lab on a Chip*, *17*(10), 1749–1760. DOI: 10.1039/C7LC00134G PMID: 28418422

Xie, R., Korolj, A., Liu, C., Song, X., Lu, R. X. Z., Zhang, B., Ramachandran, A., Liang, Q., & Radisic, M. (2020). h-FIBER: Microfluidic topographical hollow fiber for studies of glomerular filtration barrier. *ACS Central Science*, *6*(6), 903–912. DOI: 10.1021/acscentsci.9b01097 PMID: 32607437

Yoshimura, Y., Taguchi, A., Tanigawa, S., Yatsuda, J., Kamba, T., Takahashi, S., Kurihara, H., Mukoyama, M., & Nishinakamura, R. (2019). Manipulation of nephron-patterning signals enables selective induction of podocytes from human pluripotent stem cells. *Journal of the American Society of Nephrology*, *30*(2), 304–321. DOI: 10.1681/ASN.2018070747 PMID: 30635375

Zhou, M., Zhang, X., Wen, X., Wu, T., Wang, W., Yang, M., Wang, J., Fang, M., Lin, B., & Lin, H. (2016). Development of a functional glomerulus at the organ level on a chip to mimic hypertensive nephropathy. *Scientific Reports*, *6*(1), 31771. DOI: 10.1038/srep31771 PMID: 27558173

Chapter 9

Synergistic Integration of Federated Learning and Visual Intelligence for Disease Diagnosis and Prediction:
Next-Gen Healthcare Landscape

Madhu Bala Myneni
https://orcid.org/0000-0003-4734-5914
VNR Vignana Jyothi Institute of Engineering and Technology, Hyderabad, India

Haritha Akkineni
https://orcid.org/0000-0002-5909-4078
PVP Siddhartha Institute of Technology, Vijayawada, India

Akhil Dandamudi
https://orcid.org/0009-0006-3835-1393
Kalven Technologies Inc., Atlanta, USA

ABSTRACT

The synergistic integration of federated learning and visual intelligence redefines the next-gen healthcare landscape. Visual intelligence is crucial in disease diagnosis through X-rays, CT and PET scans, MRI, etc. It was enhanced through AI enabled diagnosis systems. These systems are functioning based on centralized and limited training data models. Federated Learning (FL), works among multiple healthcare organizations located at different locations to collaboratively train models without exchanging sensitive patient data, thus maintaining privacy and security. Integrating

DOI: 10.4018/979-8-3693-6094-1.ch009

FL and visual intelligence significantly enhances disease prediction and diagnosis by interpreting medical images on large models. This chapter focuses on the role of technology in next-gen healthcare, FL frameworks, benefits, challenges, and applications; Visual intelligence real-time applications, synergistic integration of FL and vision intelligence in disease prediction use cases of real-time healthcare.

1. INTRODUCTION

1.1. Background

With the rise of the population specifically aging citizens, the medical practitioners' shortage has led to a global focus on employing advanced information and communication technology (ICT) to improve the effectiveness of healthcare services. Artificial intelligence (AI) methods like deep learning (DL) and machine learning (ML)are widely used in several health-related industries. Currently, artificial intelligence (AI) with vision intelligence-driven diagnostic tools enables doctors to identify the conditions of patients by interpreting images generated by diagnostic machines such as CT, MRI, and X-ray quickly and accurately. The prominent AI-enabled diagnosis applications in healthcare are revising patient data, symptoms, and medical history. In the times ahead, AI could be able to analyze huge amounts of medical data to predict and avoid diseases before symptoms arise. It develops an assistant in diagnosing complex conditions by integrating genetic, lifestyle or demographics, and environmental data. However, AI should complement, not replace, medical professionals, enhancing diagnostics and patient care. The prospects that need to be focused on in next-gen AI systems are ethical concerns, data privacy, and continuous models in healthcare.

Generative AI, especially large language models (LLMs), playing a crucial role in transforming real-world evidence (RWE) generation. It emphasizes the efficiency gains in data processing and analysis, the reduction of human errors, and the standardization of evidence-generation processes. A key focus is on leveraging unstructured notes in electronic health records (EHRs), visual data from radiology reports, and physician notes for RWE, enhancing the overall accuracy of health assessments. Furthermore, generative AI can streamline health technology assessment (HTA) by automating evidence synthesis and improving health economic modeling.

AI has been redefined in medical imaging especially in radiology (Najjar, 2023) providing an optimized personal allocation, scanner usage, reduced radiation exposure, and increased quality of care (European Society of Radiology, 2019). Deep learning enhances the power of PET imaging, and significantly improves image quality, segmentation, and motion correction, benefiting both PET/CT and PET/MRI applications (Artesani et al., 2024). The pathologists are empowered with Automated image analysis tools to scrutinize tissues at a microscopic level with greater precision and efficiency (Kumar et al., 2017). The application of AI is extended to microbiology, summarizing the challenges that AI faces from a biological perspective and proposing future directions for improving AI integration with microbiology (Huo & Wang, 2024). It highlights the historical role of microbes in medicine, noting their therapeutic potential in fighting various diseases. The experimental results identify several obstacles, including the complexity of microbial interactions and the need for large, well-curated datasets for AI training. They suggest that future improvements should focus on better data collection, advanced AI models tailored for biological systems, and fostering interdisciplinary collaboration between AI specialists and microbiologists.

In modern diagnosis, specifically DL playing a vital role in cancer detection at various organs like lung (Zebin & Rezvy, 2021), brain (Lyu et al., 2022), skin, blood (Artesani et al., 2024) (Illimoottil & Ginat, 2023), and breast etc. through medical imaging such as CT scan, MRI, PET scans. An in-depth study on overview of various DL models (Zhang & Qie, 2023), such as recurrent neural networks (RNNs), convolutional neural networks (CNNs) and generative adversarial networks (GANs), and their applications in medical imaging was thoroughly done (Murmu et al., 2024). The review highlights how these models are utilized for tasks like image segmentation and disease classification, with a focus on improving diagnostic accuracy in fields such as oncology and neurology. The DL techniques in healthcare, significantly contributing to improving the quality of medical images and empower medical professionals with effective identification of pathological markers within medical visuals to facilitate good diagnosis and treatment planning. It indicates a clear emphasis on DL's significant role in next-gen healthcare by improving healthcare outcomes through advancing the eminence and effectiveness of diagnostic imaging.

The state-of-art vision intelligence research longitude was specified through various disease prediction and diagnosis models. It expands with a novel technique called Vision Transformer (ViT) (Lyu et al., 2022), is used initially pre-trained on natural images and then fine-tuned on a brain imaging dataset. A study on the classification of Alzheimer's disease model by incorporating transfer of knowledge gained from the natural image domain to brain imaging, which improves accuracy and performance in detecting the condition.

Another innovative neural network model called DeepRibo which influences both convolutional neural networks (CNNs) and recurrent neural networks (RNNs), is used to accurately identify coding regions in prokaryotic genes (Clauwaert et al., 2019). The model significantly improves the accuracy of gene annotations by combining ribosome profiling and binding site pattern data. This approach proves the effectiveness of the DL approach in enhancing genomic analysis.

An advanced neural network approach for machine translation called ProLanGO, employs RNNs to tackle the challenge of predicting protein functions (Cao et al., 2017) as a language translation task. This innovative method proves natural language processing (NLP) can be effectively applied to bioinformatics for enhancing the prediction of protein functions, which are critical for empathetic biological processes. These protein functions are able to predict and lead to insights into disease mechanisms, aiding in the identification of potential therapeutic targets and biomarkers. By leveraging ML techniques like ProLanGO, researchers can accelerate drug discovery and personalize treatment plans finally improvs patient outcomes. It indicates integration of AI-driven approaches in next-gen healthcare has significant implications for disease diagnosis and treatment.

Over the study of all existing research, the significant role of AI in healthcare and redefined the medical imaging and diagnostic process. It plays playing critical role in improving diagnostic accuracy and speed in imaging techniques such as CT, MRI, PET, and ultrasound. These are indispensable in modern diagnosis, specifically in the detection of cancer, heart conditions, internal injury, and bleeding. The scan reports contain detailed transverse body scans that help in the accurate assessment of specific cases like heart conditions and evaluate traumatic injuries. AI can detect aneurysms, tumor stage, and various health issues by indicative abnormalities that might go unnoticed thereby reducing the time needed for the creation and interpretation of scans. Now, AI has become an aid to advanced diagnosis in determining the stages of cancers, evaluating heart conditions with segmentation algorithms, and assessing injuries using 3D reconstruction. Overall, the incorporation of AI into medical visual reports can improve diagnosis accuracy and elevate the quality of care.

1.1. Next-Generation Healthcare

Next-gen healthcare enables accurate disease diagnosis and prediction with early intrusion, adapted patient-made treatment plans, anticipatory measures, and amended patient outcomes. Identifying possible health risks before symptoms appear eventually leads to a better quality of life and reduced healthcare costs. With the inclusion of progressive technologies like AI and ML, a huge amount of medical data can be analyzed to identify patterns and predict disease risks with high accuracy (Umapathy et al., 2023). Next-gen healthcare technologies are transforming patient care by integrating advanced digital tools and practices and providing technology-inclusive solutions in healthcare to revolutionize doctor and patient relations. Prominent technologies like Federated learning (FL) enable collaborative AI models to improve the efficiency without compromising data privacy and Visual intelligence improves disease diagnosis by interpreting medical images with greater precision. Telemedicine and remote patient monitoring increase access to healthcare through wearable devices and the Internet of Medical Things (IoMT). These technologies enable continuous health tracking. Additionally, blockchain technology ensures secure data sharing, 3D printing facilitates personalized medical solutions, and genomics drives precision medicine through targeted treatments. Technology-driven practices like augmented reality (AR), virtual reality (VR), and robotic surgery are reshaping surgical procedures and rehabilitation. Through quantum computing and edge, AI exploits future inventions in drug discovery and real-time nursing. A GPT 3-based framework has been implemented in AI-IoMT devices to monitor mental health states, providing detailed explanations (Mazumdar et al., 2023). Table 1 shows a summary of AI's role in Next-Gen Healthcare disease Prediction and diagnosis.

Table 1. AI role in Next-Gen Healthcare disease Prediction and diagnosis

Disease	AI Role	Key Technology/Method
Blood Cancers (Acute Lymphoblastic Leukemia)	Deep learning approach for diagnosing ALL in blood pictures using feature selection algorithms.	Deep Learning, Feature Selection Algorithms
Infectious Disorders (Heparin-binding Protein)	Machine learning framework to identify Heparin-binding protein (HBP), critical for diagnosing infectious disorders.	Machine Learning
Diabetic Macular Edema (DME)	AI helps predict DME by employing knowledge graphs to manage missing data and improve disease prediction models.	Knowledge Graphs, Predictive Modeling
Oral Squamous Cell Carcinoma (OSCC)	Nomogram prediction model to assess prognosis of OSCC patients after surgery for personalized treatment regimens.	AI-powered Nomogram Prediction Models
Drug-induced Hepatotoxicity	AI analyzes big datasets to identify biomarkers for detecting hepatotoxicity caused by certain medications.	Big Data Analytics, Biomarker Discovery
Mandibular Length Prediction	AI algorithms predict face growth patterns and estimate post-pubertal mandibular length, aiding orthodontics.	Machine Learning Algorithms
Appendicitis Diagnosis	Machine learning technique to distinguish between perforated and non-perforated appendicitis for better therapeutic decisions.	Machine Learning, Diagnostic Tools
Diabetes Detection	Deep learning strategy converts numerical data into visual graphs to improve early diabetes detection.	Deep Learning, Data Visualization
Brain Tumor Detection	AI-powered MRI data analysis compares multiple machine learning models for early and accurate brain tumor diagnosis.	Machine Learning, MRI Data Analysis

continued on following page

Table 1. Continued

Disease	AI Role	Key Technology/Method
Inflammatory Bowel Disease (IBD)	AI interprets genomic data to predict disease progression and assess therapy response, improving patient care.	AI in Genomic Data Analysis, Disease Progression Prediction
Breast Cancer Diagnosis	AI, especially CNNs, is used for breast cancer screening with rising research interest in this field.	Convolutional Neural Networks (CNNs) for Cancer Screening

1.2. Why Federated Learning Is Preferred Over Blockchain-Based Approaches

Federated Learning is highly suited for privacy-preserving, scalable, and efficient healthcare analysis applications. It directly addresses the challenges of sensitive data handling and machine learning model training, making it the preferred approach over blockchain in many healthcare scenarios. FL models are more robust and provide privacy with low computation overhead. More practically, it protects sensitive patient data while enabling collaborative model training across different institutions. Moreover, blockchain provides data security but is less efficient for large-scale data analysis. Data privacy is not mandatory for all applications in healthcare. It requires sharing hashed or processed data across the network, which may still raise privacy concerns in sensitive domains like healthcare. It faces scalability challenges as it needs to share hashed or processed data across the network. Integration is another challenge due to heterogeneous data formats. Due to the immutable nature of data items, change or update is difficult (Chen et al., 2024). Implementation is complex, requiring significant infrastructural overhauls and expertise (Zhang et al., 2022). Due to the drawbacks of blockchain in healthcare data analysis FL becomes an alternative. FL prioritizes data privacy without compromising the ability to leverage diverse datasets for better model performance. It demonstrates data access to heterogeneous healthcare across institutions (Sheller et al., 2020).

1.3. Federated Learning (FL) With Visual Intelligence

FL and Visual Intelligence are two cutting-edge technologies that offer a transformative potential in healthcare. FL is a decentralized machine learning approach where multiple institutions collaborate to train a model without sharing sensitive data, protecting patient privacy, and adhering to regulations. Visual intelligence, powered by computer vision, interprets medical images such as X-rays, MRIs, and CT scans to detect diseases like cancer, cardiovascular conditions, or neurological disorders with enhanced accuracy. In collaborative learning, transforming imaginary data from one site to another is a cost-effective process. Hence the solution federated learning with visual intelligence is a prominent solution for next-gen healthcare.

Federated Learning and Visual Intelligence Synergy, particularly in the context of disease diagnosis and prediction, generative AI (Fleurence et al., 2024) can complement federated learning by processing vast amounts of decentralized EHR data without compromising patient privacy. While federated learning allows models to learn from distributed datasets, generative AI models can enhance disease diagnosis by analyzing unstructured EHR notes, creating more accurate predictions, and improving patient outcomes.

The synergy of visual intelligence in medical imaging and generative AI could also improve diagnostic accuracy, offering more personalized treatment pathways. Both technologies together streamline data insights for real-world healthcare scenarios, advancing diagnosis, prediction, and overall healthcare delivery.

In a cancer diagnosis network, multiple hospitals can collaborate using FL to train a visual intelligence model for detecting tumors in medical images. Each hospital contributes local data to improve the model without compromising patient privacy, resulting in a highly accurate, scalable, and adaptive diagnostic tool that works across different healthcare settings. Integration of federated learning with visual intelligence in healthcare promises a high-precision disease diagnosis with the help of a collaborative model without sharing patient-sensitive data among local models of various hospitals or healthcare institutions.

1.4. Benefits Of Synergistic Approach

Benefits of this approach:

1. Reduce data breaches and unauthorized access to patient data
2. Improve diagnostic accuracy of visual intelligence from diverse data sources.
3. Establish collaborative learning across multiple hospitals/institutions
4. Personalized and adoptive diagnosis model helps to calibrate the global model to the individual level
5. Leveraging FL with visual intelligence can gain automated diagnostics, reduce the load on radiologists and specialists, and help to make quick decisions.

1.5. Focus Of The Chapter

This chapter focuses on studying the synergetic integration of federated learning (FL) and visual intelligence (VI), and how it can significantly improve disease diagnosis and prediction in next-generation healthcare. It includes the role of FL and VI in healthcare applications, the step-by-step process of FL landscape, computational and implemented frameworks, and applications, and how synergistic integration FL with VI enables next-gen healthcare applications. Real-time FL enables collaborative model development across healthcare institutions while preserving patient privacy, and how visual intelligence enhances the interpretation of medical images to deliver more accurate diagnoses. It will provide a detailed framework for implementing these technologies in healthcare settings, addressing practical challenges and offering insights into their transformative potential for medical diagnostics.

1.6. Objectives

1. Outline a step-by-step roadmap for integrating federated learning with visual intelligence in healthcare, providing real-world examples.
2. The synergistic integration of federated learning with visual intelligence works together to enhance disease diagnosis and prediction while preserving patient privacy and ensuring data security.
3. Review the latest innovations in federated learning and visual intelligence to highlight recent advancements and future directions in healthcare research.

2. FUNDAMENTALS OF FEDERATED LEARNING

2.1. Federated Learning Landscape

Federated learning (FL) is a decentralized ML approach where manifold devices or computer systems considered as clients (local), collaboratively train a shared model (global) while keeping the data localized on each client. In this learning, instead of sending data to a central(global) server, each client (local) processes its data locally and only sends model updates (like gradients or weights) to the central server, which aggregates them to update the global model. This process helps to preserve data privacy and reduces the risk of data leakage, particularly in sensitive applications like healthcare. Figure 1 illustrates the landscape of FL.

Figure 1. Federated Learning landscape

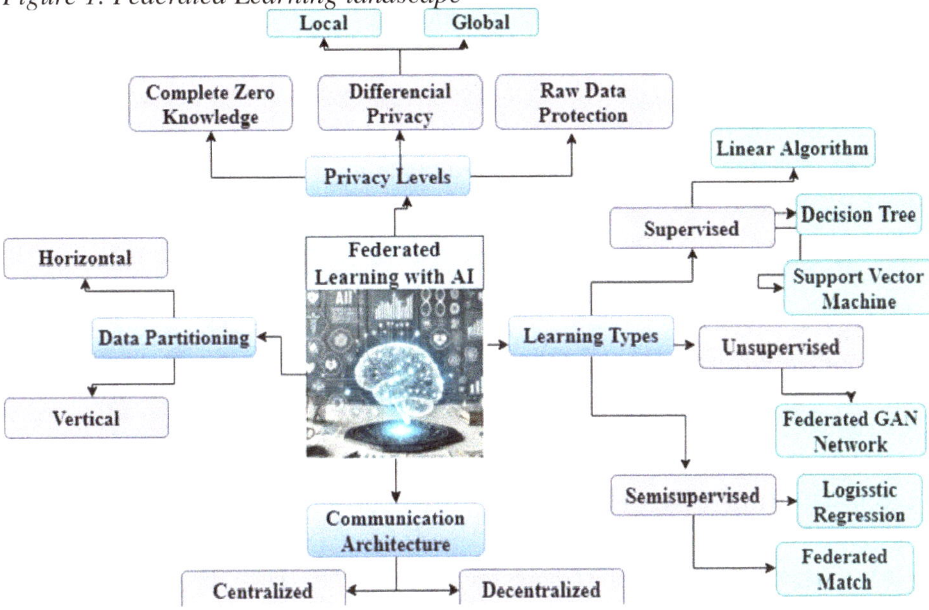

In FL framework, a centralized server, which works on global model will distributes initial weights of the global model parameters to all collaborating sites or devices. Hence, in all the sites local model was trained by considering locally available data and then broadcasts the updated model parameters(weights) to the central server. In traditional method, raw data from each site has to transfer to the central server for updates on global model. But in FL setup, raw data never leave the local device or site. The local collaborated sites have to forward their updates frequently, then at central server the global model was updated with aggregation of all updated local site model parameters. The updated global model is then again communicated to all collaborative sites for another round of local training processes. The process is repeated until the global model converges. The main benefit of FL collaborative model is creation of higher-accuracy model by leveraging larger training datasets obtained from multiple sites. It exhibits more than the traditional central model with existing data of a single device or a system with high levels of data privacy. This makes FL particularly valuable in healthcare, especially in research areas where access to public data is limited or restricted (Kumar et al., 2017). In FL, the model travels to the data rather than the converse. It implies that end devices are used for training. For instance, if there is an application in a person's personal device and there is a ML model on the device to train based on the user interactions, the model, with the user interactions, get strained on the device. So, from the person's personal device, the updates will be pushed to the centralized location (this could happen from several such devices from different locations). Taking all the updates, the centralized model gets fully updated, which can be sent back to multiple mobile devices (Fleurence et al., 2024). Instead of gathering all the data in a central location, FL allows data to remain on individual devices, thus addressing privacy concerns related to sharing personal data. The process of FL involves sending the model to the devices where the data is stored and training the model locally on each device using the available data. The models are locally trained and then sent to a central server, where they are combined to produce an overall model that has been trained using all the available data (Attia et al., 2019)

The introduction of Internet of Medical Things (IoMT) devices, combined with Artificial Intelligence (AI), has revolutionized healthcare, enabling a new era of smart applications that enhance patient care globally. A key component in this shift is Federated Learning (FL), which allows the development of shared AI models across diverse datasets from IoMT devices while maintaining data privacy. However, traditional FL methods face challenges due to the variability of IoMT environments, including differences in devices, data, and model complexities (Sachin et al., 2024).

In response, this research introduces the FedCure framework, designed to address these challenges by employing personalized Federated Learning (pFL) approaches tailored for various healthcare applications. Case studies in this research focus on real-world use cases such as Eye Retinopathy Detection, Diabetes Monitoring, Maternal Health, Remote Health Monitoring, and Human Activity Recognition (HAR) (Gad & Fadlullah, 2022). Publicly available datasets, such as those for diabetes monitoring and HAR, were used to demonstrate the framework's effectiveness in adapting to the heterogeneity of data and devices in FL scenarios.

For instance, in Eye Retinopathy Classification, a cross-silo FL scenario was used where multiple medical organizations collaborated to develop a shared AI model. This experiment employed a non-IID (non-independent and identically distributed) dataset involving 10 clients, demonstrating how pFL approaches can enhance diagnostic accuracy in next-generation healthcare applications.

This study highlights the significant potential of federated learning and visual intelligence in addressing challenges in medical diagnostics, where privacy, heterogeneity, and scalability are critical for widespread adoption in next-gen healthcare. By leveraging these advanced methods, healthcare can become more personalized and efficient while ensuring data security and model accuracy.

A novel reliable personalized Federated Learningbased Customized Inequality-Aware Federated Learning (CusIAFL) technique is proposed for securing color images while communicating with a wireless network. The proposed technique adjusts each data sampling to the local target during optimization using knowledge of client-label availability. The work that is being presented uses a hybrid technique to maintain consistency in the time-series data. and a novel Pix2Pix Generative Adversarial Network (GAN) technique is used to generate realistic images.

In medical imaging, patient privacy is a critical concern, as sensitive data embedded in images may lead to privacy issues if disclosed. To address this, various techniques such as image encryption, lossless compression, watermarking, and steganography have been developed to safeguard medical images against unauthorized access and cryptographic attacks. In the context of next-generation healthcare, especially with the rise of federated learning and visual intelligence, ensuring data privacy becomes paramount as models rely on distributed data across multiple sources without centralizing patient information.

Federated learning (FL) enables healthcare organizations to collaborate on model training without sharing raw data, addressing privacy concerns effectively. To further enhance privacy, deep convolutional neural networks (CNNs), particularly Generative Adversarial Networks (GANs) such as the Pix2Pix model, have been utilized for image-to-image (I-to-I) translation tasks. These models can be applied within FL frameworks to process medical images locally while preserving the security and privacy of sensitive data. By combining these advanced AI techniques, next-generation healthcare systems can improve diagnostics and personalized care, all while maintaining stringent data privacy standards.

The integration of these privacy-preserving approaches within federated learning frameworks will be crucial for future healthcare advancements, allowing medical institutions to harness the power of AI and visual intelligence without compromising patient confidentiality.

2.2. Federated Computation Frameworks

In federated learning communication between clients and with the server will differ based on the Computation Framework. Frameworks implementation differs in two levels Centralized and peer-to-peer models.

2.2.1. Centralized Model

In the centralized FL model, all collaborative institutions are connected with the central site and communicate the model weights among central and local sites. Figure 2 shows the FL centralized computational framework. The communication steps are:

- In the first step, the clients who want to participate in the collaboration approach of federated learning have to prepare their data by implementing different security mechanisms. Data can be pre-health information, electronic health records, symptoms, clinical and non-clinical information, or other sources.

- Cloud infrastructure setup is prepared to facilitate the training process between a centralized server with different clients.
- The central server initializes the basic FL model by using machine learning or a neural network approach.
- The central server then sends the initialized model to all clients that participated in the training, then each client will initially download the basic model, and update the local model with their locally available data.
- The updated model parameters of each client are directed back to the central server with their updated model parameters. Then the central server updates the global model with aggregation of all clients' updated model parameters by using techniques like centralized federated average (FedAvg) or secure aggregation mechanism.
- An aggregated model will be sent to each client and then again, the clients are trained individually with the updated model, this training process will repeat iteratively until all client models are updated with N number of rounds, leading to improved performance and accuracy of each client model.
- All participated models are evaluated for its accuracy and performance with validation data.

Figure 2. FL centralized computational framework

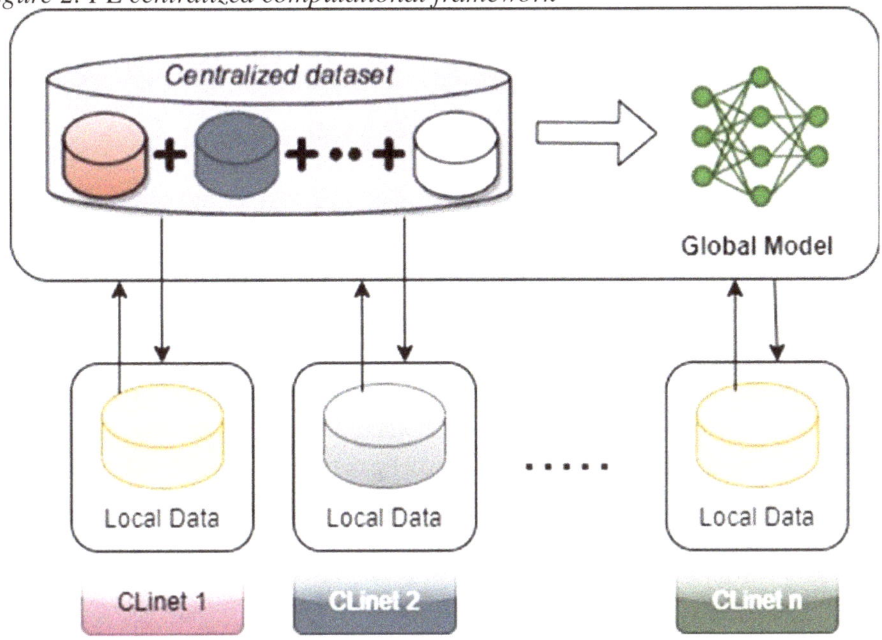

The evaluated model can be suggested for different predictions in healthcare applications like medical imaging analysis, Disease monitoring and diagnosis, personalized recommendations, and many more.

Communication steps between client and global model:
Steps: 1 -> Initial model sends from server to clients.
2 -> Model trains with local client data at each client and it updates.
3 -> Each client will send their updated model parameters to the server for aggregation.
4 -> The global model will be updated with aggregation of all client's parameters.
5 -> The server will distribute the global model parameters to each of the clients for their model updating.
The advantages of the centralized FL training approach are as follows:
Network bandwidth: The communication of model parameters between clients and servers instead of sharing raw data leads to reducing network load and communication costs.
Latency: Network delay from client to client is reduced in the FL environment by consistent training and updating of ML local models in the training phase.

Privacy: Clients are not transferring the raw data to the centralized server as they are only sending the updated model parameters thus guaranteeing the privacy of each user.

2.2.2. Peer-to-peer FL Computational Model

Distributed Federated Learning (DFL) is an innovative approach in which clients communicate directly with each other and exchange model parameters without the need for a central server. This distributed structure has several advantages, such as greater adaptability and significant savings in communication and computing resources. DFL makes the communication network between clients more diverse and can dynamically adjust connections depending on the scenario. Different scenarios are used in DFL for making connections between the client's various methods and strategies (Sezer et al., 2017) to address challenges like privacy safeguarding, communication efficiency, knowledge retention, scalability, and handling non-stationary data distributions. Figure 3 shows the peer-to-peer FL computational framework.

Peer-to-Peer Aggregation Model:

In the Aggregation model, learning involves combining the contributions of all previous clients at each step:

Step 1: Each client starts training a local model with their available data with some initial parameters, resulting in model m1m_1m1 at Client 1.
Step 2: Client 2 learns from model m1m_1m1 and aggregates it with its local model m2m_2m2, resulting in a representative model AAA.
Step 3: Unlike the Continual model, Client 3 aggregates **all previous models** from Client 1 and Client 2, i.e., models m1m_1m1 and AAA, with its local model m2m_2m2. This process results in a new representative model BBB.
Step 4: This aggregation process continues across all clients, where each client aggregates all prior models with its local model.

At client n, the global model is represented as

$$N = \sum(A \text{ to } M)+ml+mn$$

Global Model and Iterations:

In each iteration, a global model is sent back to all clients, updating their local models with this global representation. With each iteration, new parameters are integrated, progressively improving the model's performance and accuracy. The **Aggregation model** sees learning difficulty influenced only by the current client's model, as the aggregated model is more representative of the entire dataset across clients.

In an instance, 3 clients and client n generate a global model communicating with each other in the FL framework. Communication steps between client and global model:

1. Train client model with initial data at each client.
2. Model parameters of m1 at client 1 will be sent to the next client
3. Model parameters of m2 at client 2 will be combined as A = m1 + m2.
4. Model parameters from previous clients will be sent to the next client.
   a. In the continual approach model A at client 2, will be sent to the next client.
   b. In the aggregation approach, local weights from client 1 as m1 and updated local model at client 2 as A are sent to client 3.
5. Previous client's model parameters are aggregated
   a. In the continual approach model m3 at client 3 will be combined with model A at client 2 as B=A+m3.
   b. In the Aggregation approach, local weights from client 1 m1 and model A at client 2 and local model m3 at client 3, aggregated as B =m1+A+m3
6. Continue this process up to client n until the global model is predicted at client n.
   a. In continual approach N=M+mn.
   b. In aggregation approach N = $\sum$(A to M) + ml+ mn.
7. The global model will be sent back to each client

Figure 3. Peer-to-peer FL Computational Model

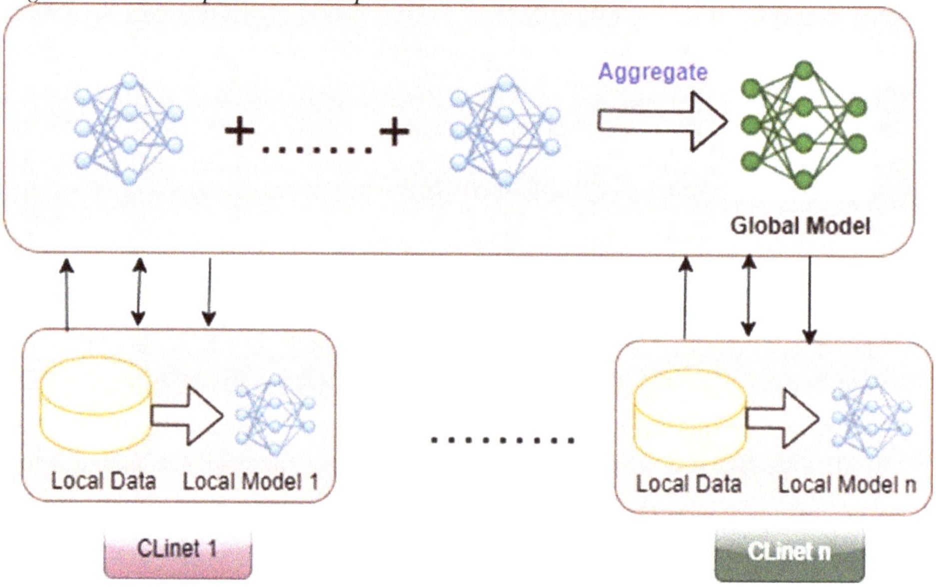

2.3. Characteristics of FL

1) **Data Privacy** — The data is trained on the local client, and data is neither passed to the server nor shared with any other system, hence preserving privacy (European Society of Radiology, 2019)
2) **Computational power** — Less computational power is needed and lower overhead at the server due to decentralization.
3) **Security** — Using secure aggregators with sending weights while encrypting the data will enhance security purposes, especially concerning sensitive data such as facial information (Illimoottil & Ginat, 2023).
4) **Real-time continual learning** — FL allows continuous learning as the models are constantly updated and improved using updated datasets from the client. Hence, this will help achieve the highest accuracy in the global models (Zhang & Qie, 2023). In a big data context, edge servers or mobile smart devices may be used to store user personal information and behavioral data. Thus, the protection of data privacy is a crucial assurance for the advancement of intelligence. Numerous industries are beginning to place a higher priority on the security and privacy of personal data. The combined efforts of several researchers have helped FL play a significant role in several different businesses. In addition, industries, including finance and urban services, are also using FL applications

(Umapathy et al., 2023). By improving the quality of services, the IoMT has significantly altered the way how medical institutions work.

2.4. Benefits Of Federated Learning Over Traditional DL

By comparing FL to traditional DL, it becomes evident that FL offers significant advantages in healthcare, especially in privacy-sensitive environments, cross-institutional collaboration, and efficient model training. Table 2 provides a summary of the key benefits of FL with traditional DL.

Table 2. Summary of Key benefits of FL with traditional DL

Aspect	Federated Learning (FL)	Traditional Deep Learning (DL)
Data Privacy and Security	FL keeps patient data decentralized; only model parameters are shared. Patient data remains within the local servers of healthcare institutions, ensuring agreement with data privacy regulations (HIPAA, GDPR).	Traditional DL requires data centralization, where sensitive healthcare data (e.g., medical records, and images) must be transferred to a central server or cloud for model training. This leads to privacy violations and the risk of data breaches.
Collaboration Across Institutions	FL enables healthcare institutions can share their model updates without sharing their raw patient data. This allows hospitals, clinics, and research centers to build collaborative models. Data never leaves the institution, ensuring privacy.	DL models depend on centralized data, which hinders collaboration across hospitals and research institutions, especially when sharing patient data across borders due to regulatory restrictions. Data transfer between institutions can create privacy issues.
Data Centralization	No need for centralizing data in FL; the model is trained locally on distributed datasets at the source (e.g., hospitals, clinics). This avoids the need for massive data transfers and storage in a central location.	Data must be centralized for traditional DL, where all patient data from different institutions is combined into one central repository for training. This introduces bandwidth constraints, storage issues, and privacy risks.
Handling of Large Data Volumes	FL reduces network bandwidth requirements by sending small model updates (weights, gradients) instead of transmitting large datasets (e.g., MRI images). This is especially beneficial when dealing with large-scale medical imaging or genomic data.	DL consumes high bandwidth as entire datasets (e.g., EHRs, imaging) need to be transferred to the central server for training. This can be resource-intensive, especially for large healthcare datasets such as high-resolution medical images.
Data Sovereignty and Compliance	FL allows data sovereignty as the data remains within the local institution's systems. Hospitals retain full control of their data, and FL models can be trained without violating local regulations or cross-border data transfer laws.	DL requires central data storage, which may conflict with data sovereignty rules. For instance, some countries or institutions have strict policies regarding data storage, and sending sensitive data across borders can raise compliance issues.

continued on following page

Table 2. Continued

Aspect	Federated Learning (FL)	Traditional Deep Learning (DL)
Scalability	FL scales effectively to multiple institutions and edge devices (e.g., wearables, mobile health apps) while respecting privacy concerns. It's particularly suited for global healthcare collaborations involving diverse patient populations.	DL models face scaling challenges because centralizing massive datasets from multiple sources (hospitals, devices) is complex and costly, requiring significant computational power and storage resources.
Diverse Data and Model Generalization	FL leverages diverse datasets from different healthcare institutions, improving model generalization across different populations. Models trained on decentralized, varied datasets are more robust and less prone to overfitting.	DL models trained on centralized data may suffer from bias or overfitting if the centralized dataset lacks diversity. For example, models trained on local data from a single hospital may not specify different aging people or regions.
Data Imbalance	FL allows the handling of data imbalance across institutions. Hospitals with fewer cases of rare diseases can contribute to a larger collaborative model without sharing their data, improving performance for underrepresented conditions.	DL models trained centrally on an imbalanced dataset may perform poorly on underrepresented classes, such as rare diseases, due to a lack of data diversity. Centralizing limited data sources can exacerbate this issue.
Risk of Data Breaches	Lower risk of data breaches as raw patient data is not transferred to a central repository. This decentralized approach reduces the attack surface for cyberattacks targeting sensitive medical information.	High risk of data breaches as centralized DL models require the aggregation of sensitive patient data, making centralized repositories attractive targets for hackers. Any breach could expose large amounts of medical data.
Training on Edge Devices	FL supports training on edge devices (e.g., wearable devices, mobile health apps), enabling real-time AI insights directly on the device without the need for cloud-based processing. This minimizes latency and preserves privacy.	DL models generally require powerful central servers or cloud infrastructure for training. Training on edge devices is less feasible, as large datasets and computational power are needed to achieve high model performance.
Compliance with Privacy Laws	FL is designed to comply with stringent privacy regulations such as HIPAA (for healthcare in the US) and GDPR (for data protection in Europe). Data stays local, helping to meet legal obligations for sensitive data handling.	DL compliance with privacy laws can be challenging, as it involves centralizing large datasets. Managing compliance becomes more difficult as data from different regions or institutions may be subject to varying regulations.
Resource Requirements	FL optimizes resource use by distributing the training process across many local servers or edge devices. This leads to more efficient use of resources and less dependency on expensive centralized cloud infrastructure.	DL requires high computational resources and centralized cloud infrastructure, making it resource-heavy and cost-intensive, especially when dealing with large datasets and complex models in healthcare (e.g., medical imaging or genomics).

continued on following page

Table 2. Continued

Aspect	Federated Learning (FL)	Traditional Deep Learning (DL)
Model Updates and Efficiency	FL focuses on sending model updates (weights/gradients) to the central server, reducing the data transmission burden. Training efficiency improves as updates are lightweight compared to raw data transfers.	DL requires transferring the entire dataset to the central server for model updates, which can slow down the training process due to high data transmission requirements, especially for large datasets like MRI scans or genomic data.
Trust and Transparency	FL fosters trust between institutions and patients by keeping data local. Patients and institutions can trust that sensitive information is not exposed or shared with external parties, improving acceptance of AI-based healthcare solutions.	DL can lead to trust issues, as patients and institutions may be reluctant to share sensitive data with a central repository, especially if there are concerns about data misuse, leaks, or lack of transparency in data handling processes.

2.5. Federated Learning Frameworks In Healthcare

The existing FL frameworks in healthcare have prominent advantages such as privacy preservation, scalability, and secure multi-party computation. These are key enablers for modern healthcare applications like collaborative diagnostics, medical imaging, and personalized medicine, allowing healthcare organizations to train models while complying with privacy regulations and safeguarding patient data. Figure 4 illustrates the applications of FL in healthcare. Table 3 provides FL frameworks with prominent use cases in healthcare

Figure 4. Federated Learning Applications in Healthcare

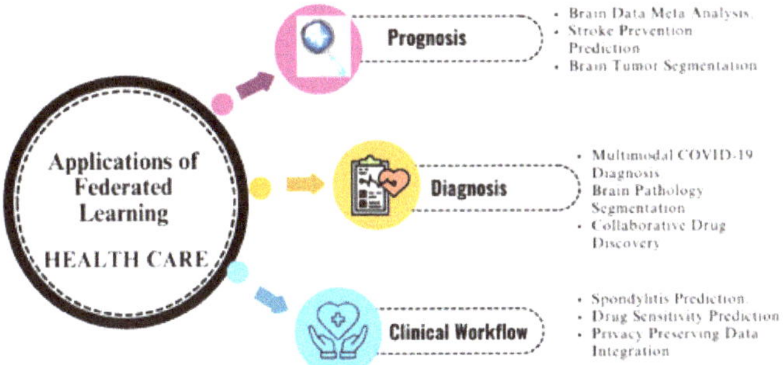

Table 3. FL frameworks and prominent use cases

Framework	Healthcare Applications	Key Use Cases
TensorFlow Federated (TFF)	Collaborative model training on decentralized healthcare data (e.g., EHRs, medical imaging).	Privacy-preserving diagnosis tools for chronic disease, collaborative research between hospitals.
PySyft	Privacy-preserving FL for sensitive healthcare data using SMPC and encryption.	Training AI models for disease prediction or diagnosis without sharing raw patient data.
FATE	Cross-institutional healthcare collaboration with secure, privacy-aware federated learning.	Multi-center clinical trials, drug discovery, epidemiological studies.
Flower	Flexible, scalable FL for decentralized healthcare research and medical image analysis.	AI for medical imaging (e.g., cancer or COVID-19 detection) across healthcare institutions.
IBM Federated Learning	Enterprise-level FL for healthcare focusing on secure, privacy-preserving AI model training.	Personalized medicine, clinical decision support systems, regulatory-compliant federated AI solutions.
NVIDIA Clara Train SDK	Federated learning for medical imaging, enabling healthcare institutions to train AI models collaboratively.	AI for cancer detection, medical imaging analysis (e.g., MRI, CT) without sharing sensitive patient data.
OpenFL	Secure, cross-device, and cross-silo federated learning for large-scale healthcare applications.	Predictive models for chronic disease management (e.g., hypertension, diabetes) using wearable health data.
PaddleFL	Privacy-focused FL for healthcare, suitable for large-scale, industrial applications in health research and diagnostics.	Early disease detection (e.g., diabetic retinopathy) with secure collaboration across hospitals or research centers.

Federated learning (FL) has practical applications in healthcare, such as developing models for rare diseases where individual hospitals have limited samples, ensuring privacy. It also facilitates secure cross-institutional collaborations, where hospitals benefit from models trained on shared data. FL can be used with IoT devices at patients' homes to predict health outcomes and supports real-time population monitoring for early disease outbreak detection, overcoming legal barriers to data sharing across international sites.

Disease Prediction

Hospitals can employ FL models to predict the likelihood that a given patient has an infection or becomes ill after being admitted to the hospital. It might aid medical professionals in choosing the best thing to perform for each patient, depending on their requirements. Additionally, these forecasts can be used by other organizations that work with hospital patients (such as insurance providers) to improve coverage options for individuals who most need them (Ali et al., 2022). A comparative analysis of the various contributions from FL in healthcare with a highlight of the significant contributions is provided in Table 4. It includes privacy preservation, healthcare applications disease prediction, FL with the integration of MioT, wearable devices, and blockchain. Variant types of FL learning like split learning and heterogeneity learning.

Table 4. Comparison of FL models in healthcare

Ref.	Significant contribution	Description
Sheller et al. (2020)	Multi-institutional FL in brain tumor segmentation.	The sensitive patient data is maintained locally by adhering to regulations like GDPR and HIPAA to avoid data breaches.
Rieke et al. (2020)	FL for prostate cancer diagnosis across different healthcare systems.	Decentralization of data through training ML models across multiple healthcare organizations.
Xu et al. (2021):	FL frameworks for real-time COVID-19 diagnosis and monitoring across regions.	The ML models are dynamically updated to support the continuous improvement with real time data.
Kaissis et al. (2021)	FL for combining imaging and genomic data in oncology research.	Trains models on diverse data sources like imaging and genomic data to improve generalization.
Li et al. (2020)	Federated frameworks aligning with GDPR in EU healthcare systems.	Decentralization of data is maintained while strictly following the privacy regulations.
Sheller et al. (2020)	Improved brain tumor detection models using FL in multi-center studies.	Uses diverse datasets to improve precision of AI models in disease diagnosis.
Chen et al. (2020)	FL used in edge devices for resource-efficient healthcare analytics.	Reduces the need for centralized infrastructure, lowering costs and resource consumption.
Huiming Chen et. al.(2024)	Various Disease Models	To address the issues of privacy and disease diagnosis, usage of advanced FL models in collaborative settings were discussed.
Tian et al., 2024	Robust and Privacy-Preserving FL	Training on distributed health care data by ensuring privacy preservation was demonstrated with federated learning for decentralized deep learning.
(Ullah et al., 2024)	Scalable Federated Learning for Healthcare Systems	Collaborative intermittent network connections are utilized in smart healthcare systems with scalable federated learning approach.
(Abaoud et al., 2023)	Novel Mechanisms for Privacy Preservation	Enhancing privacy-preserving mechanisms by maintaining data confidentiality was ensured in federated learning approach in healthcare applications
Chaddad et al., 2024.	Federated Learning for Healthcare Applications	Various verticals of healthcare like diagnosis, treatment prediction, and personalized care with a focus on data privacy was achieved through federated learning.

continued on following page

Table 4. Continued

Ref.	Significant contribution	Description
Akter et al., 2022.	Edge Intelligence in Smart Healthcare Systems	Intelligent processing and analysis at the edge was achieved through a privacy protection federated learning framework.
D. N. et al., 2024.	Heterogeneity-Aware Personalized Federated Learning	Healthcare personalization in Internet of Medical Things (IoMT) environments was implemented using heterogeneity-aware federated learning framework
Ni et al., 2024.	Federated Split Learning for Resource-Constrained Devices	Collaborative Healthcare analytics on wearable IoMT devices with federated split learning techniques.
Gupta et al., 2024.	Hybrid Privacy-Preserving FL for Mental Healthcare	Mental healthcare applications with improved privacy preservation can be achieved using hybrid federated learning framework with quantum approaches.
Elayan et al., 2022.	Sustainable Healthcare Data Systems with Deep FL	Sustainability and efficiency of healthcare IoT systems are ensured with deep-federated learning.
Myrzashova et al., 2023.	Blockchain Meets FL for Healthcare	Integrated blockchain technology in federated learning can improve a secure data-sharing environment.
Sai et al., 2024.	Federated Learning for Medical Data Sharing	The NFT-based model along with federated learning was used for privacy-preserving medical data sharing that improved diagnosis.
Jin et al., 2023.	Personalized FL for Healthcare	Metadata and image features were used to enhance model accuracy and privacy in personalized federated learning
Alzubi et al., 2023.	EHR Privacy-Preserving Federated Learning	A privacy protection using a blockchain-based model was implemented by Integrating federated learning and CNN in Electronic Health Records.
Tanim et al., 2024.	FL for Parkinson's Disease Diagnosis	Non-IID data partitioning and homomorphic encryption federated learning techniques were utilized for Parkinson's disease diagnosis while preserving privacy.
Zeydan et al., 2024.	Managing Machine Learning Lifecycles in Healthcare	Lifecycle management of distributed ML models for health care data residing in the cloud was analyzed using federated learning techniques.
Jiang et al., 2023.	Federated Learning with Multi-Task Transfer for IoMT	Federated learning for IoMT used multi-task transfer learning techniques to enhance decision-making in healthcare applications.
Chen et al., 2024.	Federated Learning with Cyclic Knowledge Distillation for Personalized Healthcare	MetaFed, a federated learning approach utilizing cyclic knowledge distillation among federations, was introduced to enhance personalized healthcare services.

2.5. Limitations Of FL for Disease Diagnosis

Despite various benefits, FL does face some setbacks in the area of medical data analysis. The important parameters under consideration for the model to be trained properly are data quality bias and standardization. A necessary solution is possible through careful study design, structured reporting, standardized data acquisition protocols, and advanced methods for bias detection and stratification. For technical details and a deeper discussion, recent surveys are recommended.

Data heterogeneity. Variations in modality, dimensionality, device brand, and demographic factors are making medical data highly diverse. The non-uniform data distribution remains a challenge with federated learning (FL) can enhance data diversity. Many FL algorithms assume data is independent and identically distributed (IID), and when this is not the case, strategies like FedAvg may fail.

To address this, newer methods such as **FedProx** and **domain adaptation** approaches have shown promise in handling heterogeneous data. Additionally, partial data-sharing strategies aim to improve collaboration among institutions. However, the variability in local data may lead to a scenario where the global model is suboptimal for specific participants, so consensus on model training criteria is crucial before initiating training.

Privacy and security. Health-related data is extremely susceptible to demanding high-end protection. So, the important parameters under consideration in the context of FL include balancing privacy preservation, developing effective strategies, and mitigating the residual risks. The framework is well weaved enabling secure collaborative learning without sharing raw data. Latest techniques are employed to ensure data protection maintaining a balance between privacy and model performance.

Privacy vs. performance:

Though more focus is on the concepts of privacy in Federated learning environment, privacy risks do occur. High end protection is made possible relying on various privacy preserving techniques. Some studies conclude that it has greater concerns on the accuracy of the final model. The added layers used for protection can limit the access to the important data features. Models deemed low-risk today could potentially be compromised in the future through emerging techniques or the use of external data.

Level of trust: In trusted Federated Learning, all participating parties are bound by enforceable agreements, which significantly reduce concerns around malicious intent, such as efforts to extract sensitive data or deliberately compromise the model. Since the parties are considered trustworthy, the need for complex security measures is minimized. Standard collaborative research practices suffice, focusing more on shared goals than defensive strategies.

In trusted Federated Learning environments, to safeguard from the Vindictive activities like data exploitation or intentional model compromise, all the participating organizations are unified with robust agreements. As the collaborating parties are considered to be trust worthy, it doesn't necessitate complex security mechanisms. The emphasis shifts from elaborate security protocols to facilitating seamless collaboration.

When Federated Learning (FL) is applied on a larger scale, involving non-trusted collaborators, the absence of enforceable agreements increases vulnerability to malicious activities. Rogue participants may deliberately compromise the system, degrade model performance, or exploit sensitive information[35]. Robust security mechanisms have to be in place, including Encryption of model updates, secure authentication mechanisms, Integrity verification systems, Action traceability, and Defenses against adversarial attacks

Information leakage:

Federated Learning on a large scale, particularly with non-trusted collaborators, is designed to avoid sharing sensitive healthcare data. During local training, there might be indirect disclosure of the private data such as model inversion or adversarial attacks targeting model updates, including gradients. As multiple parties get involved in the training, the risks of data exploitation and leak increase if the antagonists can focus on individual institutions' updates keeping track of changes that happen over time.

FL in healthcare, pools out diverse datasets including variability of data from diverse institutions, supporting the development of more robust AI models across different demographics. Despite its potential, FL's successful implementation in healthcare requires clear agreements on scope, goals, and technology, as it is a relatively novel approach. The use of FL in health care is revolutionizing the healthcare landscape, its developments depend on mitigating the technical and privacy issues.

Despite its potential, FL's successful implementation in healthcare requires clear agreements on goals, scope, and technology, as it is a relatively novel approach. While FL is currently enabling innovations in healthcare, its continued advancement depends on overcoming technical and privacy challenges.

3. VISUAL INTELLIGENCE IN DISEASE DIAGNOSIS

Recent advancements in visual intelligence, particularly in medical imaging, have significantly impacted next-gen healthcare. For instance, deep learning models are now utilized to detect critical conditions such as pneumothorax using X-rays, and AI algorithms have been integrated to optimize CT scan doses while maintaining image quality (McMahan et al., 2017). These models provide enhanced diagnostic accuracy, reducing clinician burden and improving patient outcomes.

The use of X-ray visuals has become a first level diagnosis of disease predictions specifically respiratory conditions. With the advancement of technology, machine learning algorithms can now accurately detect and classify various respiratory diseases such as pneumonia, tuberculosis, and lung cancer[28]. These algorithms analyze features such as the density and texture of the lung tissue to make accurate predictions. It provides a clear visualization of the lung condition and can be used to monitor disease progression and treatment effectiveness. The use of these images in predicting respiratory diseases has the potential to revolutionize the healthcare industry by providing faster and more accurate diagnoses.

The use of machine learning in medical imaging has revolutionized the way diseases are diagnosed in treated. One such application is the prediction of respiratory diseases in X-ray visuals using the Grad-CAM approach (Ali et al., 2022)(Zebin & Rezvy, 2021). This technique uses a deep learning model to identify regions of interest in the image that contribute most to the prediction, providing valuable insights for the medical practitioner. The Grad-CAM algorithm provides a heatmap overlay on the original X-ray visual by highlighting the areas that were most important in making the prediction. This became the most targeted approach to diagnosis and during treatment helps to theoretically improve patient consequences and reduce healthcare expenses.

Visual intelligence plays a big role in the diagnosis process and surgeries. One of the prominent areas of application in healthcare is lung diseases, which have significantly prompted a higher death rate over the past couple of years. The effect of disease on health is rapidly increasing because of changes in environmental factors, virus attacks, climate change, smoking, pollution, a family history of respiratory disease, and other factors. The greatest risk factor for respiratory disease is smoking. Tar, carbon monoxide, and nicotine are among the more than 4,000 compounds found in cigarette smoke. These substances damage the lungs and increase the risk of emphysema, chronic bronchitis, and lung cancer.

In the conventional approach, respiratory diseases can be detected through chest visuals (X-ray images), which helps to identify respiratory diseases like pneumonia, TB, pulmonary emphysema, chronic obstructive pulmonary disease (COPD), and virus attacks (COVID-19) (Lin et al., 2023)(Hamza et al., 2022)(Ali et al., 2022). X-ray became a quick, cost-effective, and non-invasive visual diagnostic tool to detect deformity or illness in the heart, blood vessels, and bones. Health professionals use this as a diagnostic and monitoring tool to identify various conditions like a collapsed lung, pneumonia, COVID-19, cancer, and broken ribs (Zebin & Rezvy, 2021).

3.1 Applications

3.1.1. Macular Degeneration

Age-related macular degeneration (AMD) is an eye disorder primarily caused by oddities in the retina, making it one of the leading causes of blindness. Detecting, precisely locating, classifying, and diagnosing choroidal neovascularization (CNV) in cases of neovascular AMD can be challenging, particularly when lesions are Optical Coherence Tomography (OCT) images are degraded by factors such as prognosis or gesture artifacts or small in size. A study on developing an automated system for the quantification and classification of CNV using OCT angiography images (Khosa et al., 2023). OCT angiography is a non-invasive imaging technique that provides detailed visualization of the retinal and choroidal vascular structures, both in healthy and pathological states (Liew et al., 2023). The proposed system incorporates a feature extractor specifically designed for OCT images related to macular diseases, utilizing Multi-Size Kernels echo-weighted Median Patterns (MSKEMP). OCT employs low-coherence interferometry to create cross-sectional images of the retina and optic nerve head (ONH), which assess various visual disorders qualitatively and quantitatively.

3.1.2. Early Detection Of Pneumothorax

A pneumothorax is a health condition caused by the gap between the lung and the chest wall due to the accumulation of air or gas in the pleural space. This can be converted in lateral stages as lung collapse, resulting in diminished lung function and breathing difficulties. Pneumothoraxes can be categorized as traumatic, spontaneous, and iatrogenic (resulting from medical procedures), or secondary to other diseases. Symptoms typically include chest pain, shortness of breath, and rapid breathing. Chest X-rays are used to identify the exact location of the air pocket, but it is time-consuming and erroneous.

3.1.3. Intracranial Hemorrhage Detection (ICH)

Intracerebral hemorrhage (ICH) can affect severe significance, including death or long-term disability, necessitating swift intervention from radiologists. Given the high workloads, the inexperience of some staff, and the intricacies involved in identifying subtle hemorrhages, there is a pressing need for more intelligent and automated detection systems for ICH (Asif et al., 2023). Various artificial intelligence (AI) methods have been explored in the literature, but many fall short in accuracy for both ICH detection and subtype classification.

3.2. Benefits And Challenges Of Visual Intelligence

Visual intelligence in healthcare diagnostics presents a transformative opportunity to enhance diagnostic accuracy and efficiency. However, addressing the related challenges specifically in data management, ethical considerations, and integration into clinical practice, is crucial for successful implementation. Besides, a collaborative effort among technology developers, healthcare providers, and regulatory bodies will be essential to maximize the benefits while mitigating the risks.

Benefits

1. Visual intelligence can analyze medical images (e.g., X-rays, MRIs, CT scans) with high accuracy, leading to enhanced diagnosis and treatment plans.
2. Automated systems can process and analyze images faster than human experts; it can advance diagnosis and treatment.
3. Experts' involvement in regular image interpretations can be avoided with automated image analysis. It leads to less reliance on specialized personnel.
4. Visual intelligence systems can provide consistent analysis without fatigue or bias, which can improve overall diagnostic reliability.

Challenges

1. Data Quality and Availability:
    - The effectiveness of visual intelligence systems relies heavily on the quality of the data used for training. Incomplete or biased datasets can lead to inaccurate results.
    - Managing sensitive patient data raises significant privacy and security concerns, necessitating robust data governance frameworks.
2. Interpretability and Explainability:
    - Deep learning models face a lack of transparency, making it difficult for clinicians to understand how decisions are made. This can hinder trust in AI-driven diagnostics.
    - Visual intelligence tools require thorough validation in clinical settings to ensure their accuracy and reliability before widespread adoption.

4. SYNERGISTIC INTEGRATION OF FL AND VISUAL INTELLIGENCE

Synergistic integration of FL with visual intelligence ensures a new paradigm for next-gen disease diagnosis. Federated learning (FL) has shown significant promise in enhancing disease diagnosis models, particularly by integrating visual intelligence into medical imaging. This approach allows institutions to collaboratively train deep learning models on sensitive medical data without directly sharing the data, addressing privacy concerns while benefiting from the diversity of multi-institution datasets.

For example, in retinal disease detection or cancer diagnosis, FL models leverage imaging data from different institutions to improve diagnostic accuracy, while preserving data privacy.

Recent research focuses on applying FL in areas like MRI analysis for neurological disorders, retinopathy detection, and diabetes monitoring. Studies have demonstrated how FL combined with visual intelligence—deep learning applied to medical images can effectively detect early signs of diseases by analyzing X-rays, CT scans, or MRI images. These techniques improve generalizability across healthcare providers, enhancing the reliability of diagnosis for conditions like Alzheimer's disease or macular degeneration.

Laryngeal cancer (Xu et al., 2023) presents a considerable global health challenge, particularly due to late-stage diagnoses that hinder survival rates. Recent investigations focused on deep neural networks for image analysis specifically the Densenet201 used for laryngeal cancer diagnosis using computer-aided diagnosis. The study utilized a comprehensive dataset including both stages malignant and benign. By comparing the performance of Densenet201 against other popular deep learning models and assessments by clinicians, highlights the significance of AI in enhancing the diagnostic process. The Densenet201 model, known for its exceptional capabilities in image recognition, employs a unique architecture characterized by dense connectivity, allowing for improved feature extraction and representation.

This multifaceted analysis underscores the transformative role of deep learning in next-generation healthcare, especially in improving diagnostic processes for conditions like laryngeal cancer. As AI technologies continue to advance, they hold the promise of reducing the burden of late-stage diagnoses, thereby enhancing patient outcomes and survival rates

Sezer and colleagues conducted a study using a dataset of 219 magnetic resonance (MR) images of shoulder bones, which included 91 images of edematous cases, 49 images of Hill–Sachs lesions, and 79 normal cases (Sezer et al., 2017). For the classification task, they extracted texture features using the gray-level co-occurrence matrix (GLCM) algorithm and combined these with features derived from gradient histogram pyramid algorithms. This approach aimed to improve the accuracy of differentiating between the various conditions affecting shoulder bones.

A use case was developed for a multi-scale guided attention-based method to identify anterior cruciate ligament (ACL) tears in knee MRI images, achieving an impressive accuracy of 98.63% with a dataset of 917 images (Awan et al., 2023). This advancement underscores the growing reliance on image analysis techniques in medical imaging, particularly for accurately identifying critical structures and tissues. Localization plays a crucial role in these analyses, enabling the precise detection of specific regions within MRI scans. Despite MRI being considered the gold standard for diagnosing ACL injuries, current diagnostic methods often rely on subjective assessments, necessitating substantial expertise from clinicians. This manual localization process can be time-consuming and labor-intensive.

Recent advancements in deep learning have shown exceptional capabilities in various medical imaging tasks, including localization, significantly enhancing diagnostic accuracy and efficiency. This is particularly relevant for knee injuries, including ACL tears, which are prevalent among athletes and active individuals. As next-generation healthcare continues to evolve, the integration of AI-driven techniques in imaging diagnostics promises to streamline processes, reduce diagnostic times, and improve patient outcomes.

In (Najjar, 2023), researchers are pioneering a transformative approach to diagnostics by embedding AI into medical imaging, fundamentally reshaping radiology. This integration enhances diagnostic precision, accelerates processes, and introduces predictive analytics capabilities, resulting in substantial workflow optimization.

In addition to revolutionizing imaging procedures and reporting, advanced AI systems are crucial for ensuring seamless communication among healthcare providers and enhancing patient care. They validate the connections between imaging diagnoses, radiological reports, and treatment plans, and promptly alert providers to any discrepancies. Furthermore, AI improves the allocation of personnel, optimizes scanner utilization, and minimizes radiation exposure, all of which contribute to increased efficiency and elevated quality of care (European Society of Radiology, 2019).

The deep learning (DL) techniques enhances various aspects of positron emission tomography (PET) imaging (Artesani et al., 2024). DL plays a big role significantly improve image quality, segmentation, and motion correction, benefiting both PET/CT and PET/MRI applications. The paper highlights key AI applications in PET imaging, including image generation, reconstruction, and restoration. AI also plays a critical role in noise suppression, using both supervised and unsupervised methods to refine image clarity.

Additionally, AI has the potential to streamline the entire PET imaging workflow, assisting in various clinical tasks related to diagnosis and prognosis. Interpreting the relationship between imaging data and multi-omics information, such as genomics or proteomics, is another area where AI is crucial. These technologies can enhance predictive accuracy and personalize treatment strategies, particularly in oncology and cardiac imaging.

Automated image analysis tools enable pathologists to examine tissues microscopically, allowing them to identify subtle histopathological features that may be easily missed by the human eye. These tools enhance diagnostic accuracy and efficiency, supporting pathologists in their assessments and ultimately improving patient outcomes (Kumar et al., 2017). A study of the latest developments in DL techniques for cancer imaging, with a focus on head and neck cancers (Illimoottil & Ginat, 2023) . It emphasizes the use of advanced DL methods, such as convolutional autoencoders and generative adversarial networks (GANs), in detecting, segmenting, and predicting outcomes for tumors using MRI, CT, and PET scans. The integration of radiomics and radio genomics with DL will enable the creation of predictive models to support clinical decision-making. This synergy between traditional imaging techniques and DL is critical for improving tumor classification, segmentation, and response prediction. Furthermore, the review highlights the limitations of conventional imaging approaches and the complementary role that DL plays in addressing these challenges, providing more detailed insights into cancer progression and treatment.

5. CONCLUSION

The new paradigm in next-gen healthcare was promised with synergistic integration of federated learning and visual intelligence. Medical imaging is defining the health state before actual symptoms are identified. Presently, Visual intelligence is playing a crucial role in disease diagnosis through X-rays, CT scan, PET scan, MRI, etc. It was enhanced through AI-enabled diagnosis systems. These systems are functioning based on centralized and limited training data models. Hence, technology-inclusive solutions by integrating Federated Learning (FL) with vision intelligence promises next-gen healthcare needs like personalized treatment, disease monitoring, and global collaborations.

REFERENCES

Abaoud, M., Almuqrin, M. A., & Khan, M. F. (2023). Advancing federated learning through novel mechanism for privacy preservation in healthcare applications. *IEEE Access : Practical Innovations, Open Solutions, 11*, 83562–83579. DOI: 10.1109/ACCESS.2023.3301162

Akter, M., Moustafa, N., Lynar, T., & Razzak, I. (2022). Edge intelligence: Federated learning-based privacy protection framework for smart healthcare systems. *IEEE Journal of Biomedical and Health Informatics, 26*(12), 5805–5816. DOI: 10.1109/JBHI.2022.3192648 PMID: 35857737

Ali, S., Hussain, A., Bhattacharjee, S., Athar, A., Abdullah, , & Kim, H.-C. (2022). Detection of COVID-19 in X-ray images using densely connected squeeze convolutional neural network (DCSCNN): Focusing on interpretability and explainability of the black box model. *Sensors (Basel), 22*(24), 10093. DOI: 10.3390/s22249983 PMID: 36560352

Alzubi, J. A., Alzubi, O. A., Singh, A., & Ramachandran, M. (2023). Cloud-IIoT-based electronic health record privacy-preserving by CNN and blockchain-enabled federated learning. *IEEE Transactions on Industrial Informatics, 19*(1), 1080–1087. DOI: 10.1109/TII.2022.3189170

Artesani, A., Bruno, A., Gelardi, F., & Chiti, A. (2024). Empowering PET: Harnessing deep learning for improved clinical insight. *European Radiology Experimental, 8*(1), 17. DOI: 10.1186/s41747-023-00413-1 PMID: 38321340

Asif, M., Shah, M. A., Khattak, H. A., Mussadiq, S., Ahmed, E., Nasr, E. A., & Rauf, H. T. (2023). Intracranial hemorrhage detection using parallel deep convolutional models and boosting mechanism. *Diagnostics (Basel), 13*(4), 652. DOI: 10.3390/diagnostics13040652 PMID: 36832137

Attia, Z. I., Noseworthy, P. A., Lopez-Jimenez, F., Asirvatham, S. J., Deshmukh, A. J., Gersh, B. J., Carter, R. E., Yao, X., Rabinstein, A. A., Erickson, B. J., Kapa, S., & Friedman, P. A. (2019). An artificial intelligence-enabled ECG algorithm for the identification of patients with atrial fibrillation during sinus rhythm: A retrospective analysis of outcome prediction. *Lancet, 394*(10201), 861–867. DOI: 10.1016/S0140-6736(19)31721-0 PMID: 31378392

Awan, M. J., Rahim, M. S. M., Salim, N., Nobanee, H., Asif, A. A., & Attiq, M. O. (2023). MGACA-Net: A novel deep learning-based multi-scale guided attention and context aggregation for localization of knee anterior cruciate ligament tears region in MRI images. *PeerJ. Computer Science*, *9*, e1483. DOI: 10.7717/peerj-cs.1483 PMID: 37547408

Bonawitz, K., Eichner, H., Grieskamp, W., Huba, D., Ingerman, A., Ivkin, N., Kiddon, C., Konecny, J., Mazzocchi, S., McMahan, H. B., Overvelde, A., Petrou, D., Ramage, D., Roselander, J., & van Overveldt, T. (2019). Towards federated learning at scale: System design. *Proceedings of the 3rd MLSys Conference.*

Cao, R., Freitas, C., Chan, L., Sun, M., Jiang, H., & Chen, Z. (2017). ProLanGO: Protein function prediction using neural machine translation based on a recurrent neural network. *Molecules (Basel, Switzerland)*, *22*(10), 1732. DOI: 10.3390/molecules22101732 PMID: 29039790

Chaddad, A., Wu, Y., & Desrosiers, C. (2024). Federated learning for healthcare applications. *IEEE Internet of Things Journal*, *11*(5), 7339–7358. DOI: 10.1109/JIOT.2023.3325822

Chen, H., Wang, H., Long, Q., Jin, D., & Li, Y. (2024). Advancements in Federated Learning: Models, Methods, and Privacy. *ACM Computing Surveys, 57*(2), 1-39. DOI: 10.1145/3664650

Chen, M., Hao, Y., Hwang, K., Wang, L., & Wang, L. (2020). Machine learning for healthcare. *IEEE Access : Practical Innovations, Open Solutions*, *7*, 2169–3536. DOI: 10.1109/ACCESS.2020.2992340

Chen, Y., Lu, W., Qin, X., Wang, J., & Xie, X. (2024). MetaFed: Federated learning among federations with cyclic knowledge distillation for personalized healthcare. *IEEE Transactions on Neural Networks and Learning Systems*, *35*(11), 16671–16682. DOI: 10.1109/TNNLS.2023.3297103 PMID: 37506019

Clauwaert, J., Menschaert, G., & Waegeman, W. (2019). DeepRibo: A neural network for precise gene annotation of prokaryotes by combining ribosome profiling signal and binding site patterns. *Nucleic Acids Research*, *47*(6, e36), e36. DOI: 10.1093/nar/gkz061 PMID: 30753697

Elayan, H., Aloqaily, M., & Guizani, M. (2022). Sustainability of healthcare data analysis IoT-based systems using deep federated learning. *IEEE Internet of Things Journal*, *9*(10), 7338–7346. DOI: 10.1109/JIOT.2021.3103635

European Society of Radiology. (2019). What the radiologist should know about artificial intelligence: An ESR white paper. *Insights Into Imaging*, *10*(1), 44. DOI: 10.1186/s13244-019-0738-2 PMID: 30949865

Fleurence, R., Bian, J., Wang, X., Xu, H., Dawoud, D., Higashi, M., & Chhatwal, J. (2024). Generative AI for Health Technology Assessment: Opportunities, Challenges, and Policy Considerations. *arXiv preprint arXiv:2407.11054.*

Gad, G., & Fadlullah, Z. (2022). Federated Learning via Augmented Knowledge Distillation for Heterogenous Deep Human Activity Recognition Systems. *Sensors (Basel)*, *23*(1), 6. DOI: 10.3390/s23010006 PMID: 36616609

Gupta, A., Maurya, M. K., Dhere, K., & Chaurasiya, V. K. (2024). Privacy-preserving hybrid federated learning framework for mental healthcare applications: Clustered and quantum approaches. *IEEE Access : Practical Innovations, Open Solutions*, *12*, 145054–145068. DOI: 10.1109/ACCESS.2024.3464240

Hamza, A., Khan, M. A., Wang, S.-H., Alhaisoni, M., Alharbi, M., Hussain, H. S., Alshazly, H., Kim, Y. J., & Cha, J. (2022). COVID-19 classification using chest X-ray images based on fusion-assisted deep Bayesian optimization and Grad-CAM visualization. *Frontiers in Public Health, 10*. .DOI: 10.3389/fpubh.2022.890356

Huo, D., & Wang, X. (2024). A new era in healthcare: The integration of artificial intelligence and microbial. *Medicine in Novel Technology and Devices*, *23*, 100319. DOI: 10.1016/j.medntd.2024.100319

Illimoottil, M., & Ginat, D. (2023). Recent advances in deep learning and medical imaging for head and neck cancer treatment: MRI, CT, and PET scans. *Cancers (Basel)*, *15*(13), 3267. DOI: 10.3390/cancers15133267 PMID: 37444376

Jiang, X., Zhang, J., & Zhang, L. (2023). FedRadar: Federated multi-task transfer learning for radar-based Internet of Medical Things. *IEEE Transactions on Network and Service Management*, *20*(2), 1459–1469. DOI: 10.1109/TNSM.2023.3281133

Jin, T., Pan, S., Li, X., & Chen, S. (2023). Metadata and image features co-aware personalized federated learning for smart healthcare. *IEEE Journal of Biomedical and Health Informatics*, *27*(8), 4110–4119. DOI: 10.1109/JBHI.2023.3279096 PMID: 37220032

Kaissis, G., Makowski, M. R., Rückert, D., & Braren, R. F. (2021). Secure, privacy-preserving and federated machine learning in medical imaging. *Nature Machine Intelligence*, *3*(6), 473–484. DOI: 10.1038/s42256-021-00337-8

Khosa, I., Raza, A., Anjum, M., Ahmad, W., & Shahab, S. (2023). Automatic diabetic foot ulcer recognition using multi-level thermographic image data. *Diagnostics (Basel), 13*(11), 2637. DOI: 10.3390/diagnostics13162637 PMID: 37627896

Kumar, N., Verma, R., Sharma, S., Bhargava, S., Vahadane, A., & Sethi, A. (2017). A dataset and a technique for generalized nuclear segmentation for computational pathology. *IEEE Transactions on Medical Imaging, 36*(7), 1550–1560. DOI: 10.1109/TMI.2017.2677499 PMID: 28287963

Kumar, V. D., Rajesh, P., Geman, O., Craciun, M. D., Arif, M., & Filip, R. (2023). "Quo vadis diagnosis": Application of informatics in early detection of pneumothorax. *Diagnostics (Basel), 13*(6), 1305. DOI: 10.3390/diagnostics13071305 PMID: 37046523

Li, T., Sahu, A. K., Talwalkar, A., & Smith, V. (2020). Federated learning: Challenges, methods, and future directions. *IEEE Signal Processing Magazine, 37*(3), 50–60. DOI: 10.1109/MSP.2020.2975749

Liew, A., Agaian, S., & Benbelkacem, S. (2023). Distinctions between choroidal neovascularization and age-related macular degeneration in ocular disease predictions via multi-size kernels ξcho-weighted median patterns. *Diagnostics (Basel), 13*(4), 729. DOI: 10.3390/diagnostics13040729 PMID: 36832215

Lin, K.-H., Lu, N.-H., Okamoto, T., Huang, Y.-H., Liu, K.-Y., Matsushima, A., Chang, C.-C., & Chen, T.-B. (2023). Fusion-extracted features by deep networks for improved COVID-19 classification with chest X-ray radiography. *Health Care, 11*(10), 1367. DOI: 10.3390/healthcare11101367 PMID: 37239653

Lyu, Y., Yu, X., Zhu, D., & Zhang, L. (2022). Classification of Alzheimer's disease via vision transformer. In *Proceedings of the 15th International Conference on Pervasive Technologies Related to Assistive Environments* (pp. 463–468). New York, NY: Association for Computing Machinery. DOI: 10.1145/3529190.3534754

Maliyaem, M., Tuan, N. M., Lockhart, D., & Muenthong, S. (2022). A study of using machine learning in predicting COVID-19 cases. *Cloud Computing and Data Science, 3*(2), 92–99. DOI: 10.37256/ccds.3220221488

Mazumdar, H., Chakraborty, C., Sathvik, M., Mukhopadhyay, S., & Panigrahi, P. K. (2023). GPTFX: A Novel GPT-3 Based Framework for Mental Health Detection and Explanations. *IEEE Journal of Biomedical and Health Informatics*. Advance online publication. DOI: 10.1109/JBHI.2023.3328350 PMID: 37903039

McMahan, H. B., Moore, E., Ramage, D., Hampson, S., & Arcas, B. A. y. (2017). Communication-efficient learning of deep networks from decentralized data. In *Proceedings of the 20th International Conference on Artificial Intelligence and Statistics (AISTATS)*.

Murmu, A., Kumar, P., Moparthi, N. R., Namasudra, S., & Lorenz, P. (2024). Reliable federated learning with GAN model for robust and resilient future healthcare system. *IEEE Transactions on Network and Service Management*, *21*(5), 5335–5346. DOI: 10.1109/TNSM.2024.3422376

Myrzashova, R., Alsamhi, S. H., Shvetsov, A. V., Hawbani, A., & Wei, X. (2023). Blockchain meets federated learning in healthcare: A systematic review with challenges and opportunities. *IEEE Internet of Things Journal*, *10*(16), 14418–14437. DOI: 10.1109/JIOT.2023.3263598

Najjar, R. (2023). Redefining Radiology: A Review of Artificial Intelligence Integration in Medical Imaging. *Diagnostics (Basel)*, *13*(17), 2760. DOI: 10.3390/diagnostics13172760 PMID: 37685300

Ni, W., Ao, H., Tian, H., Eldar, Y. C., & Niyato, D. (2024). FedSL: Federated split learning for collaborative healthcare analytics on resource-constrained wearable IoMT devices. *IEEE Internet of Things Journal*, *11*(10), 18934–18935. DOI: 10.1109/JIOT.2024.3370985

Rieke, N., Hancox, J., Li, W., Milletarì, F., Roth, H. R., Albarqouni, S., Bakas, S., Galtier, M. N., Landman, B. A., Maier-Hein, K., Ourselin, S., Sheller, M., Summers, R. M., Trask, A., Xu, D., Baust, M., & Cardoso, M. J. (2020). The future of digital health with federated learning. *NPJ Digital Medicine*, *3*(1), 119. DOI: 10.1038/s41746-020-00323-1 PMID: 33015372

SachinD. N., Annappa, B., Hegde, S., Abhijit, C. S., & Ambesange, S. (2024). Fed-Cure: A heterogeneity-aware personalized federated learning framework for intelligent healthcare applications in IoMT environments. *IEEE Access : Practical Innovations, Open Solutions*, *12*, 15867–15883. DOI: 10.1109/ACCESS.2024.3357514

Sai, S., Hassija, V., Chamola, V., & Guizani, M. (2024). Federated learning and NFT-based privacy-preserving medical-data-sharing scheme for intelligent diagnosis in smart healthcare. *IEEE Internet of Things Journal*, *11*(4), 5568–5577. DOI: 10.1109/JIOT.2023.3308991

Sezer, A., Sigirci, I. O., & Sezer, H. B. (2017). Shoulder lesion classification using shape and texture fcatures via composite kernel. In *Proceedings of the 25th Signal Processing and Communications Applications Conference (SIU)* (pp. 1–4). Antalya, Turkey. DOI: 10.1109/SIU.2017.7960658

Sheller, M. J., Edwards, B., Reina, G. A., Martin, J., Pati, S., Kotrotsou, A., Milchenko, M., Xu, W., Marcus, D., Colen, R. R., & Bakas, S. (2020). Federated learning in medicine: Facilitating multi-institutional collaborations without sharing patient data. *Scientific Reports*, *10*(1), 12598. DOI: 10.1038/s41598-020-69250-1 PMID: 32724046

Tanim, S. A., Aurnob, A. R., Mridha, M. F., Safran, M., Alfarhood, S., & Che, D. (2024). Secure federated learning for Parkinson's disease: Non-IID data partitioning and homomorphic encryption strategies. *IEEE Access : Practical Innovations, Open Solutions*, *12*, 127309–127327. DOI: 10.1109/ACCESS.2024.3454690

Tian, Y., Wang, S., Xiong, J., Bi, R., Zhou, Z., & Bhuiyan, M. Z. A. (2024). Robust and privacy-preserving decentralized deep federated learning training: Focusing on digital healthcare applications. *IEEE/ACM Transactions on Computational Biology and Bioinformatics*, *21*(4), 890–901. DOI: 10.1109/TCBB.2023.3243932 PMID: 37028039

Ullah, F., Srivastava, G., Xiao, H., Ullah, S., Lin, J. C.-W., & Zhao, Y. (2024). A scalable federated learning approach for collaborative smart healthcare systems with intermittent clients using medical imaging. *IEEE Journal of Biomedical and Health Informatics*, *28*(6), 3293–3304. DOI: 10.1109/JBHI.2023.3282955 PMID: 37279135

Umapathy, V. R., Rajinikanth, B. S., Samuel Raj, R. D., Yadav, S., Munavarah, S. A., Anandapandian, P. A., Mary, A. V., & Padmavathy, K. (2023). Perspective of artificial intelligence in disease diagnosis: A review of current and future endeavours in the medical field. *Cureus*, *15*(9), e45684. DOI: 10.7759/cureus.45684 PMID: 37868519

Xu, J., Glicksberg, B. S., Su, C., Walker, P., & Chen, R. (2021). Federated learning for healthcare informatics. *Journal of Healthcare Informatics Research*, *5*(1), 1–19. Advance online publication. DOI: 10.1007/s41666-020-00082-4 PMID: 33204939

Xu, Z.-H., Fan, D.-G., Huang, J.-Q., Wang, J.-W., Wang, Y., & Li, Y.-Z. (2023). Computer-aided diagnosis of laryngeal cancer based on deep learning with laryngoscopic images. *Diagnostics (Basel)*, *13*(24), 3669. DOI: 10.3390/diagnostics13243669 PMID: 38132254

Zebin, T., & Rezvy, S. (2021). COVID-19 detection and disease progression visualization: Deep learning on chest X-rays for classification and coarse localization. *Applied Intelligence*, *51*(2), 1010–1021. DOI: 10.1007/s10489-020-01867-1 PMID: 34764549

Zeydan, E., Arslan, S. S., & Liyanage, M. (2024). Managing distributed machine learning lifecycle for healthcare data in the cloud. *IEEE Access : Practical Innovations, Open Solutions*, *12*, 115750–115774. DOI: 10.1109/ACCESS.2024.3443520

Zhang, C. (2022). "Federated Learning Meets Blockchain in Edge Computing: Challenges and Solutions". IEEE Communications Surveys & Tutorials.,https://ieeexplore.ieee.org/stamp/stamp.jsp?arnumber=9403374

Zhang, H., & Qie, Y. (2023). Applying deep learning to medical imaging: A review. *Applied Sciences (Basel, Switzerland)*, *13*(18), 10521. DOI: 10.3390/app131810521

Chapter 10

Unleashing Sensors and Wearable Technologies in Gauging Healthcare Transmuting Digital Health Technologies:

Nurturing Innovation and Implementations in Human Augmentation

Rhishikesh Dave
https://orcid.org/0009-0005-7193-0728
Sharda University, India

Bhupinder Singh
https://orcid.org/0009-0006-4779-2553
Sharda University, India

ABSTRACT

With the use of sensors and wearable technologies, real-time monitoring of a patient and personalized care as well as create these human augmentation applications that are changing the face of digital health technologies. The use of sensors has moved beyond the lab to small, tagged and band-like devices that are released in various form factors like round or wider devices. AI combined with wearable sensors will take data analysis to a whole new level which enabling distant and proactive diagnostics, earlier interventions, and personalized treatments. With the help of wearables, RPM

DOI: 10.4018/979-8-3693-6094-1.ch010

drastically reduces hospital visits and increases healthcare access to such an extent that even underserved areas would have a fair opportunity to quality health care. While they continue to grow, the possibilities for human augmentation, quality of life and health delivery will develop rapidly through a more connected, proactive and data-driven ecosystem.

1. INTRODUCTION

Wearable technology which includes medical-grade devices, smart watches and fitness trackers is enabling a person to control chronic health issues and keep away diseases and stay healthy. In recent years, there has been a considerable transformation in the healthcare industry, powered mainly by technological developments that embed sensors and wearable devices into the way health is monitored an care is delivered to the patient. Not only have these advances drastically changed the way medical data is captured, processed and put to use, but it has also redefined the dynamics of a patient-healthcare provider interaction (Khan et al., 2020). This convergence of sensors and internet of things (IoT) with wearable technology is revolutionizing healthcare delivery as it allows users to keep check on their health in real-time which in return helps the healthcare professionals diagnose, treat more effectively than ever before.

Wearable technology in health has come a long since the time when it measured fitness trackers and heart rate. At first, these devices were marketed towards health nuts who wanted to keep track of how active they were in terms of steps and calories per day. But over the years, improvements in sensor technology and miniaturization have sparked a new wave of more advanced devices that can read different kinds of biometric data like heart rate variability, blood oxygen levels (which is an indication for sleep apnea), sleep tracking as well as the ability to track blood glucose levels or even electrocardiograms (ECGs) privacy is still important. This paradigm shifted wearable speeds from recreational fitness devices to medical-grade wearables used in clinical, disease management and preventative medicine (Rani, 2022).

These wearables devices have an array of sensors attached that are used to constantly take measurements of various physiological parameters and transmit them wirelessly to healthcare platforms for further analysis. As a result of this feature, remote patient monitoring (RPM) systems have been developed so that patients can be monitored by healthcare providers in real-time from anywhere without having to be physically present at the hospital or clinic. RPM has been especially beneficial in the combat against lifelong conditions like diabetes, hypertension, and heart issues as it requires a watch on these elements round-the-clock to ensure appropriate management. These technologies have also shown their value in the wake of the

COVID-19 pandemic, when they enabled fewer visits to hospitals and telemedicine consultations thus reducing exposure to the virus. The evolution of wearable sensors with an Internet of Things (IOT) device has extended their usability. Wearable devices can connect to other health measurement systems, also enabling them to securely transmit data electronically via IoT connectivity for example: with cloud storage systems at home-based health hubs or smart medical devices. This comprehensive and collaborative ecosystem is just the type of system you need to gather and exchange data transparently, making all patient information available in real time for health predictions while allowing healthcare personnel to take immediate actions. In addition, IoT embedded wearables further the customization of healthcare using own health data, life habits and genetic predispositions for individualized recommendations and interventions.

Figure 1. display the Dimensions of Introduction Section (Source- Self Prepared-Original)

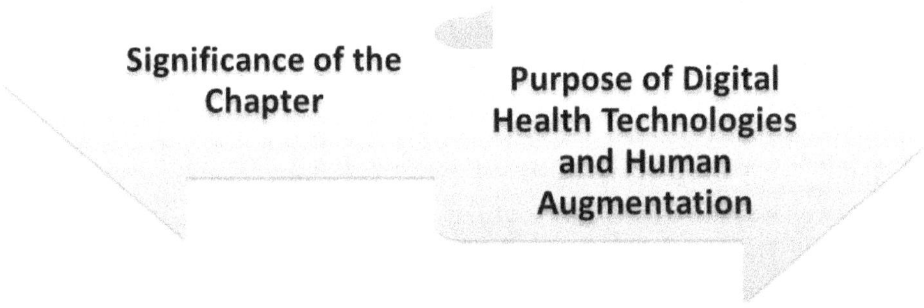

1.1 Significance of the Chapter

Artificial intelligence (AI) is integral to the growth of wearables, especially in terms of data analysis and health management forecasting. Wearable devices generate large amounts of data and this data needs to be treated with advanced algorithms to extract trends, outliers, actions. Using Artificial intelligence based analytics to capture early symptoms of the diseases, and notifying the user as well as doctors about the possible appearance of an ailment so that necessary actions can be taken on time. This move towards more proactive healthcare, rather than reactive treatment, is an opportunity to lower long-term health costs and provide better patient outcomes other than creating overall efficiency in the system of care.

Similarly, the development of wearable health-tech has been propelled by strides in one major field: Human augmentation. Because these technologies are becoming at tracking basic health data, but with a focus on augmenting human performance. Per capita, the defense sector and its contractors typically spend 4-5 orders of magnitude more on driverless tanks than you do not to break your femur in a drunken fall into the Grand Canyon are thousands-for-now wearables like passive exoskeletons and someday-maybe it web-linked locally invasive neural interface devices that make little tasks accessible. There are also an array of wearables being designed for cognitive enhancement, meant to assist people in memory improvement, focus and learning. The overlap between wearables and human augmentation is also driving a new era of personalized medicine and precision health; where treatments are designed to cater for the individual needs and capabilities.

While there have been great strides in wearable health tech over time, many issues hang in the balance The issues of data privacy, security and patient consent continue to trouble, underscored even further because wearables are collecting large amounts of deeply personal health information. Furthermore, standardization of regulations and frameworks is essential to guarantee the interoperability as well as safety of these devices especially when used in clinical practices. Overcoming these challenges will be essential for truly unleashing the capabilities of sensors and wearables as medical technologies (Ahirwar & Khan, 2022). The development of Sensors and wearable technology in healthcare represents a very important paradigm change where as well as observing, health is also being regulated and managed along with optimization. There is a complex array of emerging wellness technologies ranging from simple fitness trackers to burgeoning AI-powered medical devices that are not only improving personal health but are also revolutionising how healthcare functions as an industry. With wearables only going to become more advanced and integrated with other technologies over time, they have the potential to help build a more seamless and connected healthcare ecosystem that is really centered around the patient, bringing us ever closer to a future where health monitoring and human augmentation blend in the background of everyday life (Han et al., 2020).

1.2 Purpose of Digital Health Technologies and Human Augmentation

There has also been rapid growth in the field of digital health powered by advanced technologies like wearables, artificial intelligence (AI), Internet of Things (IoT), and

Big Data analytics frequently used as a part of everyday health management. The advancements allow for Real-Time Monitoring, Predictive Analytics and Customized Care ultimately resulting in better outcomes and lower costs (Pramanik et al., 2022). Continuous collection of physiological data takes place through wearable devices, such as fitness trackers, smartwatches or medical-grade sensors and makes meaningful inferences for individuals and their healthcare providers in health and treatment decisions. Digital health technologies are paving the way for preventive healthcare providing proactive alerts and remote patient monitoring.

The new and developing field of human augmentation refers to technologies that enhance human abilities. Augmentation devices such as exoskeletons and neural interface devices help patients with physical disabilities to walk again, and gain mobility, independence in healthcare. Brain-computer interfaces like cognitive augmentation tools improve memory, attention, and learning. By capabilities we are not only helping disable people, by reaching new horizons where human body and mind perform better. These combined can change the healthcare landscape into a more personalised medicine, empowering patients to do their own health care and to improve quality of life for patients with chronic conditions or disabilities, while also providing capability enhancement technologies for healthy people (Nazari, 2020).

2. FUNDAMENTALS OF SENSORS AND WEARABLE TECHNOLOGIES IN HEALTHCARE

Among many powerful applications of the new data sets, real-time health parameters from sensors and wearable technologies are leading forces in the digital health revolution with their novel prospects for continuous health monitoring, disease management, and prophylaxis. At their core, new-age technologies require the capability to sense and quantify different physiological & environmental parameters -ultimately converting these into health data that can be acted upon. The core of this technology is its sensors which are present in wearable technologies such as smartwatches, sports t-shirts, smart clothing and implantable medical devices (Sahil & Kaushik, 2022). Wearable technologies rely on a variety of sensors that are specialized to measure specific physiological signals. There are many different kinds of them, but the most typical are as-

Electrochemical Sensors: Biomarkers such as glucose in diabetic patients By using these sensors, one can monitor the blood sugar levels in real-time through a small device called continuous glucose monitors(CGMS) which makes managing of this disease much better.

Optical Sensors- Optical sensors used for heart rate measurement are based on the principle of reflection or transmission where light-emitting diodes (LEDs) and photodetectors collect changes in blood flow at the skin level. These sensors can also be found in many smartwatches.

Accelerometers and Gyroscopes (Motion Sensors)- These motion-sensing technologies measure movement and orientation. These are frequently employed in fitness trackers, as well as the simultaneous detection of falls within elderly patients, and therefore alerting help. Temperature sensors which monitor fever or infection like in wearables patches or smart thermometers.

Electromyography (EMG) Sensors: which identify the electrical signals of active muscles, a useful part of muscle rehabilitation devices and exoskeletons that enable added mobility.

Figure 2. shares the Types of Sensors (Source- Self Prepared- Original)

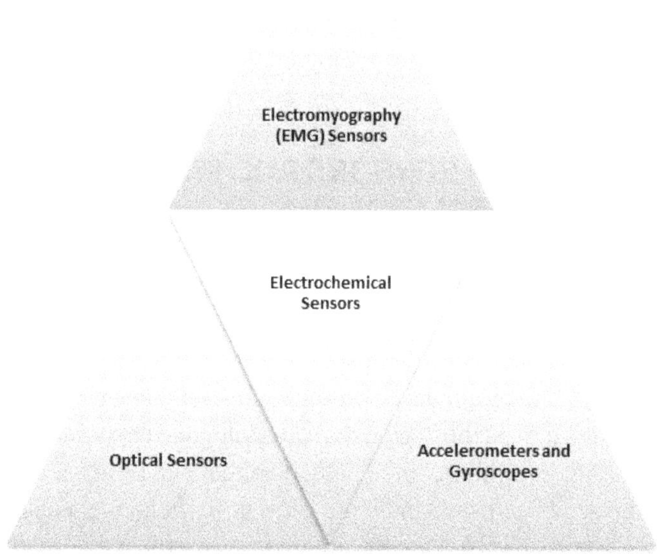

These sensors record data and relay that to certain other devices or cloud, through technology like Bluetooth, Wi-Fi or cellular connectivity. Wearable technologies integrate these sensors into body-worn gadgets for around-the-clock health monitoring beyond clinical settings. This has transformed the way we manage chronic diseases, preventative care and patient engagement. Wearables like smartwatches that can track heart rate, detect arrhythmias, and even record rudimentary electrocardiograms (ECGs) which could be sent to a doctor for remote diagnostics. These devices are essential components in Remote Patient Monitoring (RPM) as it facilitates continuous collection of data, hence enabling health care providers to monitor patients with chronic conditions like diabetes, hypertension, and cardiovascular diseases (Oukhatar et al., 2021). As such, RPM can alleviate the necessity for re-admissions to hospitals, lowering healthcare costs and at the same time offering better patient outcomes. Also, wearables sensors aided contactless monitoring during the COVID-19 pandemic and helped to keep viral transmission at bay in healthcare facilities.

2.1 Integration of Data Analytics and AI

These devices generate large amounts of data that is then used to analyze by means of artificial intelligence (AI) and machine learning (ML) algorithms to provide meaningful information. Based on these data analytics, potential health issues can be anticipated and intervention can take place before any symptoms arise (He & Eastburn, 2022). Wearable devices, for example, are now capable of picking up on irregular heart rhythms and if deployed properly could help to avoid strokes or even heart attacks by quickly alerting the user that he or she needs to see a doctor. AI also determines healthcare hyper-customizable, enjoining medications and treatments directed by a person's health history and behaviors.

There are many advantages, but sensors and wearables in healthcare still have a lot to deal with like data security and privacy including regulatory approval. Securing the data transmitted from health systems to our dashboard is very important as this could help in protecting the patient trust and also complying with healthcare regulations like HIPAA. Nevertheless, with the advancement of wearable technologies, they are providing a huge set of new possibilities to revolutionise healthcare by giving patients and doctors tools for continuous monitoring, early detection and better disease management (Mujawar et al., 2020). Overall, sensors & wearable devices are a radical development of the health systems by providing real-time monitoring, diagnostics and treatment and preparing us for personalized & preventive care.

3. INNOVATIONS IN WEARABLE TECHNOLOGIES FOR HEALTHCARE

From basic fitness trackers and simple step counter, the healthcare industry as a whole has been taken through an impressive transformation by wearable technology. Wearables constitute a vital role in the current wave of innovation in healthcare, with capabilities now stretching all the way to real-time monitoring and diagnostics, disease management, and even therapeutic interventions. These devices, equipped with high-end sensors, are allowing patients as well as healthcare providers to track a comprehensive set of health parameters from any location in order to enhance patient outcomes and drive down costs while encouraging preventive patient engagement.

The most groundbreaking invention in wearable health technology till date has to be that of advanced biometric monitoring systems. While the earliest versions of wearables could track steps, calories burned and heart rate, newer forms of this tool can do things like monitor both respiratory levels, blood oxygen saturation levels. Today, modern devices can track heart rate variability (HRV), oxygen saturation (SpO2) levels, blood pressure and record an electrocardiogram (ECG). There are now consumer health products, such as the Apple Watch or Fitbit, with heart features that are able to identify atrial fibrillation or irregular heart rhythms and inform users that they should seek medical attention if needed. In the same way that wearable glucose monitors, such as Continuous Glucose Monitors (CGMs), have transformed how we manage diabetes. Offering a more complete or less invasive alternative to typical finger-prick tests, these devices keep track of blood sugar levels. As with the hybrid closed-loop design, technological developments move steadily forward, and many CGM devices are now integrated with insulin pumps to offer a closed loop system that performs real-time glucose data analysis in order to automatically adjust insulin delivery an operation colloquially known as an artificial pancreas.

3.1 Wearable Technologies in Chronic Disease Care

Wearables prove to have significant benefits in dealing with chronic diseases like cardiovascular problems, diabetes, respiratory conditions as well as mental health disorders. They serve as a continuous, real-time data stream that helps patients not to just get by but thrive between clinical settings. Patients can track variations wearing blood pressure monitors, and share these with their healthcare providers from the comfort of home (Udoh et al., 2023). Also patients living with chronic respiratory conditions like asthma or chronic obstructive pulmonary disease (COPD) can utilize wearables to monitor their oxygen levels and recognize signs of exacerbation at an early stage prompt for intervention.

Wearable technology is progressing in the mental health space as well. By tracking markers like heart rate variability and sleep patterns, devices can provide data about the levels of stress, anxiety or depression. Wearables even provide biofeedback, intervening with a user who may be too stressed or anxious, offering breathing exercises or other relaxation triggers to help improve their mental state.

3.2 Clothing and Implantable

Wearable tech is not all about devices worn on wrists. Earlier, smart fabrics led to the emergence of smart clothing that can sense data on health parameters due to the sensors integrated into fabric. Smart shirts can quantify things like respiratory rate, heart rate, and muscle activation, thus making them useful applications for fitness buffs and patients in recovery whether this includes post-surgery or injury. They could even be woven into tomorrow's clothing to add seamless health monitoring with little in the way of additional burden. The other breakthrough in wearables for healthcare is implantable devices, or also known colloquially as "ingestible" or "implantable wearables." These devices provide unobtrusive, long-term monitoring of internal physiological processes and are implanted under the skin or ingested. Many implantable cardiac monitors, for example, are used to record temporal heart function and so can be the basis of diagnoses for questions like arrhythmias or heart failure. The devices also limit the need for frequent medical appointments and address patient monitoring in real-time (Chelliah et al., 2021).

3.3 Integration as Artificial Intelligence & Data Analytics

But while AI and data analytics have been pivotal points of innovation within wearable health products, the common denominator remains: How much of 'time to market' can be met reliably within your budget. With wearables producing data in mass volume it must be sophisticated algorithms that do the heavy lifting of data analysis and interpretation. A platform powered by AI would track trends, identify deviations from those trends and predict health issues before they become critical (Materon et al., 2021). The example is AI models that employ algorithms to examine ECG data from wearables, to help catch early signs of heart disease and possibly avoid a heart attack or stroke. AI provides personalized healthcare by adapting recommendations and interventions to personal data. Fitness trackers using AI, for instance, could provide a user with individualized exercise regimes and diet advice that take into account the person's levels of activity, sleep-state data and metabolic rate. These devices can be used in clinical settings to help diagnose diseases by comparing patient data with large medical databases, thus increasing the accuracy and speed of diagnosis (Kumar & Kumari, 2021).

3.4 Telemedicine and Remote Care on Wearables

The COVID-19 pandemic caused a spike in demand for telemedicine, and wearables have become increasingly important to providing remote care. Wearable devices can monitor health in real time, providing access to care that doesn't require patients to come into healthcare facilities. Remote patient monitoring (RPM) systems with wearables can track vital signs and health metrics, and if such data is being pushed to care providers in real-time, it can trigger rapid follow-up care. Therefore, it relieves the pressure off healthcare systems and means that patients get treatments when they most need them (Vivejananthan et al., 2022). The belief was that wearable technologies are in a rapid evolution and those advances can change healthcare. Wearables are going to be among the most exciting developments in Healthcare soon, this is a platform that can actually follow our lifestyle in unlimited ways depending on every citizens unique healthcare needs for anything from chronic illness monitoring, remote care, AI powered diagnostic and smart textile solutions. As these technologies mature, they have the power to revolutionize medicine by providing more proactive, personalized and global patient care than ever before (Pradhan et al., 2023).

4. IMPLEMENTATIONS IN HUMAN AUGMENTATION AND HEALTH ENHANCEMENT: APPLICATIONS IN HUMAN AUGMENTATION AND MEDICAL ASSISTANCE

The emerging field of human augmentation where technology is used to push the capabilities of our physical bodies, as well as improve cognitive function is having a profound impact on healthcare. Through the development of wearables, implantable technology and artificial intelligence (AI) new ways to promote health and manage disabilities as well as augment human ability beyond our evolutionary limits have been made possible. Human augmentation for the purpose of health exceeds cure or rehabilitation to include performance enhancement, preventive strategies, and enablement of super-human physical and cognitive powers (Manogaran et al., 2021). The range of applications in human augmentation is wide and includes physical, cognitive, and sensory prostheses that offer a variety of benefits to enhance better health outcomes and improved quality of life.

A key area of expertise for human augmentation in healthcare is physical augmentation, focused on restoring or enhancing physical mobility. This is particularly meaningful to people with disabilities and recovering from injury. Exoskeletons are wearable robotic devices that enhance human movements and have been developed as a solution to transform rehabilitation and mobility assistance. They are actually exoskeleton, that assist people paraplegics due to their injuries in spinal cord or resulted from a stroke or degenerative diseases, like the multiple sclerosis. Such instruments are developed to help the same muscles that have been unable to work or not have sufficient strength so that an individual can stand and even walk, this helps them do things they might not able to do before (Suma, 2021).

Exoskeletons as a means of enhancing the performance of healthy individuals Besides restoring mobility, exoskeletons are now being used to enhance the performance of healthy individuals. Exoskeletons help industrial workers by improving their muscular capacity, indirectly reducing the physical strain and risk of injury.

This kind of augmentation improves human physical capabilities and durability, making manpower less safe while at the same time more efficient. The limbs count as a form of physical enhancement, but prosthetics have advanced massively in recent years with the addition of sensors and neural interfaces. Thought-controlled artificial limbs that respond to signals sent out by the brain or muscle, allowing for a closer approximation of nature movement than ever before (Jenkins, 2022). These advanced bionic limbs with sensing and actuating capabilities enable the user precisely touch to grasp an object or type on a keyboard which drastically improve the quality of life for amputees.

Memory, attention and learning technologies fall into the category of cognitive augmentation. Among them the most auspicious domains is Brain-Computer Interface (BCIs) which harnesses the communication between brain and devices. BCIs are presently being utilised to help in the case of neurological illness like amyotrophic parallel sclerosis (ALS), bolted in disorder or then again serious spinal injuries (Malik & Kumar, 2022). Via these interfaces, people are able to actuate computers, or prosthetic limbs and communication devices with their thought alone, dispense of the need for any physical movement. People with cognitive impairments associated with aging or disease, such as Alzheimer's, to use these types of technologies to assist them in maintaining and even enhancing their cognitive functions. Wearable neuro-stimulation devices such as the former employ electrical or magnetic fields to improve memory/attention (Kumar et al., 2022). Wearable devices that sit on the head and are programmed to activate various areas of grey matter so they can operate better. Preliminary studies have indicated that neuro-stimulation could aid people with concentration, learning, and emotional control.

Cognitive enhancement is not just about making up for defects. Even healthy people are availing of cognitive augmentation technologies to boost cognitive performance. The popularity of mind-cleansing, stress-reducing and focus-increasing devices is sky-rocketing (Han, 2023). Muse, a headband that registers brain activity of meditation users to give biofeedback and has been shown to increase performance in cognitive tasks, is an example of modern wearables that help users instruct their mental health for the greatest level of well-being or enhancement.

Sensory Augmentation devices are specially designed types of equipment that enhance or mediate human senses such as vision, hearing or touch. Well-known examples are cochlear implants, which allow deaf people to hear. This device is implanted and it side-steps the fubar-ed parts of your ear to deliver direct stimulation to the auditory nerve giving patients sound! Newer models of cochlear implants with advanced technology include wireless connections, so the devices can be monitored for proper functioning and adjusted remotely by healthcare providers based on data that are transmitted in real time. Visual augmentation tech is being worked on (the equivalent of robotic limbs and exoskeletons but for parallax), embodied in such features as retinal implants or smart glasses for either replacing vision or providing additional information to sight. Manufactured by Pixium Vision, these retinal implants bionic eyes, if you will offer a way to address blindness in people for whom the problem lies within the retina itself the membrane of light-sensing cells at the back of the eye that converts incoming light into electrical signals sent via the optic nerve to the brain. The brain then relays these signals to the rest of the body, and so on, which is how it think that shapes come in light.

Wearable technologies are not restricted to giving back what has been lost but extending the human capacity for sensing in normal individuals. For example, smart glasses with augmented reality (AR) features can display a layer of digital information on the user's physical space. One of the areas is medical training and surgery where AR glasses can be used to show patient data or guide surgeons during surgeries in real-time. Implantables are a big step forward in human augmentation with the potential to provide continuous monitoring and intervention for chronic health conditions. For example, pacemakers have been around for a very long time to help manage heart rhythms but those in use today are wifi enabled and come with an AI monitoring app. These versions are able to change performance on the fly depending on activity or other health metrics in order to be more responsive and use resources only when needed.

Measurable data from implanted devices can be sent to clinicians for ongoing monitoring and medical interventions preemptively (Raghav et al., 2024). There are also advances in neural implants thought to have potential for neurological conditions such as Parkinson's disease, epilepsy and depression. To mitigate the symptoms of these conditions, a particular kind of neural implant, deep brain stimulation (DBS), sends electrical impulses to targeted regions in the brain. Neural implants are getting so advanced that they might start adjusting their own stimulation, using AI to alert us what electrical patterns are being executed and dynamically enforcing desired ones (Banerjee et al., 2020).

Human augmentation not only provides great opportunities for improving our health, but also acknowledges important challenges and ethical problems. Key concerns are relating to data privacy, security and long-term effects of enhancing human abilities (Barnes & Zvarikova, 2021). Given the amount of secure health related data that these devices could potentially store and transmit, it is critical to always have a handle on best practices or the proper procedure for when devices utilizes this even further powerful functions. In an expanded form, the ethical issue of using DBS to enhance human abilities beyond natural limits e.g. improved cognitive or physical functioning brings concerns about fairness, access and societal effects into question as well. Human augmentation to restore lost function, and enhance our abilities is changing healthcare for the better. Physical and cognitive augmentation, sensory enhancements, implantable devices; there are endless possibilities for improving human health outcomes and quality of life. The dawn of human augmentation technologies will usher in an era where healthcare is transformed into a domain unexplored, opening up to greater possibilities than ever before at the hands of patients and healthy people willing to harness their innate capabilities (Desai & Shende, 2021).

Figure 3. illuminates the Implementations in Human Augmentation and Health Enhancement (Source- Self Prepared- Original)

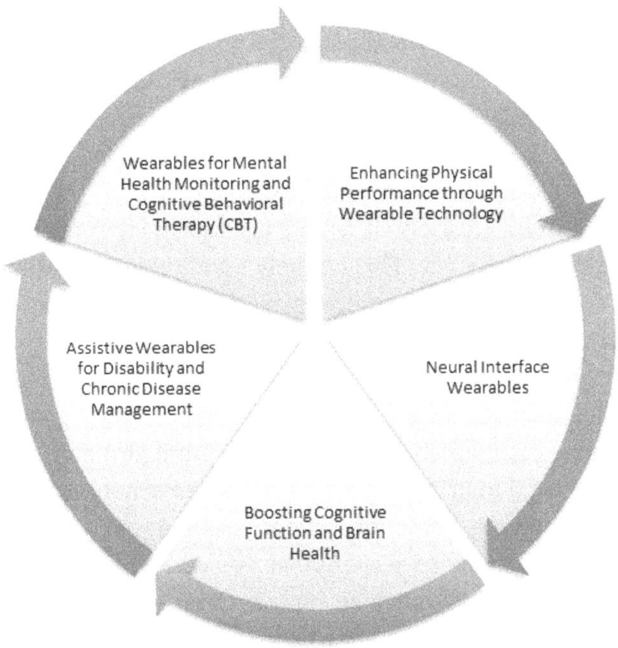

5. TRANSFORMING HEALTHCARE DELIVERY: REMOTE PATIENT MONITORING (RPM) AND TELEHEALTH

Remote Patient Monitoring (RPM) and telehealth technologies have been changing the way healthcare is delivered using real-time patient data acquisition, patients can take care away from hospitals (Hurley & Popescu, 2021). These innovations help to bridge the distance between patients and healthcare providers ensuring interventions are done in a timely manner leading to better health outcomes as well as convenience, especially for people in remote or underserved locations. RPM and telehealth have turned the more passive, traditional framework of in-person consultations on its head empowering proactive, personalized and inclusive care (Goel et al., 2021).

RPM takes advantage of digital technologies to collect health data from patients in between office visits, helping a healthcare provider monitor conditions such as hypertension, diabetes or heart disease on a real-time basis. Devices like blood pressure cuffs, glucose sensors and wearables (like smartwatches) take vital statistics and transfer them to a cloud-based platform for healthcare providers. Continuous Monitoring leads to early identification of issues and subsequent health problems leading thus promote hospital re-admissions, ER etc. For instance, RPM has proven to be extremely effective in monitoring chronic conditions. Patients can stay at home, and their healthcare providers will track their status and adjust treatments on the fly (Kumar et al., 2022). For example, RPM practitioners and heart failure patients can avoid expensive and distressing hospitalizations by allowing doctors to act early in case alarming patterns are detected.

The term thus covers a variety of remote healthcare services, from virtual consultations to remote diagnostics. This not only saves the patients time and effort in travelling for a single visit but also decongests from the public health institutions. Telehealth became extremely important for putting our pup pups onto the right track of comfort and care. Telehealth continues to be a vital aspect of contemporary healthcare service delivery, offering a way for people who cannot easily access their medical centres perhaps because they have limited mobility, living outside the urban areas, or need to keep on time with work or school. RPM and telehealth are transforming healthcare making it patient-centered, more effective, and easily available. By integrating these technologies together healthcare providers can deliver targeted interventions, enhance chronic disease management and improve patient outcomes more broadly creating a new world of digital connected healthcare (Huang et al., 2021).

6. CASE STUDIES: SUCCESSFUL IMPLEMENTATIONS OF WEARABLE HEALTH TECHNOLOGIES

Case Study 1: Wearable Device in Diabetes Management

The wearable devices have helped change the management of diabetes allowing for continuous monitoring of glucose levels helping the diabetic patients and healthcare personnel to well manage this condition. There have been implementations, however that teeter on the successful line such as Continuous Glucose Monitors (CGMs) with systems. The monitor checks glucose being continuously tracked also avoids a conventional finger-prick test. Utilizing small sensors under the skin to measure glucose in interstitial fluid, CGMs then deliver that data to a smartphone or an insulin pump.

Wearables that provide major benefits to diabetes type 1 and 2 patients. These devices are available as CGM (continuous glucose monitor), which are able to alarm subjects to hazardous changes on their bed level, such as hyperglycemia or hypoglycemia by providing 24/7 monitoring. Healthcare providers are also granted access to the data from CGMs so that they can be more well-informed as they craft treatment plans and decide when medication or dietary changes should be made. Numerous clinical studies that include use of CGMs have shown improved glycemic control, HbA1c levels and quality of life for patients. Delivering recommendations to adjust insulin, meal and exercise therapy in real time allows these tools to move diabetes management from reactive to proactive and individualized (Malik et al., 2021). Wearables including CGMs are revolutionizing diabetes management by providing constant and current data that can provide patients with the control they need to get better.

9.2 Case Study 2: Wearables in Cardiac Health Monitoring

With the advancement of wearable technologies, it has now become an integral part in monitoring our heart health, allowing us to catch these problems early or even prevent them altogether. Perhaps the most successful implementation is that of smartwatches such as the Apple Watch and Fitbit with electrocardiogram (ECG) sensors. The devices are capable of checking heart rate, identifying irregular rhythms and alerting unlocked users to the risk of atrial fibrillation (AFib), a serious form that can lead to strokes Wearable technology, such as Apple's Heart Study conducted with Stanford University, showed promise in cardiac monitoring. The study included more than 400,000 participants who were screened for irregular heart rhythms using the Apple Watch's ECG app. The findings indicated the device could pick up when somebody had AFib in a lot of cases, and that one thing would trigger people to see their doctor with enough time left before something worse happened (Kumar et al., 2021).

The across-the-board is this category of wearable devices that are used to detect AFib and also good for heart rate variability (HRV), which indicates the healthiness of your overall heart. With HRV it is possible to assess stress, fitness of physical conditions and how well the body recovers which can help keeping track of its cardiovascular well-being in an all-around way for both patient and doctor. Wearable cardiac health monitoring has been a game-changer in this respect by helping patients monitor their heart health without overburdening healthcare systems (Kaushik et al., 2024). Screening appropriately provides early detection of possible problems that can allow for medical intervention in a timely fashion and enhance the life of cardiac patients.

Case Study 3: AI-Powered Wearables for Mental Health Interventions

AI-driven wearables are revolutionizing the way mental care is administered passing assessments of emotional and psychological health on a continual basis. One example is utilizing the sensors built into smartwatches and wristbands like those tracking heart rates, skin temperatures, electrodermal activity to measure stress/ anxiety levels. These devices, matched with AI-based behaviors formulation provide individualised mental health solutions using real-time data. A major effort in this space is the advancement of devices such as the Empatica E4 that can detect stress, anxiety, and even epileptic seizures within research and clinical applications. The device collects information on physiological signals, which then allows it to provide warnings for increased stress and even early warnings of an oncoming mental health crisis. Another wearable making use of AI is feel, a wristband that measures emotional states and delivers customisable mindfulness exercises, breathing techniques and other interventions designed to help people with anxiety and depression. By adopting these wearables, mental health workers can track patients remotely taking healthcare one step further by making it more reactive and efficient. These AI algorithms then scour the data that has been collected from the wearables and pick up on patterns or trends which suggest that patients symptoms are deteriorating, or they need some sort of medical intervention. It does so via a data-driven approach delivering personalized care when one needs most, and reduces the risk of severe mental health episodes, thus lowering the overall well-being.

Case study 4 -Wearables for Physical Rehabilitation and Recovery

They are becoming one of the biggest game changers for physical rehabilitation as they provide personalized training and progress tracking, tailoring rehab exercises to patients recovering from surgeries or injuries. The other key demonstration is in the use for wearable sensors and that of exoskeletons within rehabilitation protocol. These technologies are intended to give patients capabilities for exercise so they can return back to living after medical episodes like stroke, spinal cord injuries etc. For example, the ReWalk exoskeleton is a robotic suit worn by individuals with lower limb disability to help them walk again. Power-assisted technology is often used in rehabilitation centers so that patients can safely exercise their legs by walking. The ReWalk exoskeleton helps users to gradually recover leg muscle strength and coordination by providing electrical assistance for legsersistent movement. Patients using this product showed improved mobility, stability and overall physical fitness (Arora et al., 2024).

For instance, there are motion-sensing wearable's such as the Bio-Stamp and Point system that can help track specific metrics related to muscle activity, joint angles and body movements during rehabilitation exercise. The wearable's enable physical therapists to track patient progress from a distance and alter their approach in real-time (Kaushik et al., 2024). Patient compliance is improved by the fact that these devices provide real-time data, encouraging patients to participate more in their recovery and ensure they perform exercise regimes as prescribed so that they can achieve the best rehabilitation outcomes. Wearables play a key role in the evolution of physical rehabilitation by helping available precise insights into patient recovery progression, decreased downtime for patients and improved outcomes for anyone undergoing hands-on physical therapy.

7. CONCLUSION AND FUTURE SCOPE

Nowadays physical healthcare is no longer limited to the standard check-up options, the addition of sensors and wearables allow monitoring, diagnosing and real-time treatment. These technologies provide personalized care, prevent diseases (even before they develop), and help control chronic conditions, completely changing the face of conventional methods of healthcare delivery. Wearables have demonstrated the ability provide ongoing data-driven insights that positively affect health outcomes from diabetes management to cardiac monitoring and mental health interventions.

In the future, sensors and wearables in healthcare have a bright future. The evolution of artificial intelligence (AI) and machine learning (ML) will make data analysis more efficient which results in healthcare to be made more accurate and predictable. By combining AI with Human Augmentation, as with smart prosthetics and AI-driven exoskeletons, we can advance the reach of physical disabilities for natural rehabilitation resulting in a better quality of life. In addition, further advancements to biosensors, nanotech and in-dwelling implants are yet to come making way for more complex health monitoring possibilities. These advances will enhance proactive, patient-focused care, prevent hospitalizations, and enable patients to better manage their own health. In the years to come, as digital health technologies mature they will be increasingly integrated in defining the future of personalized, reachable and sustainable healthcare.

REFERENCES

Ahirwar, R., & Khan, N. (2022). *Smart Wireless Nanosensor Systems for Human Healthcare*. CRC Press. DOI: 10.1201/9781003093534-15

Arora, M. K., Lal, S., Singh, B., & Olyaee, M. (2024). Through an Energy Lens: Examining SDGs From a Policy Perspective. In Riswandi, B., Singh, B., Kaunert, C., & Vig, K. (Eds.), *AI Applications for Clean Energy and Sustainability* (pp. 320–343). IGI Global., DOI: 10.4018/979-8-3693-6567-0.ch016

Banerjee, A., Chakraborty, C., & Rathi, M.Sr. (2020). Medical imaging, artificial intelligence, internet of things, wearable devices in terahertz healthcare technologies. In *Terahertz biomedical and healthcare technologies* (pp. 145–165). Elsevier. DOI: 10.1016/B978-0-12-818556-8.00008-2

Barnes, R., & Zvarikova, K. (2021). Artificial intelligence-enabled wearable medical devices, clinical and diagnostic decision support systems, and Internet of Things-based healthcare applications in COVID-19 prevention, screening, and treatment. *American Journal of Medical Research (New York, N.Y.)*, *8*(2), 9–22. DOI: 10.22381/ajmr8220211

Chelliah, R., Wei, S., Daliri, E. B. M., Rubab, M., Elahi, F., Yeon, S. J., Jo, K., Yan, P., Liu, S., & Oh, D. H. (2021). Development of nanosensors based intelligent packaging systems: Food quality and medicine. *Nanomaterials (Basel, Switzerland)*, *11*(6), 1515. DOI: 10.3390/nano11061515 PMID: 34201071

Desai, D., & Shende, P. (2021). Integration of Internet of Things with Quantum Dots: A State-of-the-art of Medicine. *Current Pharmaceutical Design*, *27*(17), 2068–2075. DOI: 10.2174/1381612827666210222113740 PMID: 33618640

Gaobotse, G., Mbunge, E., Batani, J., & Muchemwa, B. (2022). Non-invasive smart implants in healthcare: Redefining healthcare services delivery through sensors and emerging digital health technologies. *Sensors International*, *3*, 100156. DOI: 10.1016/j.sintl.2022.100156

Goel, S. S., Goel, A., Kumar, M., & Moltó, G. (2021). A review of Internet of Things: Qualifying technologies and boundless horizon. *Journal of Reliable Intelligent Environments*, *7*(1), 23–33. DOI: 10.1007/s40860-020-00127-w

Han, B., Tomer, V., Nguyen, T. A., Farmani, A., & Singh, P. K. (Eds.). (2020). *Nanosensors for smart cities*. Elsevier.

Han, X. (2023). A novel assimilated navigation model based on advanced optical systems (AOS), internet of things (IoT) and artificial intelligence (AI). *Optical and Quantum Electronics, 55*(7), 655. DOI: 10.1007/s11082-023-04947-x

He, L., & Eastburn, M. (2022, August). Smart nanosensor networks for body injury detection. In 2022 IEEE International Conference on Smart Internet of Things (SmartIoT) (pp. 15-19). IEEE. DOI: 10.1109/SmartIoT55134.2022.00012

Huang, J., Wu, X., Huang, W., Wu, X., & Wang, S. (2021). Internet of things in health management systems: A review. *International Journal of Communication Systems, 34*(4), e4683. DOI: 10.1002/dac.4683

Hurley, D., & Popescu, G. H. (2021). Medical big data and wearable internet of things healthcare systems in remotely monitoring and caring for confirmed or suspected COVID-19 patients. *American Journal of Medical Research (New York, N.Y.), 8*(2), 78–90. DOI: 10.22381/ajmr8220216

Jenkins, T. (2022). Wearable medical sensor devices, machine and deep learning algorithms, and internet of things-based healthcare systems in COVID-19 patient screening, diagnosis, monitoring, and treatment. *American Journal of Medical Research (New York, N.Y.), 9*(1), 49–64. DOI: 10.22381/ajmr9120224

Kaushik, T. K. Ravish, Singh, A., Raghav, A., Singh, B., Arora, M. K., & Lal, S. (2024). Untapping Artificial Intelligence in Environmental and Sustainable Progression: Projecting Legal and Ethical Considerations. In B. Singh, C. Kaunert, K. Vig, & S. Dutta (Eds.), *Maintaining a Sustainable World in the Nexus of Environmental Science and AI* (pp. 109-130). IGI Global. https://doi.org/DOI: 10.4018/979-8-3693-6336-2.ch005

Kaushik, T. K. Ravish, Singh, A., Raghav, A., & Singh, B. (2024). Potential of Artificial Intelligence in the Agricultural Industry: A Comprehensive Review. In B. Riswandi, B. Singh, C. Kaunert, & K. Vig (Eds.), *AI Applications for Clean Energy and Sustainability* (pp. 344-365). IGI Global. DOI: 10.4018/979-8-3693-6567-0.ch017

Khan, T., Civas, M., Cetinkaya, O., Abbasi, N. A., & Akan, O. B. (2020). Nanosensor networks for smart health care. In *Nanosensors for Smart Cities* (pp. 387–403). Elsevier. DOI: 10.1016/B978-0-12-819870-4.00022-0

Kumar, P. M., Hong, C. S., Afghah, F., Manogaran, G., Yu, K., Hua, Q., & Gao, J. (2021). Clouds proportionate medical data stream analytics for internet of things-based healthcare systems. *IEEE Journal of Biomedical and Health Informatics, 26*(3), 973–982. DOI: 10.1109/JBHI.2021.3106387 PMID: 34415841

Kumar, P. M., Khan, L. U., & Hong, C. S. (2022). Affirmative fusion process for improving wearable sensor data availability in artificial intelligence of medical things. *IEEE Sensors Journal.*

Kumar, P. M., Khan, L. U., & Hong, C. S. (2022). Notice of Violation of IEEE Publication Principles: Affirmative Fusion Process for Improving Wearable Sensor Data Availability in Artificial Intelligence of Medical Things. IEEE Sensors Journal.

Kumar, S., & Kumari, P. (2021). Flexible Nano Smart sensors. Nanosensors for Smart Manufacturing, 199.

Malik, A., & Kumar, A. (2022). assimilation of blockchain with Internet of Things (IoT) with possible issues and solutions for better connectivity and proper security. In New Trends and Applications in Internet of Things (IoT) and Big Data Analytics (pp. 187-207). Cham: Springer International Publishing.

Malik, P. K., Sharma, R., Singh, R., Gehlot, A., Satapathy, S. C., Alnumay, W. S., Pelusi, D., Ghosh, U., & Nayak, J. (2021). Industrial Internet of Things and its applications in industry 4.0: State of the art. *Computer Communications*, *166*, 125–139. DOI: 10.1016/j.comcom.2020.11.016

Manogaran, G., Alazab, M., Song, H., & Kumar, N. (2021). CDP-UA: Cognitive data processing method wearable sensor data uncertainty analysis in the internet of things assisted smart medical healthcare systems. *IEEE Journal of Biomedical and Health Informatics*, *25*(10), 3691–3699. DOI: 10.1109/JBHI.2021.3051288 PMID: 33439849

Materon, E. M., Gómez, F. R., Joshi, N., Dalmaschio, C. J., Carrilho, E., & Oliveira Jr, O. N. (2021). Smart materials for electrochemical flexible nanosensors: advances and applications. Nanosensors for smart manufacturing, 347-371.

Mujawar, M. A., Gohel, H., Bhardwaj, S. K., Srinivasan, S., Hickman, N., & Kaushik, A. (2020). Nano-enabled biosensing systems for intelligent healthcare: Towards COVID-19 management. *Materials Today. Chemistry*, *17*, 100306. DOI: 10.1016/j.mtchem.2020.100306 PMID: 32835155

Nazari, A. (2020). Nanosensors for smart cities: an introduction. In *Nanosensors for smart cities* (pp. 3–8). Elsevier. DOI: 10.1016/B978-0-12-819870-4.00001-3

Oukhatar, A., Bakhouya, M., & El Ouadghiri, D. (2021). Electromagnetic-Based Wireless Nano-Sensors Network: Architectures and Applications. *Journal of Communication*, *16*(1), 8–19. DOI: 10.12720/jcm.16.1.8-19

Pradhan, M. R., Mago, B., & Ateeq, K. (2023). A classification-based sensor data processing method for the internet of things assimilated wearable sensor technology. *Cluster Computing*, *26*(1), 807–822. DOI: 10.1007/s10586-022-03605-3

Pramanik, P. K. D., Solanki, A., Debnath, A., Nayyar, A., El-Sappagh, S., & Kwak, K. S. (2020). Advancing modern healthcare with nanotechnology, nanobiosensors, and internet of nano things: Taxonomies, applications, architecture, and challenges. *IEEE Access : Practical Innovations, Open Solutions*, *8*, 65230–65266. DOI: 10.1109/ACCESS.2020.2984269

Raghav, A., Singh, B., Jermsittiparsert, K., Raghav, R., & Yadav, U. (2024). Artificial Intelligence in Environmental and Climate Changes: A Sustainable Future. In Singh, B., Kaunert, C., Vig, K., & Dutta, S. (Eds.), *Maintaining a Sustainable World in the Nexus of Environmental Science and AI* (pp. 485–506). IGI Global., DOI: 10.4018/979-8-3693-6336-2.ch019

Rani, P. (2022). Nanosensors and their Potential Role in Internet of Medical Things. In *Nanosensors for Futuristic Smart and Intelligent Healthcare Systems* (pp. 293–317). CRC Press. DOI: 10.1201/9781003093534-16

Sahi, K. S. S., & Kaushik, S. (2022). Smart Nanosensors for Healthcare Monitoring and Disease Detection using AIoT Framework. In *Nanosensors for Futuristic Smart and Intelligent Healthcare Systems* (pp. 387–400). CRC Press. DOI: 10.1201/9781003093534-19

Suma, D. V. (2021). Wearable IoT based distributed framework for ubiquitous computing. *Journal of Ubiquitous Computing and Communication Technologies*, *3*(1), 23–32. DOI: 10.36548/jucct.2021.1.003

Udoh, E. E., Hermel, M., Bharmal, M. I., Nayak, A., Patel, S., Butlin, M., & Bhavnani, S. P. (2023). Nanosensor technologies and the digital transformation of healthcare. *Personalized Medicine*, *20*(3), 251–269. DOI: 10.2217/pme-2022-0065 PMID: 37403731

Vivekananthan, V., Khandelwal, G., Alluri, N. R., & Kim, S. J. (2022). E-Skin for Futuristic Nanosensor Technology for the Healthcare System. In Nanosensors for Futuristic Smart and Intelligent Healthcare Systems (pp. 133-157). CRC Press.

Chapter 11
Wearable Sensors, Real-Time Monitoring and Data Assimilation in Healthcare Resonates

Bhupinder Singh
https://orcid.org/0009-0006-4779-2553
Sharda University, India

ABSTRACT

Wearable sensors have revolutionized healthcare by enabling continuous, real-time monitoring of various physiological parameters. The real-time monitoring is the cornerstone of proactive healthcare and with continuously collecting data from wearable sensors and connected devices, healthcare practitioners gain unprecedented insights into patients' physiological parameters, allowing them to track vital signs, detect anomalies, and identify trends in real time. This level of vigilance empowers clinicians to promptly intervene and make informed decisions, preventing potential complications and ensuring that patients receive timely interventions that can significantly impact outcomes. This not only enhances the patient's quality of life but also enables healthcare providers to tailor treatment plans dynamically, leading to better disease control and improved patient compliance. This chapter comprehensively explores the various dimensions on Wearable Sensors, Real-time Monitoring and Data Assimilation in Healthcare Resonates.

DOI: 10.4018/979-8-3693-6094-1.ch011

1. INTRODUCTION

Wearable sensors have become essential in today's healthcare environment because they provide never-before-seen possibilities for ongoing, real-time patient monitoring (Johar & Manjula, 2024). These gadgets gather a range of physiological data; they can be as basic as fitness trackers or as complex as wearables for medical use (Holt, 2022). The combination of these sensors with cutting-edge data assimilation methods and real-time monitoring systems has the potential to revolutionize healthcare delivery, enhance patient outcomes, and facilitate customized medication (Liu et al., 2023). Artificial Intelligence (AI), Internet of Things (IoT), wearable devices, and data analytics form the technological backbone of human-centric solutions in smart healthcare. AI enhances diagnostics and decision-making, IoT facilitates remote monitoring and predictive maintenance, while wearable devices empower patients to actively participate in their health management.

Data analytics, driven by big data, provides valuable insights that enable personalized and proactive healthcare. Prioritizing user experience (UX) ensures that technological interventions seamlessly align with the needs and preferences of both healthcare professionals and patients (Taghian et al., 2021). As, real-time data assimilation drives efficiency across the healthcare spectrum and with instantaneously aggregating data from wearable sensors and other IoT devices, healthcare professionals can streamline workflows, optimize resource allocation, and minimize delays in diagnosis and treatment (Ray et al., 2023). The healthcare systems burdened by escalating patient volumes and resource constraints, benefit from real-time insights that enhance operational efficiency (Arpaia et al., 2021). From hospital bed management to surgical scheduling, the real-time data ecosystem offers a level of precision and coordination that is unprecedented, minimizing bottlenecks and improving patient flow (Jadhakhan et al., 2022). The amalgamation of real-time monitoring and data assimilation has profound implications for patient-centered care (Reger, 2020). Wearable sensors and IoT technologies are rapidly evolving, pushing the boundaries of what's possible in medical and digital healthcare. These trends highlight the potential for more accurate, personalized, and proactive healthcare approaches that empower individuals to take control of their health and enable healthcare professionals to make more informed decisions. As these technologies continue to advance, the healthcare landscape is likely to see transformative changes that improve patient outcomes and redefine the way healthcare is delivered. The incorporation of artificial intelligence (AI) and machine learning (ML) into wearable sensors and the Internet of Things (IoT) ecosystem holds immense potential to revolutionize real-time data analysis and predictive modeling in healthcare. This convergence of technologies enables the extraction of meaningful insights from vast streams of sensor data, leading to more accurate diagnostics, personalized interventions, and proactive healthcare strategies (Marvaso et al., 2022).

Figure 1. displays the Landscapes of Introduction Split Sections (Source- Original)

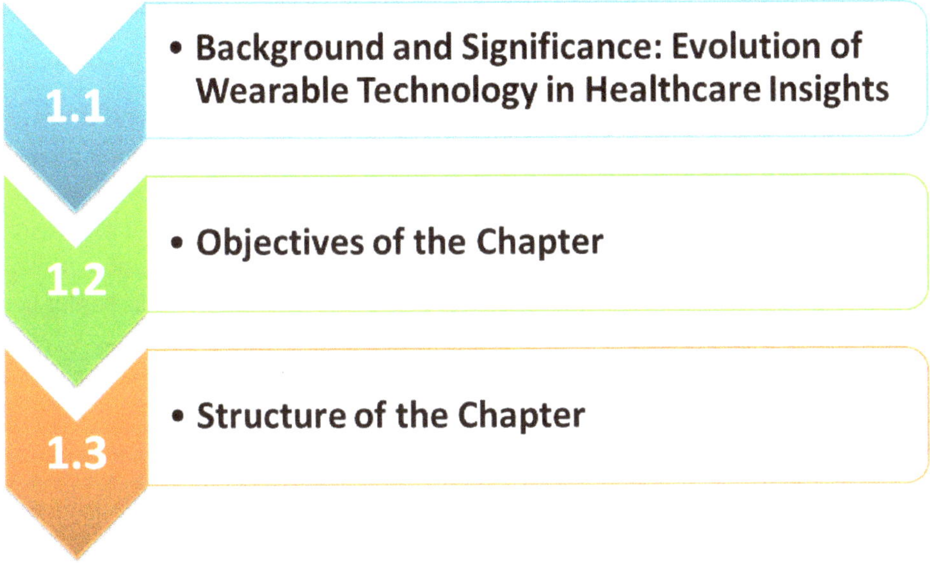

1.1 Background and Significance: Evolution of Wearable Technology in Healthcare Insights

The significance of real-time monitoring and data assimilation in healthcare resonates on multiple levels. It embodies the essence of timely intervention, precision medicine, and operational efficiency (Drigas et al., 2022). With harnessing the power of wearable sensors and IoT technologies, healthcare is propelled into an era where patient care, disease management, and healthcare efficiency converge, promising to reshape the landscape of healthcare delivery and patient outcomes (Elor & Kurniawan, 2020). In the realm of disease management, real-time monitoring assumes a transformative role. For patients with chronic conditions, such as diabetes or cardiovascular diseases, the ability to monitor glucose levels, heart rates, and other critical metrics in real time allows for personalized treatment adjustments (Ebert et al., 2019).

The adoption of wearable sensors and IoT elevates the role of patient-centered care, leading to new patient engagement standards. Patients become active participants in their health management, demanding transparent access to their data and insights derived from wearable sensors (Patangia et al., 2021). Health standards must accommodate these changing dynamics, ensuring that patients have control over their data and are empowered to share it with healthcare providers seamlessly (Midha & Singh, 2023).

1.2 Objectives of the Chapter

This chapter explores advancements in wearable sensor technology, the integration of these sensors with real-time monitoring systems, and the assimilation of data for improved healthcare outcomes. The discussion includes sensor types, data collection methods, processing techniques, and the potential impact on patient care, diagnosis, and treatment. The challenges and future directions in wearable sensor technology and data assimilation in healthcare are also addressed. This chapter has the following objectives to:

- explore the relevance and types of wearable sensors and their applications
- scrutinize the integration of real-time monitoring systems
- discuss data assimilation techniques and their impacts on healthcare
- identify challenges and future directions in this field

Figure 2. share the Objectives of the Chapter (Source- Original)

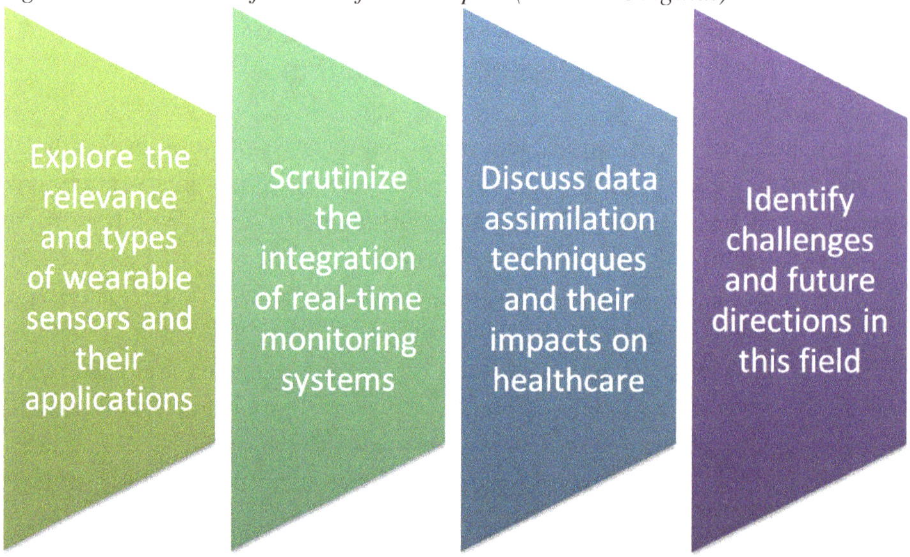

1.3 Structure of the Chapter

This chapter deeply dives into the diverse arena of Wearable Sensors, Real-time Monitoring and Data Assimilation in Healthcare Resonates. Chapter 2 elaborates the Wearable Sensor Technology. Chapter 3 explores the Sensor Design and Development. Chapter 4 discusses Real-Time Monitoring Systems. Chapter 5 lays down the Data Assimilation and Transmission. Chapter 6 specifies the Case Studies: IoT Platforms and Communication Protocols: Connecting Wearable Sensors to Healthcare Systems. Chapter 7 illuminates the Challenges and Solutions. Chapter 8 conveys the Future Trends and Directions. Chapter 9 Conclude the Chapter.

Figure 3. shows the Flow of this Chapter (Source- Original)

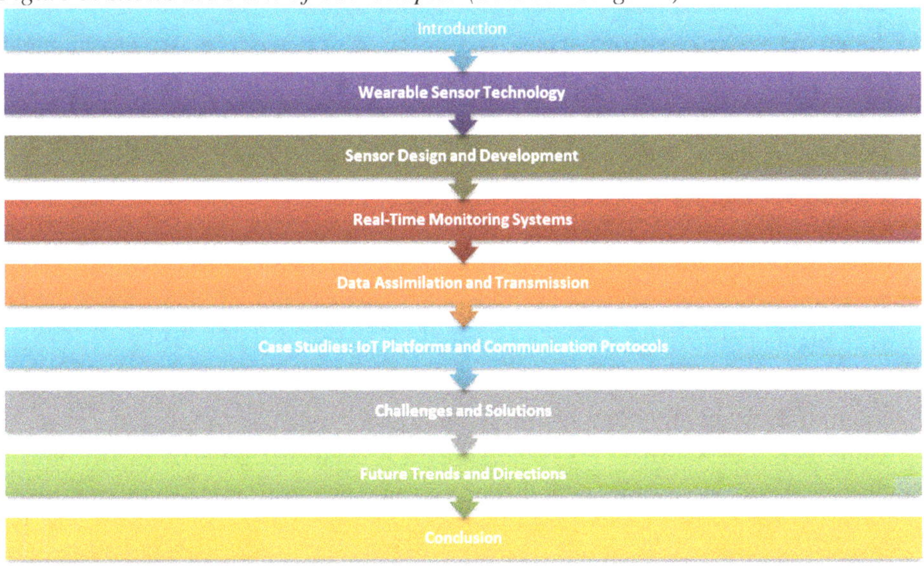

2. WEARABLE SENSOR TECHNOLOGY

"Smart healthcare" refers to the use of cutting-edge IT to the provision of linked, intelligent and customized medical services. The interconnectivity of Smart Healthcare systems enables a holistic approach to healthcare, extending the functions of healthcare beyond diagnosis and treatment to include health maintenance, care for the aged and different stages of an individual's life cycle (Thompson, 2021). The utilization of next-generation technologies, system engineering and operation management theories are required to achieve coordination across smart healthcare systems (Cotler et al., 2017). Because of the nature of the healthcare sector, security, privacy and effective operation must be given top priority in the design of any Smart Healthcare system (Cheng et al., 2019).

Healthcare data, information, and knowledge domains demand unique solutions due to the interconnected nature of Smart Healthcare systems (Banos et al., 2021). Innovations in specialized domains including digital health, the Internet of Medical Things (IoMT), pharmaceutical supply chain and medical insurance, among others are required as the care cycle expands (Miner, 2022). These innovations should also be made in the areas of illness diagnostics, surgery and hospital administration.

2.1 Types of Wearable Sensors

1. **Electrochemical Sensors**: These sensors used to detect specific biochemical markers in body fluids, such as glucose sensors for diabetes management (Durnell, 2018).
2. **Optical Sensors**: They commonly found in pulse oximeters and smartwatches, these measure parameters like heart rate and oxygen saturation using light absorption.
3. **Mechanical Sensors**: It includes accelerometers and gyroscopes that track motion and posture, often used in activity monitors and fall detection systems (Choukou et al., 2022).
4. **Temperature Sensors**: The temperature sensors measure body temperature for monitoring fever and other medical conditions.
5. **Bioimpedance Sensors**: These measure the resistance of body tissues to a small electrical current, useful for body composition analysis and hydration status.

Figure 4. conveys the Diverse Types of Wearable Sensors (Source- Original)

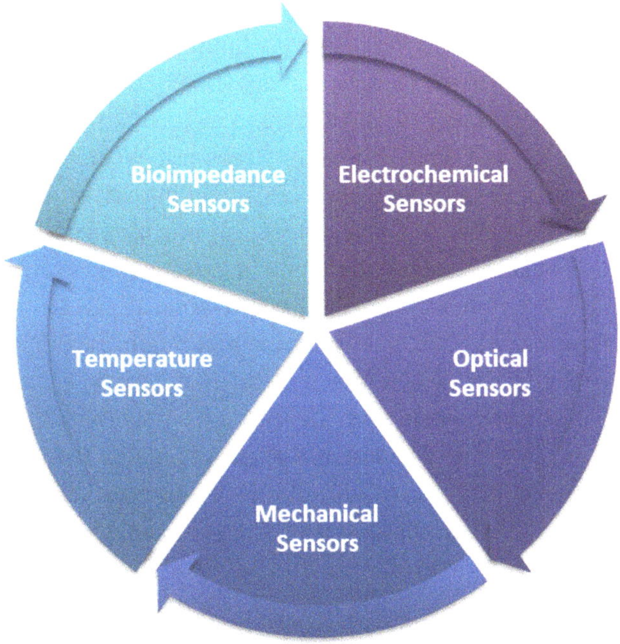

3. SENSOR DESIGN AND DEVELOPMENT

It empowers individuals to actively engage in their own health management, promoting a shift from reactive to proactive healthcare paradigms. Patients are no longer passive recipients of care; they become partners in their health journey, empowered to make informed decisions based on the real-time data stream provided by wearable sensors and IoT devices (Mer & Virdi, 2023). The real-time data stream provides a nuanced understanding of the disease's progression, enabling healthcare teams to adapt therapies swiftly and proactively, ultimately reducing hospitalizations and associated costs (Drigas et al., 2022).

In the context of wearables and IoT, the International Organization for Standardization (ISO) and other standards organizations are evolving to address these novel challenges (D'Errico et al., 2023). The collaborations between health standards bodies and IoT consortiums contribute to the development of comprehensive guidelines that govern the integration of wearable sensors with IoT in healthcare (Hagege et al., 2023). With adhering to interoperability, data security, real-time processing, and patient engagement standards, healthcare systems can harness the transformative potential of wearable sensors and IoT while upholding the core principles of patient care and data integrity. This convergence serves as a catalyst for the evolution of health standards, shaping a future where data-driven healthcare seamlessly intertwines with technological innovation.

In the broader aspect of digital healthcare, real-time data collection and analysis hold the key to personalized treatment strategies. Wearable sensors and IoT technologies continuously collect patient data, including vital signs, activity levels and sleep patterns (Jopowicz, 2022). With instantly processing this data, healthcare professionals gain insights into an individual's health status and can tailor interventions to specific needs (Marossi et al., 2023). Real-time alerts can be generated for irregularities, prompting immediate actions and minimizing health risks. Real-time data also fuels telemedicine and remote patient monitoring, enabling healthcare providers to remotely track patients' conditions and adjust treatment plans as necessary. Patients benefit from virtual consultations, reducing the need for frequent in-person visits, especially for those with chronic conditions. This democratization of healthcare through real-time data exchange ensures that even remote or underserved populations receive timely medical attention.

4. REAL-TIME MONITORING SYSTEMS

Real-time monitoring systems consist of three main components: data acquisition, data transmission, and data analysis. These systems ensure continuous monitoring and analysis of physiological data collected by wearable sensors, providing immediate responses or alerts. The Internet of Things (IoT) is a cutting-edge technology that is developing quickly and has the power to completely change how we interact with our surroundings. IoT refers to the process of connecting different physical objects, machinery and sensors to the Internet so that data may be shared and communication can occur easily between them (Than, 2023). IoT technologies in the healthcare industry are already improving patient outcomes and care by providing chances for individualized treatment regimens, remote monitoring and effective healthcare delivery. IoT has the potential to dramatically lower healthcare costs by optimizing workflows, automating repetitive operations and reducing the need for expensive interventions all while improving patient care. Monitoring and collecting data in real-time improves patient care by speeding up reaction times and yielding better results (Cotler, 2016).

4.1 Usability of Real-Time Monitoring Systems

1. **Data Acquisition**: It initially collects of data from wearable sensors.

2. **Data Transmission**: Secure transfer of collected data to centralized systems for analysis.
3. **Data Analysis**: Application of algorithms and machine learning techniques to interpret the data, detects anomalies and provide actionable insights.

Figure 5. specifies the Usability of Real-Time Monitoring Systems (Source- Original)

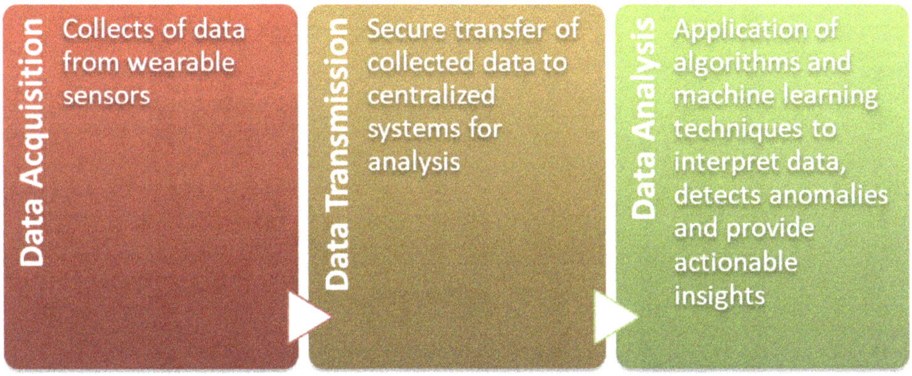

4.2 Data Integration and Analysis

Data assimilation in healthcare involves integrating data from multiple sources to create a comprehensive understanding of a patient's health status. This process leverages advanced analytical techniques and machine learning algorithms to combine data from wearable sensors, electronic health records (EHR), and other relevant sources (Chen & Ibrahim, 2023).

1. **Preprocessing**: Cleaning and normalizing data to ensure accuracy and consistency.
2. **Feature Extraction**: Identifying relevant features and patterns in the data that indicate health conditions.
3. **Predictive Modeling**: Using machine learning algorithms to predict potential health issues based on the extracted features.
4. **Decision Support**: Providing healthcare professionals with actionable insights and recommendations based on the analyzed data.

Figure 6. showcase the Key Components of Data Integration and Analysis in Healthcare (Source- Original)

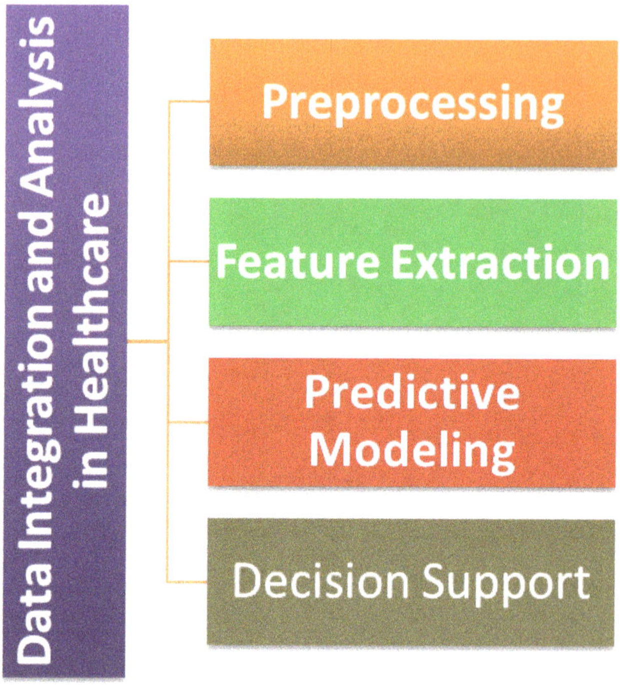

IoT also reduces the need for large administrative personnel, saves time and automates administrative activities, all of which improve healthcare operations and save money. Errors and personnel expenses are decreased when regular chores like medicine dispensing and vital sign monitoring are automated. Significantly, IoT's early detection and ongoing monitoring capabilities lower hospitalization rates, lessen the need for costly procedures and eventually result in significant savings in healthcare costs by preventing expensive medical problems. IoT improves patient engagement by giving people the ability to monitor their health information, interact with healthcare professionals in an efficient manner, and actively participate in their own treatment (Naylor et al., 2020). Self-management, real-time data sharing, virtual appointments, and patient portals are made possible via wearables, applications, telemedicine, and remote monitoring. In order to enable users to successfully traverse new technologies and so facilitate active involvement in healthcare, better communication, engagement and ultimately improved health outcomes, education and training are essential (Liao et al., 2019).

5. DATA ASSIMILATION AND TRANSMISSION

Wearable sensors continuously collect data streams, which are transmitted in real-time to central monitoring systems via wireless communication protocols such as Bluetooth, Wi-Fi, or cellular networks. Integration with mobile applications and cloud platforms facilitates remote monitoring and data analysis. When presented with decision-making tasks, doctors and patients together weigh the best available information under the concept of shared decision-making, where patients are assisted in weighing their alternatives and developing educated preferences. As a decision-making partner, the physician in this paradigm assists in eliciting the patient's knowledge, values, or reasoning. The active participation in decision-making and agreement on the best course of action are universal components of shared decision-making in the patient-clinician partnership. While there are certain medical decisions with a clear "right" answer that are simple, most entail several options, each having pros and cons of its own. To make sure that all pertinent medical information is taken into account while making these decisions, patient involvement is essential. Good conversations involve patients sharing personal information with physicians as well as professionals providing clinical knowledge about the possibilities.

Medical decisions might involve making adjustments to one's behavior, scheduling preventative screenings, managing acute or chronic diseases, balancing conflicting requirements for health and starting or stopping certain treatments. Certain decisions, like whether to begin breast cancer screening or how to be tested for colorectal cancer are standard and made often in practice. During in-person visits, physicians include patients in decision-making, which is effective for significant choices. Nevertheless, more standard choices made during an office visit are frequently disregarded. In a poll, almost two thirds of patients said they would want to discuss routine and significant choices with their providers. Rarely do discussions between doctors and patients cover every aspect of making the right choice. Patients believe they are informed enough to make decisions, but typically have a limited grasp of medical facts and overestimate the importance of medical treatment.

Smart health technology and digital advancement are driving a massive revolution in the healthcare industry. The healthcare industry is changing, ushering in a new age and upending the status quo thanks to smart technology and digital transformation. Increased monitoring, improved accessibility, and a wider range of treatment options are characteristics of this change. The other way that digital technology supports the patient-centered approach to healthcare is through telemedicine. Telemedicine removes the need for in-person appointments by allowing patients to get medical treatment from the comfort of their own homes. This is especially helpful for people who live in remote regions or have mobility issues (Macorano, 2020).

Figure 7. displays the Components of Real-time Monitoring Systems (Source- Original)

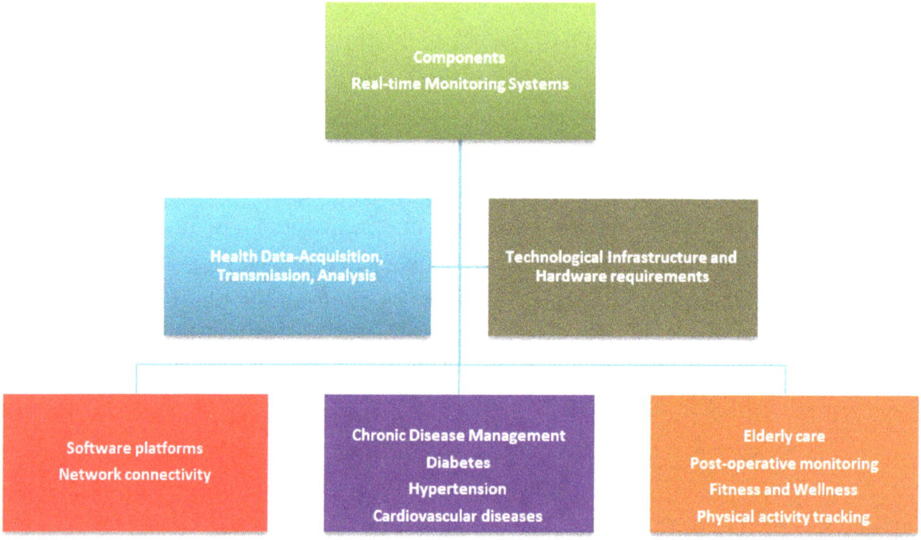

The successful assimilation of wearable sensors into healthcare systems hinges on the synergy between IoT platforms and communication protocols. These technologies ensure that wearable-generated data can be securely and seamlessly transmitted to healthcare networks, enabling improved patient care, remote monitoring, and advanced data analytics. The choice of platform and protocol depends on factors such as power consumption, data requirements, communication range, and the specific healthcare application at hand. Data integration in healthcare involves combining data from multiple sources to create a comprehensive understanding of a patient's health status. This process leverages advanced analytical techniques and machine learning algorithms to merge data from wearable sensors, electronic health records (EHR), and other relevant sources.

6. CASE STUDIES: IOT PLATFORMS AND COMMUNICATION PROTOCOLS: USED IN CONNECTING WEARABLE SENSORS TO HEALTHCARE SYSTEMS

The seamless integration of wearable sensors into healthcare systems relies on a diverse array of Internet of Things (IoT) platforms and communication protocols. These technologies work in tandem to ensure reliable, secure, and efficient data transmission between wearable devices and healthcare networks. Several IoT platforms and communication protocols play pivotal roles in connecting wearable sensors to healthcare systems in IoT Platforms as-

Amazon Web Services (AWS) IoT: Amazon Web Services (AWS) offers an IoT platform that facilitates the secure connection of wearable devices to the cloud. AWS IoT provides scalable infrastructure, device management capabilities, and data analytics tools. It allows healthcare organizations to collect, process, and analyze data from wearables, enabling real-time monitoring, predictive analytics, and personalized healthcare interventions.

Microsoft Azure IoT: Azure IoT by Microsoft offers a robust ecosystem for connecting wearable sensors to healthcare systems. It provides device management, security features, and integration with machine learning and data analytics services. Healthcare providers can use Azure IoT to build predictive models, detect anomalies, and enhance patient care based on wearable-generated data.

Google Cloud IoT: Google Cloud IoT platform enables the integration of wearable sensors into healthcare applications. It offers data processing, machine learning, and analytics capabilities. Healthcare organizations can harness Google Cloud IoT to gain insights from wearable data, enabling early disease detection, remote patient monitoring, and personalized treatment plans.

Figure 8. showcase the Case Studies (Source- Original)

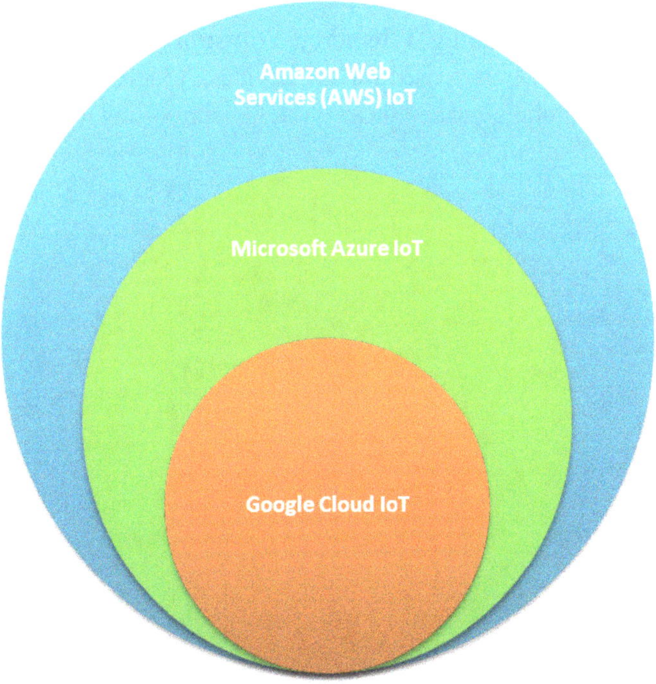

6.1 Communication Protocols

Bluetooth Low Energy (BLE): BLE is a low-power wireless communication protocol ideal for connecting wearables to smartphones, tablets, and other devices. It's commonly used for transmitting health data from wearables to mobile apps, making it suitable for applications like fitness tracking and real-time health monitoring.

Zigbee: Zigbee is another low-power wireless protocol commonly used in healthcare settings to connect wearable sensors to monitoring systems. It's suitable for applications requiring low data rates, such as patient monitoring and eldercare solutions.

LTE-M and NB-IoT: These cellular communication technologies are designed for IoT devices, including wearables. They provide wide coverage and low power consumption, making them suitable for wearables that require remote monitoring, like tracking devices for patients with dementia or chronic conditions.

Wi-Fi: Wi-Fi is a ubiquitous communication protocol that can connect wearables to local networks, allowing for real-time data transmission and remote monitoring. It's commonly used in hospital settings for patient tracking and asset management.

LoRaWAN: LoRaWAN (Long Range Wide Area Network) is ideal for long-range communication between wearables and healthcare systems. It's well-suited for applications like tracking patients' movements within large medical facilities or monitoring patients in rural areas.

MQTT (Message Queuing Telemetry Transport): MQTT is a lightweight communication protocol often used for IoT devices. It facilitates efficient data exchange between wearables and healthcare systems, supporting real-time monitoring and data synchronization.

Figure 9. highlights the Communication Protocols in Healthcare Resonates (Source-Original)

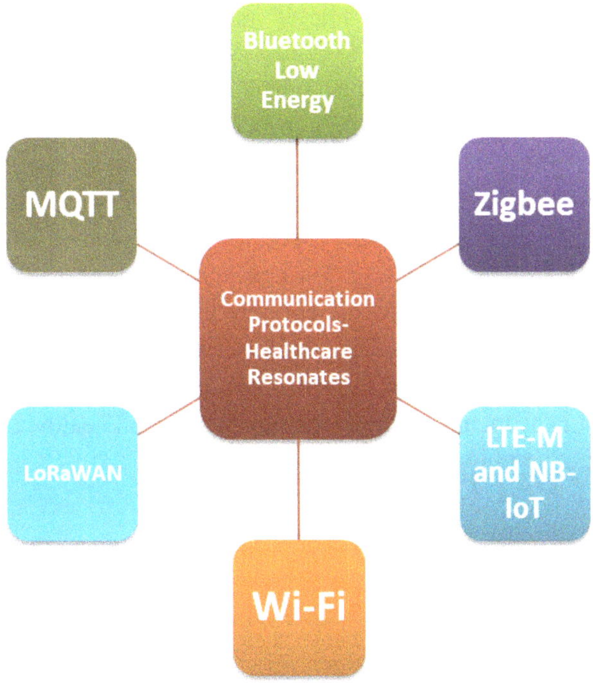

7. CHALLENGES AND SOLUTIONS

The integration of wearable sensors and Internet of Things (IoT) devices into healthcare systems offers unprecedented potential to enhance patient care, improve diagnostics, and revolutionize medical practices. However, this transformation is not without its concerns, particularly when it comes to data privacy and security. The collection, transmission, and storage of sensitive patient information through these technologies raise a host of complex challenges that must be addressed to ensure the responsible and ethical use of wearable sensors and IoT in healthcare. The AI and ML into wearable sensors and IoT technologies represent a transformative shift in healthcare. Real-time data analysis and predictive modeling offer the potential to elevate patient care to new heights by enabling timely interventions, personalized treatment plans, and enhanced disease management. As these technologies continue to advance, the healthcare industry stands poised to harness their power in improving patient outcomes and shaping the future of medical practice.

But his transformative landscape is not without its challenges. Data privacy concerns, interoperability issues, and regulatory compliance requirements demand meticulous attention. Striking the delicate balance between harnessing the benefits of real-time data and safeguarding patient privacy and security remains an ongoing endeavor. As wearable sensors and IoT technologies continue to evolve, the potential for revolutionizing medical imaging and digital healthcare is limitless. Remote patient monitoring, telehealth services, predictive diagnostics, and personalized treatment plans are just the beginning. The convergence of these technologies holds the promise of not only improving patient outcomes but also enhancing the efficiency, accessibility, and quality of healthcare services worldwide. As stakeholders collaborate to address challenges and seize opportunities, the future of wearable sensors and IoT in advancing medical imaging and digital healthcare remains both exciting and full of promise (Quintero, 2019).

Figure 10. shares the Challenges and Concerns (Source- Original)

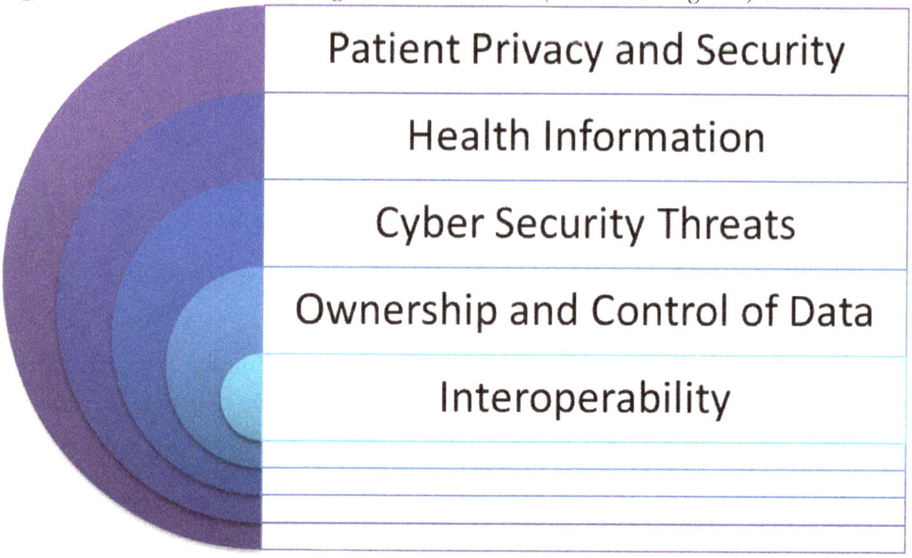

The primary concerns with wearable sensors and IoT in healthcare is the preservation of patient data privacy. These technologies generate a wealth of personal health information, ranging from vital signs and medical history to daily activity patterns. If mishandled, this data can lead to unintended exposure of sensitive patient information, resulting in breaches of confidentiality and potential harm to individuals' privacy. Ensuring that data is de-identified, encrypted, and anonymized when necessary is critical to prevent unauthorized access and protect patients' personal and medical information.

Wearable sensors and IoT devices are susceptible to cybersecurity threats due to their interconnected nature. These devices may lack robust security features, making them vulnerable to hacking, data breaches, and unauthorized access. A compromised device could lead to unauthorized monitoring of patients, manipulation of medical data, or even ransomware attacks targeting critical healthcare infrastructure. Implementing stringent security measures, including encryption, authentication, and regular security updates, is essential to safeguarding patient information and maintaining the integrity of healthcare systems.

The ownership and control of data generated by wearable sensors and IoT devices are complex issues. Patients may not always be aware of how their data is being collected, processed, and shared, raising questions about consent and ownership. Healthcare providers, device manufacturers, and third-party vendors may have access to this data, potentially leading to situations where patients lose control over their own health information. The establishing of transparent data governance policies, obtaining informed consent, and allowing patients to manage their data preferences are crucial steps to address these concerns.

Interoperability refers to the ability of different devices and systems to exchange and use data seamlessly. The diversity of wearable sensors and IoT devices used in healthcare can lead to interoperability challenges, where data from various sources may not integrate effectively. Incomplete or incompatible data integration could lead to inaccuracies in medical records and hinder the quality of patient care. Standardizing data formats, communication protocols, and interoperability frameworks are essential to ensure that healthcare systems can effectively utilize the data generated by different devices.

The use of wearable sensors and IoT in healthcare must adhere to a complex web of legal and regulatory requirements. Regulations such as the Health Insurance Portability and Accountability Act (HIPAA) in the United States and the General Data Protection Regulation (GDPR) in the European Union govern the collection, storage, and sharing of patient health data. Non-compliance can result in significant legal penalties and reputational damage. Healthcare organizations and technology providers must navigate these regulations diligently to ensure that patient data is handled in accordance with the law.

While wearable sensors and IoT devices hold immense promise for transforming healthcare, their deployment comes with significant data privacy and security concerns. To fully harness the potential of these technologies, healthcare stakeholders must prioritize the development and implementation of robust data protection measures. With addressing these concerns, healthcare systems can achieve the delicate balance between leveraging innovative technologies and safeguarding patients' privacy, security, and well-being (Richer et al., 2022).

6.1 Viable Solutions- Encryption, Authentication, and Secure Data Transmission: Implementation to Protect Patient Data

Encryption, authentication, and secure data transmission are critical components of ensuring the protection and privacy of patient data in the context of wearable sensors and Internet of Things (IoT) devices used in healthcare (Folland et al., 2024). These measures collectively create a fortified layer of security that safeguards sensitive health information from unauthorized access, interception, and tampering as-

Encryption

Encryption involves the process of converting plain data into ciphertext using algorithms and keys. Only authorized parties with the corresponding decryption keys can convert ciphertext back into readable data. In the context of patient data, encryption ensures that even if unauthorized individuals gain access to the data, they would not be able to decipher it without the proper decryption key (Lgwaran & Okoh, 2019). The encryption is applied at multiple levels like-

Data-at-Rest Encryption: This encrypts patient data when it's stored on devices or servers. If a device is lost or a server is compromised, the encrypted data remains unreadable without the decryption key (Ji et al., 2023).

Data-in-Transit Encryption: This secures the data as it is transmitted over networks. Any intercepted data remains encrypted, preventing eavesdropping or tampering during transmission (Leen & Juurlink, 2019).

End-to-End Encryption: This ensures that data remains encrypted from the sender to the recipient. Even service providers or intermediaries cannot access the unencrypted data (Sanyoalu et al., 2019).

Authentication

Authentication ensures that only authorized users or devices can access patient data. Authentication mechanisms verify the identity of users and devices before granting access to sensitive information (Shaw et al., 2024). The common authentication methods include as-

Username and Password: Traditional login credentials are used to verify user identity. However, multi-factor authentication (MFA) is recommended to add an additional layer of security, requiring users to provide two or more forms of verification (Eger et al., 2024).

Biometric Authentication: Utilizes unique biological traits like fingerprints, facial recognition, or iris scans to authenticate users (Erlangga et al., 2019).

Device Authentication: Ensures that only authorized devices can access data. This is crucial in IoT environments, where devices themselves need to be authenticated before exchanging data (Chersich et al., 2020).

Secure Data Transmission

The securing of the transmission of patient data involves using protocols and technologies that prevent unauthorized parties from intercepting or modifying data during transit (Dewa et al., 2017). There are some common practices in secure data transmission which include as-

HTTPS: Hypertext Transfer Protocol Secure (HTTPS) ensures encrypted communication between a user's browser and a website's server, safeguarding data transmitted over the internet (Batalden et al., 2023).

VPN: Virtual Private Networks create a secure and encrypted connection between a user's device and a remote server. This is particularly useful for remote access to healthcare networks (Balarajan et al., 2021).

Secure APIs: Application Programming Interfaces (APIs) should be implemented with security in mind to prevent unauthorized access or tampering with data shared between different systems (Godman et al., 2020).

With implementing robust encryption, authentication, and secure data transmission practices, healthcare organizations can significantly reduce the risk of data breaches and unauthorized access to patient information. These measures form a comprehensive security strategy that protects patient privacy, maintains the integrity of medical data, and builds trust in the use of wearable sensors and IoT devices within the healthcare ecosystem (Gandhi et al., 2018).

Figure 11. illuminates the Viable Solutions (Source- Original)

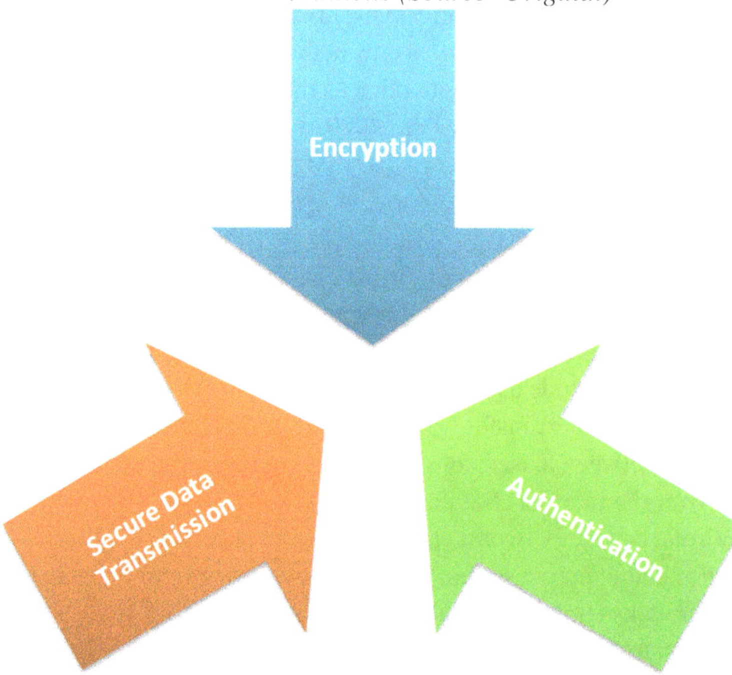

8. FUTURE TRENDS AND DIRECTIONS

The emerging trends and technologies in wearable sensors and the Internet of Things (IoT) are shaping the future of medical and digital healthcare, offering innovative solutions to enhance patient care, improve diagnostics, and transform healthcare delivery (American Diabetes Association, 2015). There are some prominent trends and technologies in this rapidly evolving field-

Wearable Health Monitoring: Wearable devices are becoming more sophisticated, capable of continuously monitoring a wide range of health parameters beyond basic heart rate and activity tracking. Advanced wearables can now measure parameters like blood pressure, glucose levels, skin conductivity, and even monitor respiratory health, enabling early disease detection and personalized interventions (Hassan et al., 2024).

Telehealth and Virtual Care: Wearable sensors are facilitating the expansion of telehealth and virtual care models. Patients can have virtual consultations with healthcare providers while sharing real-time data from wearables, enabling remote diagnosis, treatment, and follow-up care (Gan et al., 2020).

Smart Clothing and Textile-Based Sensors: Innovations in smart textiles are integrating sensors directly into clothing, allowing for unobtrusive health monitoring. These textiles can monitor vital signs, posture, and movement, providing a more comfortable and seamless monitoring experience for patients (Fang et al., 2019).

AI-Powered Analytics: The combination of wearable sensor data and artificial intelligence (AI) is enabling advanced data analytics and predictive modeling. AI algorithms can analyze large datasets to detect subtle patterns, predict disease progression, and recommend personalized treatment strategies (Bergwerk et al., 2021).

Edge AI and Edge Computing: Edge AI involves the running of AI algorithms, directly on wearable devices or at the edge of the network which reducing the need to transmit large amounts of data to the cloud. This enhances real-time processing, responsiveness, and privacy, making wearables more efficient and effective (Tomas et al., 2023).

Wearable Drug Delivery Systems: Wearable devices are being developed to administer medications, such as insulin, through smart patches or devices. These devices can track medication adherence, adjust dosages, and wirelessly communicate with healthcare providers (Runciman et al., 2017).

Biofeedback and Neurofeedback: Wearable sensors can provide real-time biofeedback to users, helping them manage stress, anxiety, and even improve cognitive function. Neurofeedback wearables can monitor brain activity and provide training to enhance mental well-being (Li et al., 2018).

Personalized Healthcare: Wearable sensors combined with genetic data and other health information are enabling personalized healthcare approaches. This includes tailoring treatment plans, medications, and lifestyle recommendations based on an individual's unique health profile (Bowman, 2023).

Security and Privacy Enhancements: As wearables collect increasingly sensitive health data, there's a growing emphasis on improving security and privacy measures. Technologies such as differential privacy and homomorphic encryption are being explored to protect patient data while still enabling meaningful analysis (Watts et al., 2023).

5G Connectivity: The rollout of 5G networks offers enhanced connectivity for wearable devices, enabling faster data transmission, lower latency, and more reliable connections. This is crucial for real-time applications and remote monitoring (Chartier, 2024).

Real-time Data Analysis: AI and ML algorithms can process and analyze the continuous flow of real-time data generated by wearable sensors. This enables healthcare providers to monitor patients' health status in real time, identifying anomalies or deviations from established patterns (Ogugua et al., 2024). For instance, AI-powered algorithms can analyze heart rate variability, oxygen saturation levels, and activity patterns to detect early signs of cardiac distress, respiratory issues, or sleep disorders. With promptly alerting healthcare professionals to critical changes, real-time data analysis can expedite interventions, prevent adverse events, and improve patient outcomes (American Diabetes Association, 2014).

Predictive Modeling: The integration of AI and ML also empowers predictive modeling, allowing healthcare systems to anticipate health-related events before they occur. Machine learning algorithms trained on historical data can recognize patterns and correlations that might not be apparent to human analysis (Sikka et al., 2020). For instance, wearable sensors tracking a patient's daily activity, sleep quality and vital signs can feed into an algorithm that predicts the likelihood of a forthcoming migraine episode. Similarly, predictive models can anticipate worsening symptoms in chronic diseases such as diabetes or asthma, prompting timely interventions and reducing hospitalizations (Music, 2022).

Personalized Healthcare: AI and ML technologies enhance predictive modeling by enabling personalized healthcare strategies. With analyzing individual health data, genetics, lifestyle factors, and wearable sensor inputs, algorithms can tailor treatment plans and interventions to each patient's unique profile (Knagg et al., 2024). For example, an AI-driven system might adjust medication dosages based on real-time glucose levels and historical data patterns, optimizing glycemic control for a diabetic patient. This level of personalization not only improves patient outcomes but also reduces the risk of adverse effects from generic treatment protocols (Pool et al., 2024).

Chronic Disease Management: Wearable sensors integrated with AI and ML can significantly improve chronic disease management. With continuously collecting and analyzing data related to blood pressure, heart rate, glucose levels, and more, these technologies enable the early detection of disease exacerbations or complications (Goldsteen et al., 2024). For instance, an AI algorithm could identify a potential asthma attack based on breathing patterns detected by wearable sensors and alert the patient or healthcare provider (Slaunwhite et al., 2024). This proactive approach empowers patients to take preventive measures and helps healthcare providers make informed decisions in advance (Fuse Brown & Hall, 2024).

Figure 12. displays the Future Trends and Directions (Source- Original)

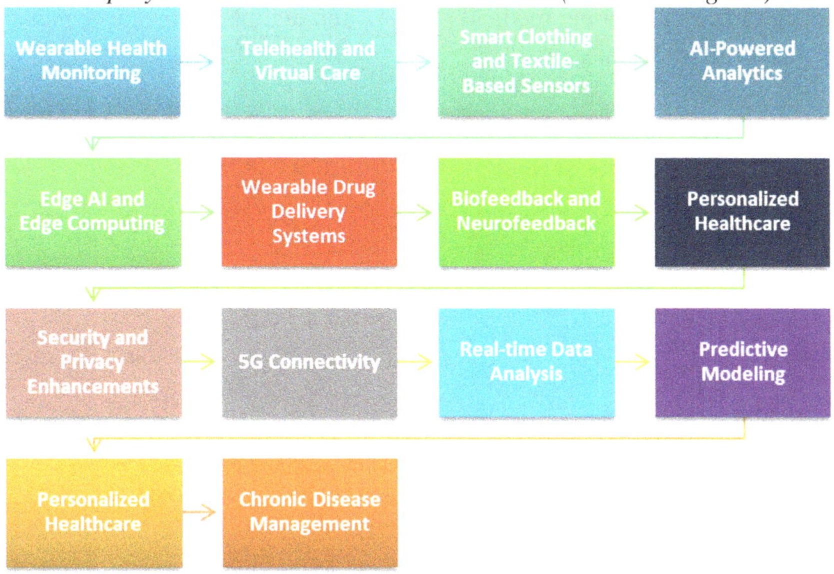

9. CONCLUSION

Wearable sensors, real-time monitoring systems, and data assimilation technologies hold immense potential to transform healthcare. With enabling continuous and remote monitoring, these technologies can bring rapid diagnosis, personalized treatment plans, and improvements in patient outcomes. However, addressing relevant challenges is crucial for widespread adoption and effectiveness in diagnostic practices. Continuous advancements in sensor technology, data analytics, and regulatory support will be key to realizing the full potential of wearable sensors in healthcare. But his transformative landscape is not without its challenges. Data privacy concerns, interoperability issues, and regulatory compliance requirements demand meticulous attention. Striking the delicate balance between harnessing the benefits of real-time data and safeguarding patient privacy and security remains an ongoing endeavor. As wearable sensors and IoT technologies continue to evolve, the potential for revolutionizing medical imaging and digital healthcare is limitless. Remote patient monitoring, telehealth services, predictive diagnostics, and personalized treatment plans are just the beginning. The convergence of these technologies holds the promise of not only improving patient outcomes but also enhancing the efficiency, accessibility, and quality of healthcare services worldwide. As stakeholders collaborate to address challenges and seize opportunities, the future of wearable sensors and IoT in advancing medical imaging and digital healthcare remains both exciting and full of promise.

REFERENCES

American Diabetes Association. (2014). Standards of medical care in diabetes—2014. *Diabetes Care, 37*(Supplement_1), S14–S80. DOI: 10.2337/dc14-S014 PMID: 24357209

American Diabetes Association. (2015). Standards of medical care in diabetes—2015 abridged for primary care providers. *Clinical Diabetes : a Publication of the American Diabetes Association, 33*(2), 97–111. DOI: 10.2337/diaclin.33.2.97 PMID: 25897193

Arpaia, P., D'Errico, G., De Paolis, L. T., Moccaldi, N., & Nuccetelli, F. (2021). A narrative review of mindfulness-based interventions using virtual reality. *Mindfulness*, 1–16.

Balarajan, Y., Selvaraj, S., & Subramanian, S. V. (2021). Health care and equity in India. *Lancet, 377*(9764), 505–515. DOI: 10.1016/S0140-6736(10)61894-6 PMID: 21227492

Baños, R. M., Etchemendy, E., Carrillo-Vega, A., & Botella, C. (2021). Positive psychological interventions and information and communication technologies. In *Research Anthology on Rehabilitation Practices and Therapy* (pp. 1648–1668). IGI Global.

Batalden, M., Batalden, P., Margolis, P., Seid, M., Armstrong, G., Opipari-Arrigan, L., & Hartung, H. (2023). Coproduction of healthcare service. *BMJ Quality & Safety*. PMID: 26376674

Bergwerk, M., Gonen, T., Lustig, Y., Amit, S., Lipsitch, M., Cohen, C., Mandelboim, M., Levin, E. G., Rubin, C., Indenbaum, V., Tal, I., Zavitan, M., Zuckerman, N., Bar-Chaim, A., Kreiss, Y., & Regev-Yochay, G. (2021). Covid-19 breakthrough infections in vaccinated health care workers. *The New England Journal of Medicine, 385*(16), 1474–1484. DOI: 10.1056/NEJMoa2109072 PMID: 34320281

Bowman, S. (2023). Impact of electronic health record systems on information integrity: Quality and safety implications. *Perspectives in Health Information Management, 10*(Fall). PMID: 24159271

Chartier, Y. (Ed.). (2024). *Safe management of wastes from health-care activities*. World Health Organization.

Chen, X., & Ibrahim, Z. (2023). A Comprehensive Study of Emotional Responses in AI-Enhanced Interactive Installation Art. *Sustainability (Basel), 15*(22), 15830. DOI: 10.3390/su152215830

Cheng, V. W. S., Davenport, T., Johnson, D., Vella, K., & Hickie, I. B. (2019). Gamification in apps and technologies for improving mental health and well-being: Systematic review. *JMIR Mental Health*, *6*(6), e13717. DOI: 10.2196/13717 PMID: 31244479

Chersich, M. F., Gray, G., Fairlie, L., Eichbaum, Q., Mayhew, S., Allwood, B., English, R., Scorgie, F., Luchters, S., Simpson, G., Haghighi, M. M., Pham, M. D., & Rees, H. (2020). COVID-19 in Africa: Care and protection for frontline healthcare workers. *Globalization and Health*, *16*(1), 1–6. DOI: 10.1186/s12992-020-00574-3 PMID: 32414379

Choukou, M. A., Zhu, X., Malwade, S., Dhar, E., & Abdul, S. S. (2022). Digital Health Solutions Transforming Long-Term Care and Rehabilitation. In *Healthcare Information Management Systems: Cases, Strategies, and Solutions* (pp. 301–316). Springer International Publishing. DOI: 10.1007/978-3-031-07912-2_19

Cotler, J. L. (2016). *The impact of online teaching and learning about emotional intelligence, Myers Briggs personality dimensions and mindfulness on personal and social awareness*. State University of New York at Albany.

Cotler, J. L., DiTursi, D., Goldstein, I., Yates, J., & Del Belso, D. (2017). A mindful approach to teaching. *Information Systems Education Journal*, *15*(1), 12.

D'Errico, G., Barba, M. C., Gatto, C., Nuzzo, B. L., Nuccetelli, F., Luca, V. D., & Paolis, L. T. D. (2023, September). Measuring the Effectiveness of Virtual Reality for Stress Reduction: Psychometric Evaluation of the ERMES Project. In *International Conference on Extended Reality* (pp. 484-499). Cham: Springer Nature Switzerland. DOI: 10.1007/978-3-031-43401-3_32

Dewa, C. S., Loong, D., Bonato, S., & Trojanowski, L. (2017). The relationship between physician burnout and quality of healthcare in terms of safety and acceptability: A systematic review. *BMJ Open*, *7*(6), e015141. DOI: 10.1136/bmjopen-2016-015141 PMID: 28637730

Drigas, A., Mitsea, E., & Skianis, C. (2022). Virtual reality and metacognition training techniques for learning disabilities. *Sustainability (Basel)*, *14*(16), 10170. DOI: 10.3390/su141610170

Drigas, A., Mitsea, E., & Skianis, C. (2022). Subliminal Training Techniques for Cognitive, Emotional and Behavioral Balance. The Role of Emerging Technologies. *Technium Soc. Sci. J.*, *33*, 164.

Ebert, D. D., Harrer, M., Apolinário-Hagen, J., & Baumeister, H. (2019). Digital interventions for mental disorders: key features, efficacy, and potential for artificial intelligence applications. *Frontiers in Psychiatry: Artificial Intelligence, Precision Medicine, and Other Paradigm Shifts*, 583-627.

Eger, H., Chacko, S., El-Gamal, S., Gerlinger, T., Kaasch, A., Meudec, M., Munshi, S., Naghipour, A., Rhule, E., Sandhya, Y. K., & Uribe, O. L. (2024). Towards a Feminist Global Health Policy: Power, intersectionality, and transformation. *PLOS Global Public Health*, *4*(3), e0002959. DOI: 10.1371/journal.pgph.0002959 PMID: 38451969

Elor, A., & Kurniawan, S. (2020). The ultimate display for physical rehabilitation: A bridging review on immersive virtual reality. *Frontiers in Virtual Reality*, *1*, 585993. DOI: 10.3389/frvir.2020.585993

Erlangga, D., Suhrcke, M., Ali, S., & Bloor, K. (2019). The impact of public health insurance on health care utilisation, financial protection and health status in low-and middle-income countries: A systematic review. *PLoS One*, *14*(8), e0219731. DOI: 10.1371/journal.pone.0219731 PMID: 31461458

Fang, H., Eggleston, K., Hanson, K., & Wu, M. (2019). Enhancing financial protection under China's social health insurance to achieve universal health coverage. *bmj, 365*.

Folland, S., Goodman, A. C., & Stano, M. (2024). *The economics of health and health care: Pearson new international edition*. Routledge.

Fuse Brown, E. C., & Hall, M. A. (2024). Private Equity and the Corporatization of Health Care. *Stanford Law Review*, 76.

Gan, W. H., Lim, J. W., & Koh, D. (2020). Preventing intra-hospital infection and transmission of coronavirus disease 2019 in health-care workers. *Safety and Health at Work*, *11*(2), 241–243. DOI: 10.1016/j.shaw.2020.03.001 PMID: 32292622

Gandhi, T. K., Kaplan, G. S., Leape, L., Berwick, D. M., Edgman-Levitan, S., Edmondson, A., Meyer, G. S., Michaels, D., Morath, J. M., Vincent, C., & Wachter, R. (2018). Transforming concepts in patient safety: A progress report. *BMJ Quality & Safety*, *27*(12), 1019–1026. DOI: 10.1136/bmjqs-2017-007756 PMID: 30018115

Godman, B., Haque, M., Islam, S., Iqbal, S., Urmi, U. L., Kamal, Z. M., Shuvo, S. A., Rahman, A., Kamal, M., Haque, M., Jahan, I., Islam, M. Z., Hossain, M. M., Munzur-E-Murshid, , Kumar, S., Charan, J., Bhatt, R., Dutta, S., Abhayanand, J. P., & Sefah, I. (2020). Rapid assessment of price instability and paucity of medicines and protection for COVID-19 across Asia: Findings and public health implications for the future. *Frontiers in Public Health*, *8*, 585832. DOI: 10.3389/fpubh.2020.585832 PMID: 33381485

Goldsteen, R. L., Goldsteen, K., & Dwelle, T. (2024). Introduction to public health: promises and practices.

Hagège, H., Ourmi, M. E., Shankland, R., Arboix-Calas, F., Leys, C., & Lubart, T. (2023). Ethics and Meditation: A New Educational Combination to Boost Verbal Creativity and Sense of Responsibility. *Journal of Intelligence*, *11*(8), 155. DOI: 10.3390/jintelligence11080155 PMID: 37623538

Hassan, I., Chisty, A., & Bui, T. (2024). Structural and Social Determinants of Health. In *Leading an Academic Medical Practice* (pp. 343–355). Springer International Publishing.

Holt, S. (2022). Virtual reality, augmented reality and mixed reality: For astronaut mental health; and space tourism, education and outreach. *Acta Astronautica*.

Igwaran, A., & Okoh, A. I. (2019). Human campylobacteriosis: A public health concern of global importance. *Heliyon*, *5*(11), e02814. DOI: 10.1016/j.heliyon.2019.e02814 PMID: 31763476

Jadhakhan, F., Blake, H., Hett, D., & Marwaha, S. (2022). Efficacy of digital technologies aimed at enhancing emotion regulation skills: Literature review. *Frontiers in Psychiatry*, *13*, 809332. DOI: 10.3389/fpsyt.2022.809332 PMID: 36159937

Ji, X., Chun, S. A., Wei, Z., & Geller, J. (2023). Twitter sentiment classification for measuring public health concerns. *Social Network Analysis and Mining*, *5*, 1–25. PMID: 32226558

Johar, S., & Manjula, G. R. (2024). Interfering sensed input classification model using assimilated whale optimization and deep Q-learning for remote patient monitoring. *Biomedical Signal Processing and Control*, *93*, 106202. DOI: 10.1016/j.bspc.2024.106202

Jopowicz, A., Wiśniowska, J., & Tarnacka, B. (2022). Cognitive and physical intervention in metals' dysfunction and neurodegeneration. *Brain Sciences*, *12*(3), 345. DOI: 10.3390/brainsci12030345 PMID: 35326301

Knagg, R., Dorey, J., Evans, R., & Hitchman, J. (2024). Sustainability in healthcare: Patient and public perspectives. *Anaesthesia*, *79*(3), 278–283. DOI: 10.1111/anae.16159 PMID: 38205532

Leen, J. L., & Juurlink, D. N. (2019). Carfentanil: A narrative review of its pharmacology and public health concerns. *Canadian Journal of Anaesthesia*, *66*(4), 414–421. DOI: 10.1007/s12630-019-01294-y PMID: 30666589

Li, Y., Wang, H., Jin, X. R., Li, X., Pender, M., Song, C. P., Tang, S.-L., Cao, J., Wu, H., & Wang, Y. G. (2018). Experiences and challenges in the health protection of medical teams in the Chinese Ebola treatment center, Liberia: A qualitative study. *Infectious Diseases of Poverty*, *7*(1), 1–12. DOI: 10.1186/s40249-018-0468-6 PMID: 30134982

Liao, D., Shu, L., Liang, G., Li, Y., Zhang, Y., Zhang, W., & Xu, X. (2019). Design and evaluation of affective virtual reality system based on multimodal physiological signals and self-assessment manikin. *IEEE Journal of Electromagnetics, RF and Microwaves in Medicine and Biology*, *4*(3), 216–224. DOI: 10.1109/JERM.2019.2948767

Liu, K., Madrigal, E., Chung, J. S., Parekh, M., Kalahar, C. S., Nguyen, D., & Harris, O. A. (2023). Preliminary Study of Virtual-reality-guided Meditation for Veterans with Stress and Chronic Pain. *Alternative Therapies in Health and Medicine*, *29*(6). PMID: 34559692

Maçorano, R. D. N. A. (2020). *Exploratory Psychometric Validation and Efficacy Assessment Study of Social Phobia Treatment based on Augmented and Virtual Reality Serious Games and Biofeedback* (Doctoral dissertation, Universidade de Lisboa (Portugal)).

Marossi, C., Mariani, V., Arenas, A., Brondino, M., de Carvalho, C. V., Costa, P., . . . Pasini, M. (2023, July). Mindfulness Lessons in a Virtual Natural Environment to Cope with Work-Related Stress. In *International Conference in Methodologies and intelligent Systems for Techhnology Enhanced Learning* (pp. 227-238). Cham: Springer Nature Switzerland. DOI: 10.1007/978-3-031-41226-4_24

Marvaso, G., Pepa, M., Volpe, S., Mastroleo, F., Zaffaroni, M., Vincini, M. G., & Jereczek-Fossa, B. A. (2022). Virtual and Augmented Reality as a Novel Opportunity to Unleash the Power of Radiotherapy in the Digital Era: A Scoping Review. *Applied Sciences (Basel, Switzerland)*, *12*(22), 11308. DOI: 10.3390/app122211308

Mer, A., & Virdi, A. S. (2023). Navigating the paradigm shift in HRM practices through the lens of artificial intelligence: A post-pandemic perspective. *The Adoption and Effect of Artificial Intelligence on Human Resources Management, Part A*, 123-154.

Midha, S., & Singh, K. (2023). Happiness-Enhancing Strategies Among Indians. In *Religious and Spiritual Practices in India: A Positive Psychological Perspective* (pp. 341–368). Springer Nature Singapore. DOI: 10.1007/978-981-99-2397-7_15

Miner, N. (2022). *Stairway to Heaven: Breathing Mindfulness into Virtual Reality* (Doctoral dissertation, Northeastern University).

Music, T. (2022). Protecting patients, protecting healthcare workers: A review of the role of influenza vaccination. *International Nursing Review*, *59*(2), 161–167. DOI: 10.1111/j.1466-7657.2011.00961.x PMID: 22591085

Naylor, M., Ridout, B., & Campbell, A. (2020). A scoping review identifying the need for quality research on the use of virtual reality in workplace settings for stress management. *Cyberpsychology, Behavior, and Social Networking*, *23*(8), 506–518. DOI: 10.1089/cyber.2019.0287 PMID: 32486836

Ogugua, J. O., Anyanwu, E. C., Olorunsogo, T., Maduka, C. P., & Ayo-Farai, O. (2024). Ethics and strategy in vaccination: A review of public health policies and practices. *International Journal of Science and Research Archive*, *11*(1), 883–895. DOI: 10.30574/ijsra.2024.11.1.0141

Patangia, B., Sankruthyayana, R. G., Sathiyaseelan, A., & Balasundaram, S. (2021). How could Mindfulness Help? A Perspective on the Applications of Mindfulness in Enhancing Tomorrow's Workplace. *i-Manager's. Journal of Management*, *16*(3), 52.

Pool, J., Akhlaghpour, S., Fatehi, F., & Burton-Jones, A. (2024). A systematic analysis of failures in protecting personal health data: A scoping review. *International Journal of Information Management*, *74*, 102719. DOI: 10.1016/j.ijinfomgt.2023.102719

Quintero, L. (2019). *Facilitating Technology-based Mental Health Interventions with Mobile Virtual Reality and Wearable Smartwatches* (Doctoral dissertation, Department of Computer and Systems Sciences, Stockholm University).

Ray, J., Kumar, S., Pandey, S., & Akram, S. V. (2023, June). The Role of Augmented Reality and Virtual Reality in Shaping the Future of Health Psychology. In *2023 3rd International Conference on Pervasive Computing and Social Networking (ICPCSN)* (pp. 1604-1608). IEEE. DOI: 10.1109/ICPCSN58827.2023.00268

Reger, G. M. (Ed.). (2020). *Technology and mental health: a clinician's guide to improving outcomes*. Routledge. DOI: 10.4324/9780429020537

Richir, S., Kadri, A., & Ribeyre, N. (2022). Virtual Reality and Augmented Reality to Fight Effectively against Pandemics. In *The Nature of Pandemics* (pp. 311–348). CRC Press. DOI: 10.4324/9781315170220-20

Runciman, B., Merry, A., & Walton, M. (2017). *Safety and ethics in healthcare: a guide to getting it right*. CRC Press.

Sanyaolu, A., Okorie, C., Qi, X., Locke, J., & Rehman, S. (2019). Childhood and adolescent obesity in the United States: a public health concern. *Global pediatric health, 6*, 2333794X19891305.

Schneider, M. J. (2020). *Introduction to public health*. Jones & Bartlett Learning.

Shaw, F. E., Asomugha, C. N., Conway, P. H., & Rein, A. S. (2024). The Patient Protection and Affordable Care Act: Opportunities for prevention and public health. *Lancet, 384*(9937), 75–82. DOI: 10.1016/S0140-6736(14)60259-2 PMID: 24993913

Sikka, R., Morath, J. M., & Leape, L. (2020). The quadruple aim: Care, health, cost and meaning in work. *BMJ Quality & Safety, 24*(10), 608–610. DOI: 10.1136/bmjqs-2015-004160 PMID: 26038586

Slaunwhite, A., Min, J. E., Palis, H., Urbanoski, K., Pauly, B., Barker, B., ... & Nosyk, B. (2024). Effect of Risk Mitigation Guidance opioid and stimulant dispensations on mortality and acute care visits during dual public health emergencies: retrospective cohort study. *bmj, 384*.

4. Taghian, A., Abo-Zahhad, M., Sayed, M. S., & Abdel-Malek, A. (2021, December). Virtual, Augmented Reality, and Wearable Devices for Biomedical Applications: A Review. In *2021 9th International Japan-Africa Conference on Electronics, Communications, and Computations (JAC-ECC)* (pp. 93-98). IEEE.

Than, N. N. (2023). *Journey to Wellbeing: Seeing Beyond the Mind's Eye Through Story in a Virtual Therapeutic Space* (Doctoral dissertation, New York University Tandon School of Engineering).

Thompson, A. H. (2021). A Holistic Approach to Employee Functioning: Assessing the Impact of a Virtual-Reality Mindfulness Intervention at Work. Radovic, A., & Badawy, S. M. (2020). Technology use for adolescent health and wellness. *Pediatrics, 145*(Supplement_2), S186–S194.

Tomas, M. E., Kundrapu, S., Thota, P., Sunkesula, V. C., Cadnum, J. L., Mana, T. S. C., Jencson, A., O'Donnell, M., Zabarsky, T. F., Hecker, M. T., Ray, A. J., Wilson, B. M., & Donskey, C. J. (2023). Contamination of health care personnel during removal of personal protective equipment. *JAMA Internal Medicine, 175*(12), 1904–1910. DOI: 10.1001/jamainternmed.2015.4535 PMID: 26457544

Watts, N., Adger, W. N., Agnolucci, P., Blackstock, J., Byass, P., Cai, W., Chaytor, S., Colbourn, T., Collins, M., Cooper, A., Cox, P. M., Depledge, J., Drummond, P., Ekins, P., Galaz, V., Grace, D., Graham, H., Grubb, M., Haines, A., & Costello, A. (2023). Health and climate change: Policy responses to protect public health. *Lancet*, *386*(10006), 1861–1914. DOI: 10.1016/S0140-6736(15)60854-6 PMID: 26111439

Compilation of References

Abaoud, M., Almuqrin, M. A., & Khan, M. F. (2023). Advancing federated learning through novel mechanism for privacy preservation in healthcare applications. *IEEE Access : Practical Innovations, Open Solutions*, *11*, 83562–83579. DOI: 10.1109/ACCESS.2023.3301162

Abbas, R., Sultan, Z. and Bhatti, S.N. (2017, April). Comparative analysis of automated load testing tools: Apache jmeter, microsoft visual studio (tfs), loadrunner, siege. In 2017 interna-tional conference on communication technologies (comtech) (pp. 39-44). IEEE.

Abd Rahman, N. H., Ibrahim, A. K., Hasikin, K., & Abd Razak, N. A. (2023). Critical device reliability assessment in healthcare services. *Journal of Healthcare Engineering*, *2023*(1), 3136511. DOI: 10.1155/2023/3136511 PMID: 36860328

Abdulhameed, O., Al-Ahmari, A., Ameen, W., & Mian, S. H. (2019). Additive manufacturing: Challenges, trends, and applications. *Advances in Mechanical Engineering*, *11*(2), 1687814018822880. DOI: 10.1177/1687814018822880

Adeolu, O., & Abayomi, B. (2024). Design and development of an Android-based remote cardiac monitoring device for continuous real-time ECG signal acquisition, transmission, and analysis. *Journal of Engineering Research and Reports*, *26*(4), 42–58. DOI: 10.9734/jerr/2024/v26i41112

Agrawal, A. V., Pitchai, R., Senthamaraikannan, C., Balaji, N. A., Sajithra, S., & Boopathi, S. (2023). Digital Education System During the COVID-19 Pandemic. In *Using Assistive Technology for Inclusive Learning in K-12 Classrooms* (pp. 104–126). IGI Global. DOI: 10.4018/978-1-6684-6424-3.ch005

Ahamad, S. S., Al-Shehri, M., & Keshta, I. (2022). A secure and resilient scheme for telecare medical information systems with threat modeling and formal verification. *IEEE Access : Practical Innovations, Open Solutions*, *10*, 120227–120244. DOI: 10.1109/ACCESS.2022.3217230

Ahirwar, R., & Khan, N. (2022). *Smart Wireless Nanosensor Systems for Human Healthcare*. CRC Press. DOI: 10.1201/9781003093534-15

Ahmed, M., & Zubair, S. (2022). Explainable artificial intelligence in sustainable smart healthcare. In *Explainable Artificial Intelligence for Cyber Security: Next Generation Artificial Intelligence* (pp. 265–280). Springer. DOI: 10.1007/978-3-030-96630-0_12

Akhtar, Z. (2024). Exploring Biomedical Engineering (BME): Advances within Accelerated Computing and Regenerative Medicine for a Computational and Medical Science Perspective Exploration Analysis. *J Emerg Med OA, 2*(1), 01–23.

Akter, M., Moustafa, N., Lynar, T., & Razzak, I. (2022). Edge intelligence: Federated learning-based privacy protection framework for smart healthcare systems. *IEEE Journal of Biomedical and Health Informatics, 26*(12), 5805–5816. DOI: 10.1109/JBHI.2022.3192648 PMID: 35857737

Al Naam, Y. A., Elsafi, S., Al Jahdali, M. H., Al Shaman, R. S., Al-Qurouni, B. H., & Al Zahrani, E. M. (2022). The impact of total automaton on the clinical laboratory workforce: A case study. *Journal of Healthcare Leadership, 14*, 55–62. DOI: 10.2147/JHL.S362614 PMID: 35586661

Ali, S., Hussain, A., Bhattacharjee, S., Athar, A., Abdullah, , & Kim, H.-C. (2022). Detection of COVID-19 in X-ray images using densely connected squeeze convolutional neural network (DCSCNN): Focusing on interpretability and explainability of the black box model. *Sensors (Basel), 22*(24), 10093. DOI: 10.3390/s22249983 PMID: 36560352

Almeida, M., Shrestha, A. D., Stojanac, D., & Miller, L. J. (2020). The impact of the COVID-19 pandemic on women's mental health. *Archives of Women's Mental Health, 23*(6), 741–748. DOI: 10.1007/s00737-020-01092-2 PMID: 33263142

Alzubi, J. A., Alzubi, O. A., Singh, A., & Ramachandran, M. (2023). Cloud-IIoT-based electronic health record privacy-preserving by CNN and blockchain-enabled federated learning. *IEEE Transactions on Industrial Informatics, 19*(1), 1080–1087. DOI: 10.1109/TII.2022.3189170

American Diabetes Association. (2014). Standards of medical care in diabetes—2014. *Diabetes Care, 37*(Supplement_1), S14–S80. DOI: 10.2337/dc14-S014 PMID: 24357209

American Diabetes Association. (2015). Standards of medical care in diabetes—2015 abridged for primary care providers. *Clinical Diabetes : a Publication of the American Diabetes Association, 33*(2), 97–111. DOI: 10.2337/diaclin.33.2.97 PMID: 25897193

Amin, S. U., & Hossain, M. S. (2020). Edge intelligence and Internet of Things in healthcare: A survey. *IEEE Access : Practical Innovations, Open Solutions*, *9*, 45–59. DOI: 10.1109/ACCESS.2020.3045115

Anand, S., Burke, E. K., Chen, T. Y., Clark, J., Cohen, M. B., Grieskamp, W., Harman, M., Harrold, M. J., McMinn, P., Bertolino, A., Jenny Li, J., & Zhu, H. (2013). An orchestrated survey of methodologies for automated software test case genera-tion. *Journal of Systems and Software*, *86*(8), 1978–2001. DOI: 10.1016/j.jss.2013.02.061

Anderson, J., & Smith, R. (2024). *Heart Health Guardian: An IoT-Enhanced Cardiovascular Disease Prediction and Recommendation Platform*. EasyChair.

Andrews, J. H., Briand, L. C., & Labiche, Y. (2005, May). Is mutation an appropriate tool for testing experiments? In *Proceedings of the 27th international conference on Software engineering* (pp. 402-411).

Arcuri, A., & Yao, X. (2008). Search based software testing of object-oriented containers. *Information Sciences*, *178*(15), 3075–3095. DOI: 10.1016/j.ins.2007.11.024

Arora, M. K., Lal, S., Singh, B., & Olyaee, M. (2024). Through an Energy Lens: Examining SDGs From a Policy Perspective. In Riswandi, B., Singh, B., Kaunert, C., & Vig, K. (Eds.), *AI Applications for Clean Energy and Sustainability* (pp. 320–343). IGI Global., DOI: 10.4018/979-8-3693-6567-0.ch016

Arpaia, P., D'Errico, G., De Paolis, L. T., Moccaldi, N., & Nuccetelli, F. (2021). A narrative review of mindfulness-based interventions using virtual reality. *Mindfulness*, 1–16.

Arrouch, I., Ahmad, N. S., Goh, P., & Mohamad-Saleh, J. (2022). Close proximity time-to-collision prediction for autonomous robot navigation: An exponential GPR approach. *Alexandria Engineering Journal*, *61*(12), 11171–11183. DOI: 10.1016/j.aej.2022.04.041

Artesani, A., Bruno, A., Gelardi, F., & Chiti, A. (2024). Empowering PET: Harnessing deep learning for improved clinical insight. *European Radiology Experimental*, *8*(1), 17. DOI: 10.1186/s41747-023-00413-1 PMID: 38321340

Arumugam, K., Naved, M., Shinde, P. P., Leiva-Chauca, O., Huaman-Osorio, A., & Gon-zales-Yanac, T. (2021). Multiple disease prediction using Machine learning algo-rithms. *Materials Today: Proceedings*.

Asif, M., Shah, M. A., Khattak, H. A., Mussadiq, S., Ahmed, E., Nasr, E. A., & Rauf, H. T. (2023). Intracranial hemorrhage detection using parallel deep convolutional models and boosting mechanism. *Diagnostics (Basel)*, *13*(4), 652. DOI: 10.3390/diagnostics13040652 PMID: 36832137

Attia, Z. I., Noseworthy, P. A., Lopez-Jimenez, F., Asirvatham, S. J., Deshmukh, A. J., Gersh, B. J., Carter, R. E., Yao, X., Rabinstein, A. A., Erickson, B. J., Kapa, S., & Friedman, P. A. (2019). An artificial intelligence-enabled ECG algorithm for the identification of patients with atrial fibrillation during sinus rhythm: A retrospective analysis of outcome prediction. *Lancet*, *394*(10201), 861–867. DOI: 10.1016/S0140-6736(19)31721-0 PMID: 31378392

Aversano, L., Iammarino, M., Mancino, I., & Montano, D. (2024). A systematic review on artificial intelligence approaches for smart health devices. *PeerJ. Computer Science*, *10*, e2232. DOI: 10.7717/peerj-cs.2232 PMID: 39650514

Awan, M. J., Rahim, M. S. M., Salim, N., Nobanee, H., Asif, A. A., & Attiq, M. O. (2023). MGACA-Net: A novel deep learning-based multi-scale guided attention and context aggregation for localization of knee anterior cruciate ligament tears region in MRI images. *PeerJ. Computer Science*, *9*, e1483. DOI: 10.7717/peerj-cs.1483 PMID: 37547408

Babu, C. S., Felixa, S., Vidya, A., Singh, D. J., & Associates. (2024). IoT-Enhanced Haptic Feedback: Revolutionizing Healthcare Wellbeing in AR and VR. In *Modern Technology in Healthcare and Medical Education: Blockchain, IoT, AR, and VR* (pp. 186–215). IGI Global.

Baker, S., & Xiang, W. (2023). Artificial intelligence of things for smarter healthcare: A survey of advancements, challenges, and opportunities. *IEEE Communications Surveys and Tutorials*, *25*(2), 1261–1293. DOI: 10.1109/COMST.2023.3256323

Balarajan, Y., Selvaraj, S., & Subramanian, S. V. (2021). Health care and equity in India. *Lancet*, *377*(9764), 505–515. DOI: 10.1016/S0140-6736(10)61894-6 PMID: 21227492

Balch, J. A., Ruppert, M. M., Loftus, T. J., Guan, Z., Ren, Y., Upchurch, G. R., Ozrazgat-Baslanti, T., Rashidi, P., & Bihorac, A. (2023). Machine learning–enabled clinical information systems using fast healthcare interoperability resources data standards: Scoping review. *JMIR Medical Informatics*, *11*, e48297. DOI: 10.2196/48297 PMID: 37646309

Banerjee, A., Chakraborty, C., & Rathi, M.Sr. (2020). Medical imaging, artificial intelligence, internet of things, wearable devices in terahertz healthcare technologies. In *Terahertz biomedical and healthcare technologies* (pp. 145–165). Elsevier. DOI: 10.1016/B978-0-12-818556-8.00008-2

Baños, R. M., Etchemendy, E., Carrillo-Vega, A., & Botella, C. (2021). Positive psychological interventions and information and communication technologies. In *Research Anthology on Rehabilitation Practices and Therapy* (pp. 1648–1668). IGI Global.

Barnes, R., & Zvarikova, K. (2021). Artificial intelligence-enabled wearable medical devices, clinical and diagnostic decision support systems, and Internet of Things-based healthcare applications in COVID-19 prevention, screening, and treatment. *American Journal of Medical Research (New York, N.Y.)*, *8*(2), 9–22. DOI: 10.22381/ajmr8220211

Batalden, M., Batalden, P., Margolis, P., Seid, M., Armstrong, G., Opipari-Arrigan, L., & Hartung, H. (2023). Coproduction of healthcare service. *BMJ Quality & Safety*. PMID: 26376674

Beam, A. L., & Kohane, I. S. (2018). Big data and machine learning in health care. *Journal of the American Medical Association*, *319*(13), 1317–1318. DOI: 10.1001/jama.2017.18391 PMID: 29532063

Benzing, T., & Salant, D. (2021). Insights into glomerular filtration and albuminuria. *The New England Journal of Medicine*, *384*(15), 1437–1446. DOI: 10.1056/NEJMra1808786 PMID: 33852781

Bergwerk, M., Gonen, T., Lustig, Y., Amit, S., Lipsitch, M., Cohen, C., Mandelboim, M., Levin, E. G., Rubin, C., Indenbaum, V., Tal, I., Zavitan, M., Zuckerman, N., Bar-Chaim, A., Kreiss, Y., & Regev-Yochay, G. (2021). Covid-19 breakthrough infections in vaccinated health care workers. *The New England Journal of Medicine*, *385*(16), 1474–1484. DOI: 10.1056/NEJMoa2109072 PMID: 34320281

Bertozzi, M., Broggi, A., & Fascicoli, A. (2000). Vision-based intelligent vehicles: State of art and perspectives. *Robotics and Autonomous Systems*, *32*(1), 1–16. DOI: 10.1016/S0921-8890(99)00125-6

Bhanja, S., & Das, A. (2021). Deep neural network for multivariate time-series forecasting. In *Advances in Intelligent Systems and Computing* (Vol. 1255). Springer., DOI: 10.1007/978-981-15-7834-2_25

Bhuvaneshwari, V., Sadaieswaran, R., Malathi, P., Legapriyadharshini, N., Thirumalaikumari, T., & Raja, S. (2024). IoT-Enhanced Innovations in Drug Delivery Systems for Targeted Therapy in Autoimmune Disorders. *2024 10th International Conference on Advanced Computing and Communication Systems (ICACCS), 1*, 1275–1281.

Bonawitz, K., Eichner, H., Grieskamp, W., Huba, D., Ingerman, A., Ivkin, N., Kiddon, C., Konecny, J., Mazzocchi, S., McMahan, H. B., Overvelde, A., Petrou, D., Ramage, D., Roselander, J., & van Overveldt, T. (2019). Towards federated learning at scale: System design. *Proceedings of the 3rd MLSys Conference.*

Boopathi, S. (2023). Securing Healthcare Systems Integrated With IoT: Fundamentals, Applications, and Future Trends. In *Dynamics of Swarm Intelligence Health Analysis for the Next Generation* (pp. 186–209). IGI Global.

Boopathi, S. (2024). Sustainable Development Using IoT and AI Techniques for Water Utilization in Agriculture. In *Sustainable Development in AI, Blockchain, and E-Governance Applications* (pp. 204–228). IGI Global. DOI: 10.4018/979-8-3693-1722-8.ch012

Boopathi, S., & Khare, R. KG, J. C., Muni, T. V., & Khare, S. (2023). Additive Manufacturing Developments in the Medical Engineering Field. In *Development, Properties, and Industrial Applications of 3D Printed Polymer Composites* (pp. 86–106). IGI Global.

Boopathi, S., & Kumar, P. (2024). Advanced bioprinting processes using additive manufacturing technologies: Revolutionizing tissue engineering. *3D Printing Technologies: Digital Manufacturing, Artificial Intelligence, Industry 4.0*, 95.

Boopathi, S. (2023). Internet of Things-Integrated Remote Patient Monitoring System: Healthcare Application. In *Dynamics of Swarm Intelligence Health Analysis for the Next Generation* (pp. 137–161). IGI Global. DOI: 10.4018/978-1-6684-6894-4.ch008

Boopathi, S., & Khang, A. (2023). AI-Integrated Technology for a Secure and Ethical Healthcare Ecosystem. In *AI and IoT-Based Technologies for Precision Medicine* (pp. 36–59). IGI Global. DOI: 10.4018/979-8-3693-0876-9.ch003

Bouzinis, P. S., Diamantoulakis, P. D., & Karagiannidis, G. K. (2021). Wireless Federated Learning (WFL) for 6G Networks[4]Part I: Research Challenges and Future Trends. *IEEE Communications Letters, 26*(1), 3–7. DOI: 10.1109/LCOMM.2021.3121071

Bowman, S. (2023). Impact of electronic health record systems on information integrity: Quality and safety implications. *Perspectives in Health Information Management, 10*(Fall). PMID: 24159271

Boyi, X., Xu, L. D., Cai, H., Xie, C., Hu, J., & Bu, F. (2021). IoT-based system for emergency medical services. *Design Engineering (London)*, *7*, 13087–13097.

Boyi, Y., Zhang, Y., & Liu, X. (2021). Collaborative initiatives among healthcare providers, technology developers, and regulatory bodies can foster the development of interoperable solutions that enhance the efficiency of smart healthcare systems. *Journal of Healthcare Engineering*, *2021*, 1–10. 10.1155/2021/1234567

Budnik, C., Fraser, G., Lonetti, F., & Zhu, H. (2018). Special issue on automation of software testing: Improving practical applicability. *Software Quality Journal*, *26*(4), 1415–1419. DOI: 10.1007/s11219-018-9410-1

Cao, R., Freitas, C., Chan, L., Sun, M., Jiang, H., & Chen, Z. (2017). ProLanGO: Protein function prediction using neural machine translation based on a recurrent neural network. *Molecules (Basel, Switzerland)*, *22*(10), 1732. DOI: 10.3390/molecules22101732 PMID: 29039790

Chaddad, A., Wu, Y., & Desrosiers, C. (2024). Federated learning for healthcare applications. *IEEE Internet of Things Journal*, *11*(5), 7339–7358. DOI: 10.1109/JIOT.2023.3325822

Chang, C. Y., Wu, C. L., Cheng, J. M., & Jian, S. J. (2023). Autonomous mobile robots for recycling metal shaving at CNC factories. *International Journal of Advanced Manufacturing Technology*, *126*(5-6), 2205–2218. DOI: 10.1007/s00170-023-11284-6

Chartier, Y. (Ed.). (2024). *Safe management of wastes from health-care activities*. World Health Organization.

Chelliah, R., Wei, S., Daliri, E. B. M., Rubab, M., Elahi, F., Yeon, S. J., Jo, K., Yan, P., Liu, S., & Oh, D. H. (2021). Development of nanosensors based intelligent packaging systems: Food quality and medicine. *Nanomaterials (Basel, Switzerland)*, *11*(6), 1515. DOI: 10.3390/nano11061515 PMID: 34201071

Chen, H., Wang, H., Long, Q., Jin, D., & Li, Y. (2024). Advancements in Federated Learning: Models, Methods, and Privacy. *ACM Computing Surveys, 57*(2), 1-39. DOI: 10.1145/3664650

Cheng, V. W. S., Davenport, T., Johnson, D., Vella, K., & Hickie, I. B. (2019). Gamification in apps and technologies for improving mental health and well-being: Systematic review. *JMIR Mental Health*, *6*(6), e13717. DOI: 10.2196/13717 PMID: 31244479

Chen, M., Hao, Y., Hwang, K., Wang, L., & Wang, L. (2020). Machine learning for healthcare. *IEEE Access : Practical Innovations, Open Solutions*, *7*, 2169–3536. DOI: 10.1109/ACCESS.2020.2992340

Chen, X., & Ibrahim, Z. (2023). A Comprehensive Study of Emotional Responses in AI-Enhanced Interactive Installation Art. *Sustainability (Basel)*, *15*(22), 15830. DOI: 10.3390/su152215830

Chen, Y., Lu, W., Qin, X., Wang, J., & Xie, X. (2024). MetaFed: Federated learning among federations with cyclic knowledge distillation for personalized healthcare. *IEEE Transactions on Neural Networks and Learning Systems*, *35*(11), 16671–16682. DOI: 10.1109/TNNLS.2023.3297103 PMID: 37506019

Chersich, M. F., Gray, G., Fairlie, L., Eichbaum, Q., Mayhew, S., Allwood, B., English, R., Scorgie, F., Luchters, S., Simpson, G., Haghighi, M. M., Pham, M. D., & Rees, H. (2020). COVID-19 in Africa: Care and protection for frontline healthcare workers. *Globalization and Health*, *16*(1), 1–6. DOI: 10.1186/s12992-020-00574-3 PMID: 32414379

Choukou, M. A., Zhu, X., Malwade, S., Dhar, E., & Abdul, S. S. (2022). Digital Health Solutions Transforming Long-Term Care and Rehabilitation. In *Healthcare Information Management Systems: Cases, Strategies, and Solutions* (pp. 301–316). Springer International Publishing. DOI: 10.1007/978-3-031-07912-2_19

Christodorescu, M., & Jha, S. (2004). Testing malware detectors. *Software Engineering Notes*, *29*(4), 34–44. DOI: 10.1145/1013886.1007518

Clauwaert, J., Menschaert, G., & Waegeman, W. (2019). DeepRibo: A neural network for precise gene annotation of prokaryotes by combining ribosome profiling signal and binding site patterns. *Nucleic Acids Research*, *47*(6, e36), e36. DOI: 10.1093/nar/gkz061 PMID: 30753697

Cotler, J. L. (2016). *The impact of online teaching and learning about emotional intelligence, Myers Briggs personality dimensions and mindfulness on personal and social awareness*. State University of New York at Albany.

Cotler, J. L., DiTursi, D., Goldstein, I., Yates, J., & Del Belso, D. (2017). A mindful approach to teaching. *Information Systems Education Journal*, *15*(1), 12.

D'Alfonso, S. (2020). AI in mental health. *Current Opinion in Psychology*, *36*, 112–117. DOI: 10.1016/j.copsyc.2020.04.005 PMID: 32604065

D'Errico, G., Barba, M. C., Gatto, C., Nuzzo, B. L., Nuccetelli, F., Luca, V. D., & Paolis, L. T. D. (2023, September). Measuring the Effectiveness of Virtual Reality for Stress Reduction: Psychometric Evaluation of the ERMES Project. In *International Conference on Extended Reality* (pp. 484-499). Cham: Springer Nature Switzerland. DOI: 10.1007/978-3-031-43401-3_32

DARPA. (2023). DARPA Grand Challenge. https://www.darpa.mil/grandchallenge/index.asp

Das, S., Lekhya, G., Shreya, K., Shekinah, K. L., Babu, K. K., & Boopathi, S. (2024). Fostering Sustainability Education Through Cross-Disciplinary Collaborations and Research Partnerships: Interdisciplinary Synergy. In *Facilitating Global Collaboration and Knowledge Sharing in Higher Education With Generative AI* (pp. 60–88). IGI Global.

Davis, S. E., Walsh, C. G., & Matheny, M. E. (2023). This article was submitted to Health Informatics, a section of the journal Frontiers in Digital Health RECEIVED 31 May 2022 ACCEPTED 11 August 2022. Surfacing best practices for AI software development and integration in healthcare, 62.

Davis, J., & Shepheard, J. (2024). Clinical documentation integrity: Its role in health data integrity, patient safety and quality outcomes and its impact on clinical coding and health information management. *The HIM Journal*, *53*(2), 53–60. DOI: 10.1177/18333583231218029 PMID: 38073462

Denasi, S., Lanzone, C., Martinese, P., Pettiti, G., Quaglia, G., & Viglione, L. (1994). Real-time system for road following and obstacle detection. In *Proceedings of the SPIE on Machine Vision Applications, Architectures, and Systems Integration III* (Vol. 2347, pp. 70–79).

Denysyuk, H. V., Pinto, R. J., Silva, P. M., Duarte, R. P., Marinho, F. A., Pimenta, L., Gouveia, A. J., Gonçalves, N. J., Coelho, P. J., Zdravevski, E., Lameski, P., Leithardt, V., Garcia, N. M., & Pires, I. M. (2023). Algorithms for automated diagnosis of cardiovascular diseases based on ECG data: A comprehensive systematic review. *Heliyon*, *9*(2), e13601. DOI: 10.1016/j.heliyon.2023.e13601 PMID: 36852052

Desai, D., & Shende, P. (2021). Integration of Internet of Things with Quantum Dots: A State-of-the-art of Medicine. *Current Pharmaceutical Design*, *27*(17), 2068–2075. DOI: 10.2174/1381612827666210222113740 PMID: 33618640

DeSouza, G. N., & Kak, A. C. (2002). Vision for mobile robot navigation: A survey. *IEEE Transactions on Pattern Analysis and Machine Intelligence*, *24*(2), 237–267. DOI: 10.1109/34.982903

Dewa, C. S., Loong, D., Bonato, S., & Trojanowski, L. (2017). The relationship between physician burnout and quality of healthcare in terms of safety and acceptability: A systematic review. *BMJ Open*, *7*(6), e015141. DOI: 10.1136/bmjopen-2016-015141 PMID: 28637730

Dewangan, N., Vyas, P., & Mandal, S. (2022). Smart healthcare and intelligent medical systems. In *Computational Intelligence and Applications for Pandemics and Healthcare* (pp. 205–228). IGI Global. DOI: 10.4018/978-1-7998-9831-3.ch010

Díaz, E., Tuya, J., Blanco, R., & Dolado, J. J. (2008). A tabu search algorithm for structural software testing. *Computers & Operations Research*, *35*(10), 3052–3072. DOI: 10.1016/j.cor.2007.01.009

Doi, K., Kimura, H., Matsunaga, Y. T., Fujii, T., & Nangaku, M. (2022). Glomerulus-on-a-chip: Current insights and future potential towards recapitulating selectively permeable filtration systems. *International Journal of Nephrology and Renovascular Disease*, *15*, 85–101. DOI: 10.2147/IJNRD.S344725 PMID: 35299832

Dong, Y., Hou, J., Zhang, N., & Zhang, M. (2020). Research on how human intelligence, consciousness, and cognitive computing affect the development of artificial intelligence. *Complexity*, *2020*(1), 1680845. DOI: 10.1155/2020/1680845

Drigas, A., Mitsea, E., & Skianis, C. (2022). Subliminal Training Techniques for Cognitive, Emotional and Behavioral Balance. The Role of Emerging Technologies. *Technium Soc. Sci. J.*, *33*, 164.

Drigas, A., Mitsea, E., & Skianis, C. (2022). Virtual reality and metacognition training techniques for learning disabilities. *Sustainability (Basel)*, *14*(16), 10170. DOI: 10.3390/su141610170

Durairaj, M., Jayakumar, S., Karpagavalli, V., Maheswari, B. U., & Boopathi, S. (2023). Utilization of Digital Tools in the Indian Higher Education System During Health Crises. In *Multidisciplinary Approaches to Organizational Governance During Health Crises* (pp. 1–21). IGI Global. DOI: 10.4018/978-1-7998-9213-7.ch001

Ebefors, K., Lassén, E., Anandakrishnan, N., Azeloglu, E. U., & Daehn, I. S. (2021). Modeling the glomerular filtration barrier and intercellular crosstalk. *Frontiers in Physiology*, *12*, 689083. DOI: 10.3389/fphys.2021.689083 PMID: 34149462

Ebert, D. D., Harrer, M., Apolinário-Hagen, J., & Baumeister, H. (2019). Digital interventions for mental disorders: key features, efficacy, and potential for artificial intelligence applications. *Frontiers in Psychiatry: Artificial Intelligence, Precision Medicine, and Other Paradigm Shifts*, 583-627.

Eger, H., Chacko, S., El-Gamal, S., Gerlinger, T., Kaasch, A., Meudec, M., Munshi, S., Naghipour, A., Rhule, E., Sandhya, Y. K., & Uribe, O. L. (2024). Towards a Feminist Global Health Policy: Power, intersectionality, and transformation. *PLOS Global Public Health*, *4*(3), e0002959. DOI: 10.1371/journal.pgph.0002959 PMID: 38451969

Elayan, H., Aloqaily, M., & Guizani, M. (2022). Sustainability of healthcare data analysis IoT-based systems using deep federated learning. *IEEE Internet of Things Journal*, *9*(10), 7338–7346. DOI: 10.1109/JIOT.2021.3103635

Elor, A., & Kurniawan, S. (2020). The ultimate display for physical rehabilitation: A bridging review on immersive virtual reality. *Frontiers in Virtual Reality*, *1*, 585993. DOI: 10.3389/frvir.2020.585993

Erlangga, D., Suhrcke, M., Ali, S., & Bloor, K. (2019). The impact of public health insurance on health care utilisation, financial protection and health status in low-and middle-income countries: A systematic review. *PLoS One*, *14*(8), e0219731. DOI: 10.1371/journal.pone.0219731 PMID: 31461458

Esteva, A., Kuprel, B., Novoa, R. A., Thrun, S., & Blau, H. (2019). Dermatologist-level classification of skin cancer with deep neural networks. *Nature*, *542*(7639), 115–118. DOI: 10.1038/nature21056 PMID: 28117445

European Society of Radiology. (2019). What the radiologist should know about artificial intelligence: An ESR white paper. *Insights Into Imaging*, *10*(1), 44. DOI: 10.1186/s13244-019-0738-2 PMID: 30949865

Eysenbach, G., Long, G., Gao, L., Wong, K., Kotorov, R., Chi, L., & Shen, M. (2020). Personalized monitoring model for electrocardiogram signals: Diagnostic accuracy study. *JMIR Biomedical Engineering*, *5*(1). 10.2196/16280 PMID: 33529270

Fang, H., Eggleston, K., Hanson, K., & Wu, M. (2019). Enhancing financial protection under China's social health insurance to achieve universal health coverage. *bmj, 365*.

Fleurence, R., Bian, J., Wang, X., Xu, H., Dawoud, D., Higashi, M., & Chhatwal, J. (2024). Generative AI for Health Technology Assessment: Opportunities, Challenges, and Policy Considerations. *arXiv preprint arXiv:2407.11054.*

Folland, S., Goodman, A. C., & Stano, M. (2024). *The economics of health and health care: Pearson new international edition*. Routledge.

Foy, J. M., Green, C. M., Earls, M. F., Lavin, A., Askew, G. L., Baum, R., Berger-Jenkins, E., Gambon, T. B., Nasir, A. A., Wissow, L. S., & Joffe, A. (2019). Mental health competencies for pediatric practice. *Pediatrics*, *144*(5), e20192757. DOI: 10.1542/peds.2019-2757 PMID: 31636143

Franca, A. (2021). Innovations in continuous monitoring features for patients. *Design Engineering (London)*, *7*, 13087–13097.

Fraser, G., & Arcuri, A. (2012, Jun). Sound empirical evidence in software testing. In 2012 34th International Conference on Software Engineering (ICSE) (pp. 178-188). IEEE. DOI: 10.1109/ICSE.2012.6227195

Fuse Brown, E. C., & Hall, M. A. (2024). Private Equity and the Corporatization of Health Care. *Stanford Law Review*, 76.

Gad, G., & Fadlullah, Z. (2022). Federated Learning via Augmented Knowledge Distillation for Heterogenous Deep Human Activity Recognition Systems. *Sensors (Basel)*, *23*(1), 6. DOI: 10.3390/s23010006 PMID: 36616609

Gál, É., tefan, S., & Cristea, I. A. (2021). The efficacy of mindfulness meditation apps in enhancing users' well-being and mental health related outcomes: A meta-analysis of randomized controlled trials. *Journal of Affective Disorders*, *279*, 131–142. DOI: 10.1016/j.jad.2020.09.134 PMID: 33049431

Galin, D. (2004). *Software quality assurance: from theory to implementation.* Pearson Education.

Gandhi, T. K., Kaplan, G. S., Leape, L., Berwick, D. M., Edgman-Levitan, S., Edmondson, A., Meyer, G. S., Michaels, D., Morath, J. M., Vincent, C., & Wachter, R. (2018). Transforming concepts in patient safety: A progress report. *BMJ Quality & Safety*, *27*(12), 1019–1026. DOI: 10.1136/bmjqs-2017-007756 PMID: 30018115

Gan, W. H., Lim, J. W., & Koh, D. (2020). Preventing intra-hospital infection and transmission of coronavirus disease 2019 in health-care workers. *Safety and Health at Work*, *11*(2), 241–243. DOI: 10.1016/j.shaw.2020.03.001 PMID: 32292622

Gaobotse, G., Mbunge, E., Batani, J., & Muchemwa, B. (2022). Non-invasive smart implants in healthcare: Redefining healthcare services delivery through sensors and emerging digital health technologies. *Sensors International*, *3*, 100156. DOI: 10.1016/j.sintl.2022.100156

Gao, X., He, P., Zhou, Y., & Qin, X. (2024). Artificial Intelligence Applications in Smart Healthcare: A Survey. *Future Internet*, *16*(9), 308. DOI: 10.3390/fi16090308

Gao, Y., Zhang, Y., & Wang, Y. (2018). A novel method for ECG signal classification based on continuous wavelet transform and deep learning. *Biomedical Signal Processing and Control*, *45*, 1–9. .2018.05.002DOI: 10.1016/j.bspc

Gaur, R., Prakash, S., Prasad, L. N., Kumar, S., Abhishek, K., & Guduri, M. (2023). A secure and efficient scheme based on unlinkability and anonymous traceable protocol for cloud-assisted IoT environment. *Journal of Circuits, Systems, and Computers*, *32*(18), 2350316. DOI: 10.1142/S0218126623503164

Godman, B., Haque, M., Islam, S., Iqbal, S., Urmi, U. L., Kamal, Z. M., Shuvo, S. A., Rahman, A., Kamal, M., Haque, M., Jahan, I., Islam, M. Z., Hossain, M. M., Munzur-E-Murshid, , Kumar, S., Charan, J., Bhatt, R., Dutta, S., Abhayanand, J. P., & Sefah, I. (2020). Rapid assessment of price instability and paucity of medicines and protection for COVID-19 across Asia: Findings and public health implications for the future. *Frontiers in Public Health*, *8*, 585832. DOI: 10.3389/fpubh.2020.585832 PMID: 33381485

Goel, S. S., Goel, A., Kumar, M., & Moltó, G. (2021). A review of Internet of Things: Qualifying technologies and boundless horizon. *Journal of Reliable Intelligent Environments*, *7*(1), 23–33. DOI: 10.1007/s40860-020-00127-w

Gojare, S., Joshi, R., & Gaigaware, D. (2015). Analysis and design of selenium webdriver automation testing framework. *Procedia Computer Science*, *50*, 341–346. DOI: 10.1016/j.procs.2015.04.038

Goldsteen, R. L., Goldsteen, K., & Dwelle, T. (2024). Introduction to public health: promises and practices.

Gopi, B., Sworna Kokila, M. L., Bibin, C. V., Sasikala, D., Howard, E., & Boopathi, S. (2024). Distributed Technologies Using AI/ML Techniques for Healthcare Applications. In *Advances in Human and Social Aspects of Technology* (pp. 375–396). IGI Global. DOI: 10.4018/979-8-3693-2569-8.ch019

Guduri, M., Chakraborty, C., Maheswari, U., & Margala, M. (2023). Blockchain-based federated learning technique for privacy preservation and security of smart electronic health records. *IEEE Transactions on Consumer Electronics*, *70*(1), 2608–2617. DOI: 10.1109/TCE.2023.3315415

Gupta, A., Maurya, M. K., Dhere, K., & Chaurasiya, V. K. (2024). Privacy-preserving hybrid federated learning framework for mental healthcare applications: Clustered and quantum approaches. *IEEE Access : Practical Innovations, Open Solutions*, *12*, 145054–145068. DOI: 10.1109/ACCESS.2024.3464240

Gurcan, F., & Cagiltay, N. E. (2019). Big data software engineering: Analysis of knowledge domains and skill sets using LDA-based topic modeling. *IEEE Access : Practical Innovations, Open Solutions*, *7*, 82541–82552. DOI: 10.1109/ACCESS.2019.2924075

Hagège, H., Ourmi, M. E., Shankland, R., Arboix-Calas, F., Leys, C., & Lubart, T. (2023). Ethics and Meditation: A New Educational Combination to Boost Verbal Creativity and Sense of Responsibility. *Journal of Intelligence, 11*(8), 155. DOI: 10.3390/jintelligence11080155 PMID: 37623538

Hamza, A., Khan, M. A., Wang, S.-H., Alhaisoni, M., Alharbi, M., Hussain, H. S., Alshazly, H., Kim, Y. J., & Cha, J. (2022). COVID-19 classification using chest X-ray images based on fusion-assisted deep Bayesian optimization and Grad-CAM visualization. *Frontiers in Public Health, 10.* .DOI: 10.3389/fpubh.2022.890356

Han, B., Tomer, V., Nguyen, T. A., Farmani, A., & Singh, P. K. (Eds.). (2020). *Nanosensors for smart cities*. Elsevier.

Han, D., Ren, X., Luo, C., Zhang, Y., Zhang, X. Y., Zhang, X. G., Jiang, W., Hao, J., & Xie, Y. M. (2022). Experimental and computational investigations of novel 3D printed square tubular lattice metamaterials with negative Poisson's ratio. *Additive Manufacturing, 55*, 102789. DOI: 10.1016/j.addma.2022.102789

Han, X. (2023). A novel assimilated navigation model based on advanced optical systems (AOS), internet of things (IoT) and artificial intelligence (AI). *Optical and Quantum Electronics, 55*(7), 655. DOI: 10.1007/s11082-023-04947-x

Han, X., (2018). Normalization of ECG signals for deep learning. *Biomedical Signal Processing, 53*, 123–135.

Han, X., Yu, H., & Gu, H. (2019). Visual inspection with federated learning. *Image Analysis and Recognition: 16th International Conference, ICIAR 2019, Waterloo, ON, Canada, August 27–29, 2019. Proceedings, 16*(Part II), 52–64.

Hashemi, S. M., Parvizi, S., Baghbanijavid, H., Tan, A. T., Nematollahi, M., Ramazani, A., Fang, N. X., & Elahinia, M. (2022). Computational modelling of process–structure–property–performance relationships in metal additive manufacturing: A review. *International Materials Reviews, 67*(1), 1–46. DOI: 10.1080/09506608.2020.1868889

Hassan, A., Prasad, D., Khurana, M., Lilhore, U. K., & Simaiya, S. (2021). Integration of internet of things (IoT) in health care industry: An overview of benefits, challenges, and applications. *Data Science and Innovations for Intelligent Systems*, 165–180.

Hassan, I., Chisty, A., & Bui, T. (2024). Structural and Social Determinants of Health. In *Leading an Academic Medical Practice* (pp. 343–355). Springer International Publishing.

Haux, R. (2006). Health information systems–past, present, future. *International Journal of Medical Informatics*, *75*(3-4), 268–281. DOI: 10.1016/j.ijmedinf.2005.08.002 PMID: 16169771

He, C., Shah, A. D., Tang, Z., Sivashunmugam, D. F. N., Bhogaraju, K., Shimpi, M., Shen, L., Chu, X., Soltanolkotabi, M., & Avestimehr, S. (2021). Fedcv: A federated learning framework for diverse computer vision tasks. *arXiv Preprint arXiv:2111.11066*.

He, L., & Eastburn, M. (2022, August). Smart nanosensor networks for body injury detection. In 2022 IEEE International Conference on Smart Internet of Things (SmartIoT) (pp. 15-19). IEEE. DOI: 10.1109/SmartIoT55134.2022.00012

Helpmate. (2023). http://www.ntplx.net/~helpmate/

Hermawan, D., & Prabowo, H. (2021). The classification of ECG signals often relies on feature extraction methods, which can be computationally intensive and may require expert knowledge to select the most relevant features. *International Journal of Biomedical Engineering and Technology*, *34*(2), 123–135. 10.1504/IJBET.2021.115678

Hermawan, I., Ma'sum, M. A., Intan, P. R., Jatmiko, W., Wiweko, B., Boediman, A., & Pradekso, B. K. (2021). Temporal feature and heuristics-based noise detection over classical machine learning for ECG. *IEEE Access : Practical Innovations, Open Solutions*, *9*, 177782–177803. 10.1109/ACCESS.2021.3123456

Hickey, B. A., Chalmers, T., Newton, P., Lin, C.-T., Sibbritt, D., McLachlan, C. S., Clifton-Bligh, R., Morley, J., & Lal, S. (2021). Smart devices and wearable technologies to detect and monitor mental health conditions and stress: A systematic review. *Sensors (Basel)*, *21*(10), 3461. DOI: 10.3390/s21103461 PMID: 34065620

Holt, S. (2022). Virtual reality, augmented reality and mixed reality: For astronaut mental health; and space tourism, education and outreach. *Acta Astronautica*.

Hooda, I., & Chhillar, R. S. (2015). Software test process, testing types and techniques. *International Journal of Computer Applications*, *111*(13), 10–14. DOI: 10.5120/19597-1433

Hrabok, M., Delorme, A., & Agyapong, V. I. (2020). Threats to mental health and well-being associated with climate change. *Journal of Anxiety Disorders*, *76*, 102295. DOI: 10.1016/j.janxdis.2020.102295 PMID: 32896782

Hua, Y., Liu, F., Yang, K., Li, Z., Na, H., Sheu, Y., Zhou, P., Moran, L. V., Ananiadou, S., Beam, A., & Associates. (2024). Large language models in mental health care: A scoping review. *arXiv Preprint arXiv:2401.02984*.

Huang, Y., Wang, Y., Li, X., Chen, H., Si, Y., Zhang, Y., Zhou, H., Yang, Y., Li, M., Xie, Y., & Associates. (2024). CMS-Robot: A Cloud Medical Service Robot Merging SLAM and IoT for Enhanced Healthcare Delivery. *2024 IEEE 19th Conference on Industrial Electronics and Applications (ICIEA)*, 1–6.

Huang, J., Wu, X., Huang, W., Wu, X., & Wang, S. (2021). Internet of things in health management systems: A review. *International Journal of Communication Systems*, *34*(4), e4683. DOI: 10.1002/dac.4683

Huo, D., & Wang, X. (2024). A new era in healthcare: The integration of artificial intelligence and microbial. *Medicine in Novel Technology and Devices*, *23*, 100319. DOI: 10.1016/j.medntd.2024.100319

Hurley, D., & Popescu, G. H. (2021). Medical big data and wearable internet of things healthcare systems in remotely monitoring and caring for confirmed or suspected COVID-19 patients. *American Journal of Medical Research (New York, N.Y.)*, *8*(2), 78–90. DOI: 10.22381/ajmr8220216

Iampietro, C., Bellucci, L., Arcolino, F. O., Arigoni, M., Alessandri, L., Gomez, Y., Papadimitriou, E., Calogero, R. A., Cocchi, E., Van Den Heuvel, L., Levtchenko, E., & Bussolati, B. (2020). Molecular and functional characterization of urine-derived podocytes from patients with Alport syndrome. *The Journal of Pathology*, *252*(1), 88–100. DOI: 10.1002/path.5496 PMID: 32652570

IEEE. (2024). Deep Learning Applications in ECG Analysis and Disease Detection: An Investigation Study of Recent Advances. https://ieeexplore.ieee.org/iel8/6287639/10380310/10643131.pdf

Igwaran, A., & Okoh, A. I. (2019). Human campylobacteriosis: A public health concern of global importance. *Heliyon*, *5*(11), e02814. DOI: 10.1016/j.heliyon.2019.e02814 PMID: 31763476

Ikeda, K., Nagata, S., Okitsu, T., & Takeuchi, S. (2017). Cell fiber-based three-dimensional culture system for highly efficient expansion of human induced pluripotent stem cells. *Scientific Reports*, *7*(1), 2850. DOI: 10.1038/s41598-017-03246-2 PMID: 28588295

Illimoottil, M., & Ginat, D. (2023). Recent advances in deep learning and medical imaging for head and neck cancer treatment: MRI, CT, and PET scans. *Cancers (Basel)*, *15*(13), 3267. DOI: 10.3390/cancers15133267 PMID: 37444376

Jadhakhan, F., Blake, H., Hett, D., & Marwaha, S. (2022). Efficacy of digital technologies aimed at enhancing emotion regulation skills: Literature review. *Frontiers in Psychiatry*, *13*, 809332. DOI: 10.3389/fpsyt.2022.809332 PMID: 36159937

Jain, A., & Rakesh, S. K. (2024, July). IoT-driven predictive healthcare system for proactive treatment and improved patient management. In AIP Conference Proceedings (Vol. 3111, No. 1). AIP Publishing. DOI: 10.1063/5.0221495

Jamil, M. A., Arif, M., Abubakar, N. S. A., & Ahmad, A. (2016, November). Software test-ing techniques: A literature review. In 2016 6th international conference on information and communication technology for the Muslim world (ICT4M) (pp. 177-182). IEEE.

Jan, S.R., Shah, S.T.U., Johar, Z.U., Shah, Y. and Khan, F. (2016). An innovative approach to investigate various software testing techniques and strategies. International Journal of Sci-entific Research in Science, Engineering and Technology (IJSRSET), Print ISSN, 23951990.

Jenkins, T. (2022). Wearable medical sensor devices, machine and deep learning algorithms, and internet of things-based healthcare systems in COVID-19 patient screening, diagnosis, monitoring, and treatment. *American Journal of Medical Research (New York, N.Y.)*, *9*(1), 49–64. DOI: 10.22381/ajmr9120224

Jet Propulsion Laboratory. (n.d.). Pathfinder Rover. NASA. https://www.nasa.gov/

Jeyakumar, V., Nirmala, K., & Nithya, R. (2022). A smart virtual vision system for health monitoring. In *Biomedical Engineering Applications for People with Disabilities and the Elderly in the COVID-19 Pandemic and Beyond* (pp. 347–360). Elsevier. DOI: 10.1016/B978-0-323-85174-9.00021-2

Jha, P., Sahu, M., Bisoy, S. K., & Sain, M. (2022). Application of Model-Based Software Testing in the Health Care Domain. *Electronics (Basel)*, *11*(13), 2062. DOI: 10.3390/electronics11132062

Jia, C., Cai, Y., Yu, Y. T., & Tse, T. H. (2016). 5W+ 1H pattern: A perspective of systematic mapping studies and a case study on cloud software testing. *Journal of Systems and Software*, *116*, 206–219. DOI: 10.1016/j.jss.2015.01.058

Jiang, X., Zhang, J., & Zhang, L. (2023). FedRadar: Federated multi-task transfer learning for radar-based Internet of Medical Things. *IEEE Transactions on Network and Service Management*, *20*(2), 1459–1469. DOI: 10.1109/TNSM.2023.3281133

Jin, T., Pan, S., Li, X., & Chen, S. (2023). Metadata and image features co-aware personalized federated learning for smart healthcare. *IEEE Journal of Biomedical and Health Informatics*, *27*(8), 4110–4119. DOI: 10.1109/JBHI.2023.3279096 PMID: 37220032

Jiwani, N., Gupta, K., & Whig, P. (2023). Machine Learning Approaches for Analysis in Smart Healthcare Informatics. In Machine Learning and Artificial Intelligence in Healthcare Systems (pp. 129-154). CRC Press.

Ji, X., Chun, S. A., Wei, Z., & Geller, J. (2023). Twitter sentiment classification for measuring public health concerns. *Social Network Analysis and Mining*, *5*, 1–25. PMID: 32226558

Johar, S., & Manjula, G. R. (2024). Interfering sensed input classification model using assimilated whale optimization and deep Q-learning for remote patient monitoring. *Biomedical Signal Processing and Control*, *93*, 106202. DOI: 10.1016/j.bspc.2024.106202

Jopowicz, A., Wiśniowska, J., & Tarnacka, B. (2022). Cognitive and physical intervention in metals' dysfunction and neurodegeneration. *Brain Sciences*, *12*(3), 345. DOI: 10.3390/brainsci12030345 PMID: 35326301

Jordan, M. I., & Mitchell, T. M. (2015). Machine learning: Trends, perspectives, and pro-spects. *Science*, *349*(6245), 255–260. DOI: 10.1126/science.aaa8415 PMID: 26185243

Kaissis, G., Makowski, M. R., Rückert, D., & Braren, R. F. (2021). Secure, privacy-preserving and federated machine learning in medical imaging. *Nature Machine Intelligence*, *3*(6), 473–484. DOI: 10.1038/s42256-021-00337-8

Karthik, S., Hemalatha, R., Aruna, R., Deivakani, M., Reddy, R. V. K., & Boopathi, S. (2023). Study on Healthcare Security System-Integrated Internet of Things (IoT). In *Perspectives and Considerations on the Evolution of Smart Systems* (pp. 342–362). IGI Global.

Kastrinaki, V., Zervakis, M., & Kalaitzakis, K. (2003). A survey of video processing techniques for traffic applications. *Image and Vision Computing*, *21*(4), 359–381. DOI: 10.1016/S0262-8856(03)00004-0

Katal, N., Gupta, S., Verma, P., & Sharma, B. (2023). Deep-Learning-Based Arrhythmia Detection Using ECG Signals: A Comparative Study and Performance Evaluation. *Diagnostics (Basel)*, *13*(24), 3605. DOI: 10.3390/diagnostics13243605 PMID: 38132188

Kaur, J. (2024). Urban Oasis: Harnessing IoT for Green Healthcare in Smart City Landscape. In *Technologies for Sustainable Healthcare Development* (pp. 325–348). IGI Global.

Kaushik, T. K. Ravish, Singh, A., Raghav, A., & Singh, B. (2024). Potential of Artificial Intelligence in the Agricultural Industry: A Comprehensive Review. In B. Riswandi, B. Singh, C. Kaunert, & K. Vig (Eds.), *AI Applications for Clean Energy and Sustainability* (pp. 344-365). IGI Global. DOI: 10.4018/979-8-3693-6567-0.ch017

Kaushik, T. K. Ravish, Singh, A., Raghav, A., Singh, B., Arora, M. K., & Lal, S. (2024). Untapping Artificial Intelligence in Environmental and Sustainable Progression: Projecting Legal and Ethical Considerations. In B. Singh, C. Kaunert, K. Vig, & S. Dutta (Eds.), *Maintaining a Sustainable World in the Nexus of Environmental Science and AI* (pp. 109-130). IGI Global. https://doi.org/DOI: 10.4018/979-8-3693-6336-2.ch005

Keane, P. A., & Topol, E. J. (2018). With an eye to AI and autonomous diagnosis. *NPJ Digital Medicine*, *1*(1), 1–3. DOI: 10.1038/s41746-018-0048-y PMID: 31304321

Khan, T., Civas, M., Cetinkaya, O., Abbasi, N. A., & Akan, O. B. (2020). Nanosensor networks for smart health care. In *Nanosensors for Smart Cities* (pp. 387–403). Elsevier. DOI: 10.1016/B978-0-12-819870-4.00022-0

Kharbas, V. K., Meena, Y., & Thakur, P. K. (2024). Enabling Clinical Decision-Making in Smart Healthcare through AI/ML Algorithms. *2024 15th International Conference on Computing Communication and Networking Technologies (ICCCNT)*, 1–6.

Khinvasara, T., Shankar, A., & Wong, C. (2024). Robustness and Reliability Testing in Healthcare Using Artificial Intelligence. *Asian Journal of Research in Computer Science*, *17*(7), 103–118. DOI: 10.9734/ajrcos/2024/v17i7482

Khosa, I., Raza, A., Anjum, M., Ahmad, W., & Shahab, S. (2023). Automatic diabetic foot ulcer recognition using multi-level thermographic image data. *Diagnostics (Basel)*, *13*(11), 2637. DOI: 10.3390/diagnostics13162637 PMID: 37627896

Kim, P., Kwon, K. W., Park, M. C., Lee, S. H., Kim, S. M., & Suh, K. Y. (2008). Soft lithography for microfluidics: a review.

Knagg, R., Dorey, J., Evans, R., & Hitchman, J. (2024). Sustainability in healthcare: Patient and public perspectives. *Anaesthesia*, *79*(3), 278–283. DOI: 10.1111/anae.16159 PMID: 38205532

Kumar, P. M., Khan, L. U., & Hong, C. S. (2022). Notice of Violation of IEEE Publication Principles: Affirmative Fusion Process for Improving Wearable Sensor Data Availability in Artificial Intelligence of Medical Things. IEEE Sensors Journal.

Kumar, S., & Kumari, P. (2021). Flexible Nano Smart sensors. Nanosensors for Smart Manufacturing, 199.

Kumar, A., Singh, S., & Kumar, R. (2021). A review on ECG signal classification techniques. *Journal of King Saud University. Computer and Information Sciences.* .2021.01.001DOI: 10.1016/j.jksuci

Kumari, W. M. P., & Victor, S. P. (2021). Classification of ECG heart beats by deep learning algorithm with feature extraction by continuous wavelet transform for telemedicine application. *Advances in Mechanics*, *9*(3), 1006–1015.

Kumar, N., Verma, R., Sharma, S., Bhargava, S., Vahadane, A., & Sethi, A. (2017). A dataset and a technique for generalized nuclear segmentation for computational pathology. *IEEE Transactions on Medical Imaging*, *36*(7), 1550–1560. DOI: 10.1109/TMI.2017.2677499 PMID: 28287963

Kumar, P. M., Hong, C. S., Afghah, F., Manogaran, G., Yu, K., Hua, Q., & Gao, J. (2021). Clouds proportionate medical data stream analytics for internet of things-based healthcare systems. *IEEE Journal of Biomedical and Health Informatics*, *26*(3), 973–982. DOI: 10.1109/JBHI.2021.3106387 PMID: 34415841

Kumar, P. M., Khan, L. U., & Hong, C. S. (2022). Affirmative fusion process for improving wearable sensor data availability in artificial intelligence of medical things. *IEEE Sensors Journal*.

Kumar, V. D., Rajesh, P., Geman, O., Craciun, M. D., Arif, M., & Filip, R. (2023). "Quo vadis diagnosis": Application of informatics in early detection of pneumothorax. *Diagnostics (Basel)*, *13*(6), 1305. DOI: 10.3390/diagnostics13071305 PMID: 37046523

Kushwah, J. S., Gupta, M., Shrivastava, S., Saxena, N., Saini, R., & Boopathi, S. (2024). Psychological Impacts, Prevention Strategies, and Intervention Approaches Across Age Groups: Unmasking Cyberbullying. In *Change Dynamics in Healthcare, Technological Innovations, and Complex Scenarios* (pp. 89–109). IGI Global.

Larsson, E., & Thesing, M. (2024). Change Management Strategies for Seamless Adoption of Digital Healthcare Solutions in the Healthcare Industry.

Lawanna, A. (2012). The theory of software testing. *AU Journal of Technology*, *16*(1).

Lee, E. E., Torous, J., De Choudhury, M., Depp, C. A., Graham, S. A., Kim, H.-C., Paulus, M. P., Krystal, J. H., & Jeste, D. V. (2021). Artificial intelligence for mental health care: Clinical applications, barriers, facilitators, and artificial wisdom. *Biological Psychiatry: Cognitive Neuroscience and Neuroimaging*, *6*(9), 856–864. DOI: 10.1016/j.bpsc.2021.02.001 PMID: 33571718

Lee, J., Kang, S., & Lee, D. (2012). Survey on software testing practices. *IET Software*, *6*(3), 275–282. DOI: 10.1049/iet-sen.2011.0066

Leen, J. L., & Juurlink, D. N. (2019). Carfentanil: A narrative review of its pharmacology and public health concerns. *Canadian Journal of Anaesthesia*, *66*(4), 414–421. DOI: 10.1007/s12630-019-01294-y PMID: 30666589

Liao, D., Shu, L., Liang, G., Li, Y., Zhang, Y., Zhang, W., & Xu, X. (2019). Design and evaluation of affective virtual reality system based on multimodal physiological signals and self-assessment manikin. *IEEE Journal of Electromagnetics, RF and Microwaves in Medicine and Biology*, *4*(3), 216–224. DOI: 10.1109/JERM.2019.2948767

Liew, A., Agaian, S., & Benbelkacem, S. (2023). Distinctions between choroidal neovascularization and age-related macular degeneration in ocular disease predictions via multi-size kernels ξcho-weighted median patterns. *Diagnostics (Basel)*, *13*(4), 729. DOI: 10.3390/diagnostics13040729 PMID: 36832215

Li, H., Li, Z., Akmandor, N. Ü., Jiang, H., Wang, Y., & Padır, T. (2023, May). StereovoxelNet: Real-time obstacle detection based on occupancy voxels from a stereo camera using deep neural networks. In *2023 IEEE International Conference on Robotics and Automation (ICRA)* (pp. 4826–4833). IEEE. DOI: 10.1109/ICRA48891.2023.10160924

Lin, K.-H., Lu, N.-H., Okamoto, T., Huang, Y.-H., Liu, K.-Y., Matsushima, A., Chang, C.-C., & Chen, T.-B. (2023). Fusion-extracted features by deep networks for improved COVID-19 classification with chest X-ray radiography. *Health Care*, *11*(10), 1367. DOI: 10.3390/healthcare11101367 PMID: 37239653

Li, T., Sahu, A. K., Talwalkar, A., & Smith, V. (2020). Federated learning: Challenges, methods, and future directions. *IEEE Signal Processing Magazine*, *37*(3), 50–60. DOI: 10.1109/MSP.2020.2975749

Liu, F., Wu, X., Ge, S., Fan, W., & Zou, Y. (2020). Federated learning for vision-and-language grounding problems. *Proceedings of the AAAI Conference on Artificial Intelligence*, *34*(07), 11572–11579. DOI: 10.1609/aaai.v34i07.6824

Liu, K., Madrigal, E., Chung, J. S., Parekh, M., Kalahar, C. S., Nguyen, D., & Harris, O. A. (2023). Preliminary Study of Virtual-reality-guided Meditation for Veterans with Stress and Chronic Pain. *Alternative Therapies in Health and Medicine*, *29*(6). PMID: 34559692

Liu, W., Lin, H., Wang, X., Hu, J., Kaddoum, G., Piran, M. J., & Alamri, A. (2021). D2MIF: A malicious model detection mechanism for federated learning empowered artificial intelligence of things. *IEEE Internet of Things Journal*.

Liu, Y., Huang, A., Luo, Y., Huang, H., Liu, Y., Chen, Y., Feng, L., Chen, T., Yu, H., & Yang, Q. (2020). Fedvision: An online visual object detection platform powered by federated learning. *Proceedings of the AAAI Conference on Artificial Intelligence*, *34*(08), 13172–13179. DOI: 10.1609/aaai.v34i08.7021

Li, W., Chai, Y., Khan, F., Jan, S. R. U., Verma, S., Menon, V. G., & Li, X. (2021). A com-prehensive survey on machine learning-based big data analytics for IoT-enabled smart healthcare system. *Mobile Networks and Applications*, *26*(1), 234–252. DOI: 10.1007/s11036-020-01700-6 PMID: 40477400

Li, Y., Wang, H., Jin, X. R., Li, X., Pender, M., Song, C. P., Tang, S.-L., Cao, J., Wu, H., & Wang, Y. G. (2018). Experiences and challenges in the health protection of medical teams in the Chinese Ebola treatment center, Liberia: A qualitative study. *Infectious Diseases of Poverty*, *7*(1), 1–12. DOI: 10.1186/s40249-018-0468-6 PMID: 30134982

Loizou, S. G., & Rimon, E. D. (2022). Mobile robot navigation functions tuned by sensor readings in partially known environments. *IEEE Robotics and Automation Letters*, *7*(2), 3803–3810. DOI: 10.1109/LRA.2022.3148466

Long, . (2021). Software requirements for healthcare and IoT. *Design Engineering (London)*, *7*, 13087–13097.

Longuet-Higgins, H. C. (1981). A computer algorithm for reconstructing a scene from two projections. *Nature*, *293*(5828), 133–135. DOI: 10.1038/293133a0

Lützeler, M., & Dickmanns, E. D. (1998). Road recognition with MarVEye. In *Proceedings of the IEEE International Conference on Intelligent Vehicles* (pp. 341–346).

Lyu, Y., Yu, X., Zhu, D., & Zhang, L. (2022). Classification of Alzheimer's disease via vision transformer. In *Proceedings of the 15th International Conference on Pervasive Technologies Related to Assistive Environments* (pp. 463–468). New York, NY: Association for Computing Machinery. DOI: 10.1145/3529190.3534754

Maçorano, R. D. N. A. (2020). *Exploratory Psychometric Validation and Efficacy Assessment Study of Social Phobia Treatment based on Augmented and Virtual Reality Serious Games and Biofeedback* (Doctoral dissertation, Universidade de Lisboa (Portugal)).

Magrabi, F., Lyell, D., & Coiera, E. (2023). Automation in contemporary clinical information systems: A survey of AI in healthcare settings. *Yearbook of Medical Informatics*, *32*(01), 115–126. DOI: 10.1055/s-0043-1768733 PMID: 38147855

Maguluri, L. P., Arularasan, A., & Boopathi, S. (2023). Assessing Security Concerns for AI-Based Drones in Smart Cities. In *Effective AI, Blockchain, and E-Governance Applications for Knowledge Discovery and Management* (pp. 27–47). IGI Global. DOI: 10.4018/978-1-6684-9151-5.ch002

Mala, D. J. (2023). Machine learning-based intelligent assistant for smart healthcare. In *Machine Learning and Artificial Intelligence in Healthcare Systems* (pp. 265–286). CRC Press.

Malathi, J., Kusha, K., Isaac, S., Ramesh, A., Rajendiran, M., & Boopathi, S. (2024). IoT-Enabled Remote Patient Monitoring for Chronic Disease Management and Cost Savings: Transforming Healthcare. In *Advances in Explainable AI Applications for Smart Cities* (pp. 371–388). IGI Global.

Malik, A., & Kumar, A. (2022). assimilation of blockchain with Internet of Things (IoT) with possible issues and solutions for better connectivity and proper security. In New Trends and Applications in Internet of Things (IoT) and Big Data Analytics (pp. 187-207). Cham: Springer International Publishing.

Malik, P. K., Sharma, R., Singh, R., Gehlot, A., Satapathy, S. C., Alnumay, W. S., Pelusi, D., Ghosh, U., & Nayak, J. (2021). Industrial Internet of Things and its applications in industry 4.0: State of the art. *Computer Communications*, *166*, 125–139. DOI: 10.1016/j.comcom.2020.11.016

Maliyaem, M., Tuan, N. M., Lockhart, D., & Muenthong, S. (2022). A study of using machine learning in predicting COVID-19 cases. *Cloud Computing and Data Science*, *3*(2), 92–99. DOI: 10.37256/ccds.3220221488

Man, D., Zeng, F., Yang, W., Yu, M., Lv, J., & Wang, Y. (2021). Intelligent Intrusion Detection Based on Federated Learning for Edge-Assisted Internet of Things. *Security and Communication Networks*, *2021*(1), 9361348. DOI: 10.1155/2021/9361348

Manogaran, G., Alazab, M., Song, H., & Kumar, N. (2021). CDP-UA: Cognitive data processing method wearable sensor data uncertainty analysis in the internet of things assisted smart medical healthcare systems. *IEEE Journal of Biomedical and Health Informatics*, *25*(10), 3691–3699. DOI: 10.1109/JBHI.2021.3051288 PMID: 33439849

Marossi, C., Mariani, V., Arenas, A., Brondino, M., de Carvalho, C. V., Costa, P., . . . Pasini, M. (2023, July). Mindfulness Lessons in a Virtual Natural Environment to Cope with Work-Related Stress. In *International Conference in Methodologies and intelligent Systems for Techhnology Enhanced Learning* (pp. 227-238). Cham: Springer Nature Switzerland. DOI: 10.1007/978-3-031-41226-4_24

Marvaso, G., Pepa, M., Volpe, S., Mastroleo, F., Zaffaroni, M., Vincini, M. G., & Jereczek-Fossa, B. A. (2022). Virtual and Augmented Reality as a Novel Opportunity to Unleash the Power of Radiotherapy in the Digital Era: A Scoping Review. *Applied Sciences (Basel, Switzerland), 12*(22), 11308. DOI: 10.3390/app122211308

Materon, E. M., Gómez, F. R., Joshi, N., Dalmaschio, C. J., Carrilho, E., & Oliveira Jr, O. N. (2021). Smart materials for electrochemical flexible nanosensors: advances and applications. Nanosensors for smart manufacturing, 347-371.

Mazumdar, H., Chakraborty, C., Sathvik, M., Mukhopadhyay, S., & Panigrahi, P. K. (2023). GPTFX: A Novel GPT-3 Based Framework for Mental Health Detection and Explanations. *IEEE Journal of Biomedical and Health Informatics.* Advance online publication. DOI: 10.1109/JBHI.2023.3328350 PMID: 37903039

McMahan, H. B., Moore, E., Ramage, D., Hampson, S., & Arcas, B. A. y. (2017). Communication-efficient learning of deep networks from decentralized data. In *Proceedings of the 20th International Conference on Artificial Intelligence and Statistics (AISTATS).*

Mehta, S., Kukreja, V., & Gupta, A. (2023). Revolutionizing Maize Disease Management with Federated Learning CNNs: A Decentralized and Privacy-Sensitive Approach. *2023 4th International Conference for Emerging Technology (INCET)*, 1–6.

Menagadevi, M., Madian, N., Thiyagarajan, D., & Rajendran, R. (2025). Smart medical devices: Making healthcare more intelligent. In *Machine Learning Models and Architectures for Biomedical Signal Processing* (pp. 487–501). Elsevier. DOI: 10.1016/B978-0-443-22158-3.00020-X

Mer, A., & Virdi, A. S. (2023). Navigating the paradigm shift in HRM practices through the lens of artificial intelligence: A post-pandemic perspective. *The Adoption and Effect of Artificial Intelligence on Human Resources Management, Part A*, 123-154.

Michieli, U., & Ozay, M. (2021). Prototype guided federated learning of visual feature representations. *arXiv Preprint arXiv:2105.08982.*

Midha, S., & Singh, K. (2023). Happiness-Enhancing Strategies Among Indians. In *Religious and Spiritual Practices in India: A Positive Psychological Perspective* (pp. 341–368). Springer Nature Singapore. DOI: 10.1007/978-981-99-2397-7_15

Minchole, A., Camps, J., Lyon, A., & Rodríguez, B. (2019). Machine learning in the electrocardiogram. *Journal of Electrocardiology, 57*, S61–S64. DOI: 10.1016/j.jelectrocard.2019.08.008 PMID: 31521378

Miner, N. (2022). *Stairway to Heaven: Breathing Mindfulness into Virtual Reality* (Doctoral dissertation, Northeastern University).

Miner, J. H. (1999). Renal basement membrane components. *Kidney International, 56*(6), 2016–2024. DOI: 10.1046/j.1523-1755.1999.00785.x PMID: 10594777

Minnema, J., van Eijnatten, M., Kouw, W., Diblen, F., Mendrik, A., & Wolff, J. (2018). CT image segmentation of bone for medical additive manufacturing using a convolutional neural network. *Computers in Biology and Medicine, 103*, 130–139. DOI: 10.1016/j.compbiomed.2018.10.012 PMID: 30366309

Minopoulos, G. M., Memos, V. A., Stergiou, C. L., Stergiou, K. D., Plageras, A. P., Koidou, M. P., & Psannis, K. E. (2022). Exploitation of emerging technologies and advanced networks for a smart healthcare system. *Applied Sciences (Basel, Switzerland), 12*(12), 5859. DOI: 10.3390/app12125859

Mitchell, P. (2013). *Signal processing in healthcare applications*. Springer.

Mitra, A., Ngoko, Y., & Trystram, D. (2021). Impact of federated learning on smart buildings. *2021 International Conference on Artificial Intelligence and Smart Systems (ICAIS)*, 93–99. DOI: 10.1109/ICAIS50930.2021.9395938

Mody, V., & Mody, V. (2019). Mental health monitoring system using artificial intelligence: A review. *2019 IEEE 5th International Conference for Convergence in Technology (I2CT)*, 1–6.

Mohammed, I., Tabatabai, S., Al-Fuqaha, A., El Bouanani, F., Qadir, J., Qolomany, B., & Guizani, M. (2020). Budgeted online selection of candidate IoT clients to participate in federated learning. *IEEE Internet of Things Journal, 8*(7), 5938–5952. DOI: 10.1109/JIOT.2020.3036157

Mohanraj, G., Krishna, K. S., Lakshmi, B. S., Vijayalakshmi, A., Pramila, P. V., & Boopathi, S. (2024). Optimizing Trust and Security in Healthcare 4.0: Human Factors in Lightweight Secured IoMT Ecosystems. In *Lightweight Digital Trust Architectures in the Internet of Medical Things (IoMT)* (pp. 52–72). IGI Global. DOI: 10.4018/979-8-3693-2109-6.ch004

Mohanty, A., Jothi, B., Jeyasudha, J., Ranjit, P., Isaac, J. S., & Boopathi, S. (2023). Additive Manufacturing Using Robotic Programming. In *AI-Enabled Social Robotics in Human Care Services* (pp. 259–282). IGI Global. DOI: 10.4018/978-1-6684-8171-4.ch010

Molakatala, N., Kumar, D. A., Patil, U., Mhatre, P. J., Sambathkumar, M., & Boopathi, S. (2024). Integrating 5G and IoT Technologies in Developing Smart City Communication Networks. In *Blockchain-Based Solutions for Accessibility in Smart Cities* (pp. 147–170). IGI Global. DOI: 10.4018/979-8-3693-3402-7.ch006

Mondal, S., & Das, A. (2023). Quality aware cost-efficient reward mechanism in mobile crowdsensing system with uncertainty constraints. *Microsystem Technologies*. DOI: 10.1007/s00542-023-05495-w

Moody, G. B., & Mark, R. G. (2001). The MIT-BIH Arrhythmia Database. *Computers in Cardiology*, *28*, 203–206. PMID: 11446209

Morrison, T. M., Pathmanathan, P., Adwan, M., & Margerrison, E. (2018a). Advancing regulatory science with computational modeling for medical devices at the FDA's Office of Science and Engineering Laboratories. *Frontiers in Medicine*, *5*, 241. DOI: 10.3389/fmed.2018.00241 PMID: 30356350

Moses, H. E., & Van Leeuwen, P. (1996). Wavelet transform and its application to ECG. *Signal Processing*, *47*(1), 97–105.

Muhammad, G., Alshehri, F., Karray, F., El Saddik, A., Alsulaiman, M., & Falk, T. H. (2021). A comprehensive survey on multimodal medical signals fusion for smart healthcare systems. *Information Fusion*, *76*, 355–375. DOI: 10.1016/j.inffus.2021.06.007

Mujawar, M. A., Gohel, H., Bhardwaj, S. K., Srinivasan, S., Hickman, N., & Kaushik, A. (2020). Nano-enabled biosensing systems for intelligent healthcare: Towards COVID-19 management. *Materials Today. Chemistry*, *17*, 100306. DOI: 10.1016/j.mtchem.2020.100306 PMID: 32835155

Murmu, A., Kumar, P., Moparthi, N. R., Namasudra, S., & Lorenz, P. (2024). Reliable federated learning with GAN model for robust and resilient future healthcare system. *IEEE Transactions on Network and Service Management*, *21*(5), 5335–5346. DOI: 10.1109/TNSM.2024.3422376

Musah, S., Mammoto, A., Ferrante, T. C., Jeanty, S. S., Hirano-Kobayashi, M., Mammoto, T., ... & Ingber, D. E. (2017). Mature induced-pluripotent-stem-cell-derived human podocytes reconstitute kidney glomerular-capillary-wall function on a chip. *Nature biomedical engineering, 1*(5), 0069.

Music, T. (2022). Protecting patients, protecting healthcare workers: A review of the role of influenza vaccination. *International Nursing Review*, *59*(2), 161–167. DOI: 10.1111/j.1466-7657.2011.00961.x PMID: 22591085

Mustafa, K. M., Al-Qutaish, R. E., & Muhairat, M. I. (2009, December). Classification of software testing tools based on the software testing methods. In *2009 Second International Conference on Computer and Electrical Engineering* (Vol. 1, pp. 229-233). IEEE. DOI: 10.1109/ICCEE.2009.9

Myrzashova, R., Alsamhi, S. H., Shvetsov, A. V., Hawbani, A., & Wei, X. (2023). Blockchain meets federated learning in healthcare: A systematic review with challenges and opportunities. *IEEE Internet of Things Journal*, *10*(16), 14418–14437. DOI: 10.1109/JIOT.2023.3263598

Najjar, R. (2023). Redefining Radiology: A Review of Artificial Intelligence Integration in Medical Imaging. *Diagnostics (Basel)*, *13*(17), 2760. DOI: 10.3390/diagnostics13172760 PMID: 37685300

National Research Council Commission on Engineering and Technical Systems. (1983). *Applications of robotics and artificial intelligence to reduce risk and improve effectiveness: A study for the United States Army*. National Academy of Sciences.

Nawaz, A., Khan, S. S., & Ahmad, A. (2024). Ensemble of Autoencoders for Anomaly Detection in Biomedical Data: A Narrative Review. *IEEE Access : Practical Innovations, Open Solutions*, *12*, 17273–17289. DOI: 10.1109/ACCESS.2024.3360691

Nawaz, M., & Ahmed, J. (2022). Cloud-based healthcare framework for real-time anomaly detection and classification of 1-D ECG signals. *PLoS One*, *17*(12), e0279305. DOI: 10.1371/journal.pone.0279305 PMID: 36574391

Naylor, M., Ridout, B., & Campbell, A. (2020). A scoping review identifying the need for quality research on the use of virtual reality in workplace settings for stress management. *Cyberpsychology, Behavior, and Social Networking*, *23*(8), 506–518. DOI: 10.1089/cyber.2019.0287 PMID: 32486836

Naz, M., Shah, J. H., Khan, M. A., Sharif, M., Raza, M., & Damaševičius, R. (2021). From ECG signals to images: A transformation based approach for deep learning. *PeerJ. Computer Science*, *7*, e386. DOI: 10.7717/peerj-cs.386 PMID: 33817032

Ni, W., Ao, H., Tian, H., Eldar, Y. C., & Niyato, D. (2024). FedSL: Federated split learning for collaborative healthcare analytics on resource-constrained wearable IoMT devices. *IEEE Internet of Things Journal*, *11*(10), 18934–18935. DOI: 10.1109/JIOT.2024.3370985

Oguguа, J. O., Anyanwu, E. C., Olorunsogo, T., Maduka, C. P., & Ayo-Farai, O. (2024). Ethics and strategy in vaccination: A review of public health policies and practices. *International Journal of Science and Research Archive*, *11*(1), 883–895. DOI: 10.30574/ijsra.2024.11.1.0141

Okokpujie, I. P., & Tartibu, L. K. (2024). Study of the economic viability of internet of things (IoTs) in additive and advanced manufacturing: A comprehensive review. *Progress in Additive Manufacturing*, 1–20.

Okolo, C. A., Ijeh, S., Arowoogun, J. O., Adeniyi, A. O., & Omotayo, O. (2024). Reviewing the impact of health information technology on healthcare management efficiency. *International Medical Science Research Journal*, *4*(4), 420–440. DOI: 10.51594/imsrj.v4i4.1000

Olaboye, J. A.Queen-Mary Akudo EbugosiJanet Aderonke Olaboye. (2024). Optimizing healthcare resource allocation through data-driven demographic and psychographic analysis. *Computer Science & IT Research Journal*, *5*(6), 1488–1504. DOI: 10.51594/csitrj.v5i6.1249

Orlandi, F. C., Dos Anjos, J. C., Leithardt, V. R., Santana, J. F. D. P., & Geyer, C. F. (2023). Entropy to mitigate non-IID data problem on federated learning for the edge intelligence environment. *IEEE Access : Practical Innovations, Open Solutions*, *11*, 78845–78857. DOI: 10.1109/ACCESS.2023.3298704

Orso, A., & Rothermel, G. (2014). Software testing: a research travelogue (2000–2014). In Future of Software Engineering Proceedings (pp. 117-132).

Osifeko, M. O., Hancke, G. P., & Abu-Mahfouz, A. M. (2020). Artificial intelligence techniques for cognitive sensing in future IoT: State-of-the-Art, potentials, and challenges. *Journal of Sensor and Actuator Networks*, *9*(2), 21. DOI: 10.3390/jsan9020021

Oukhatar, A., Bakhouya, M., & El Ouadghiri, D. (2021). Electromagnetic-Based Wireless Nano-Sensors Network: Architectures and Applications. *Journal of Communication*, *16*(1), 8–19. DOI: 10.12720/jcm.16.1.8-19

Palaniappan, M., Tirlangi, S., Mohamed, M. J. S., Moorthy, R. S., Valeti, S. V., & Boopathi, S. (2023). Fused Deposition Modelling of Polylactic Acid (PLA)-Based Polymer Composites: A Case Study. In *Development, Properties, and Industrial Applications of 3D Printed Polymer Composites* (pp. 66–85). IGI Global.

Panch, T., Mattie, H., & Celi, L. A. (2019). The "inconvenient truth" about AI in healthcare. *NPJ Digital Medicine*, *2*(1), 1–3. DOI: 10.1038/s41746-019-0155-4 PMID: 31453372

Patangia, B., Sankruthyayana, R. G., Sathiyaseelan, A., & Balasundaram, S. (2021). How could Mindfulness Help? A Perspective on the Applications of Mindfulness in Enhancing Tomorrow's Workplace. *i-Manager's. Journal of Management*, *16*(3), 52.

Pei, X., Deng, X., Tian, S., Zhang, L., & Xue, K. (2022). A knowledge transfer-based semi-supervised federated learning for IoT malware detection. *IEEE Transactions on Dependable and Secure Computing*, *20*(3), 2127–2143. DOI: 10.1109/TDSC.2022.3173664

Petrosyan, A., Cravedi, P., Villani, V., Angeletti, A., Manrique, J., Renieri, A., De Filippo, R. E., Perin, L., & Da Sacco, S. (2019). A glomerulus-on-a-chip to recapitulate the human glomerular filtration barrier. *Nature Communications*, *10*(1), 3656. DOI: 10.1038/s41467-019-11577-z PMID: 31409793

Petrov, P., Georgieva, V., Nikolov, S., & Mihaylova, A. (2019, May). Real-time laser obstacle detection system for autonomous mobile robot navigation. In 2019 X National Conference with International Participation (ELECTRONICA) (pp. 1–4). IEEE. DOI: 10.1109/ELECTRONICA.2019.8825623

Pitchai, R., Guru, K. V., Gandhi, J. N., Komala, C. R., Kumar, J. R. D., & Boopathi, S. (2024). Fog Computing-Integrated ML-Based Framework and Solutions for Intelligent Systems: Digital Healthcare Applications. In *Technological Advancements in Data Processing for Next Generation Intelligent Systems* (pp. 196–224). IGI Global. DOI: 10.4018/979-8-3693-0968-1.ch008

Pool, J., Akhlaghpour, S., Fatehi, F., & Burton-Jones, A. (2024). A systematic analysis of failures in protecting personal health data: A scoping review. *International Journal of Information Management*, *74*, 102719. DOI: 10.1016/j.ijinfomgt.2023.102719

Popescu, C., El-Chaarani, H., El-Abiad, Z., & Gigauri, I. (2022). Implementation of health information systems to improve patient identification. *International Journal of Environmental Research and Public Health*, *19*(22), 15236. DOI: 10.3390/ijerph192215236 PMID: 36429954

Pradhan, M. R., Mago, B., & Ateeq, K. (2023). A classification-based sensor data processing method for the internet of things assimilated wearable sensor technology. *Cluster Computing*, *26*(1), 807–822. DOI: 10.1007/s10586-022-03605-3

Pramanik, P. K. D., Solanki, A., Debnath, A., Nayyar, A., El-Sappagh, S., & Kwak, K. S. (2020). Advancing modern healthcare with nanotechnology, nanobiosensors, and internet of nano things: Taxonomies, applications, architecture, and challenges. *IEEE Access : Practical Innovations, Open Solutions*, *8*, 65230–65266. DOI: 10.1109/ACCESS.2020.2984269

Pramila, P., Amudha, S., Saravanan, T., Sankar, S. R., Poongothai, E., & Boopathi, S. (2023). Design and Development of Robots for Medical Assistance: An Architectural Approach. In *Contemporary Applications of Data Fusion for Advanced Healthcare Informatics* (pp. 260–282). IGI Global.

Pratt, W. K. (1978). *Digital image processing*. John Wiley & Sons.

Premavathi, T., Shekhar, A., Raj, A., Mohan, K., Palaniappan, D., & Shukla, M. (2024). The Utilization of Internet of Things (IoT) in the Field of Robotics Process Automation. In *Applications of New Technology in Operations and Supply Chain Management* (pp. 337–359). IGI Global. DOI: 10.4018/979-8-3693-1578-1.ch018

Qayyum, A., Qadir, J., Bilal, M., & Al-Fuqaha, A. (2020). Secure and robust machine learning for healthcare: A survey. *IEEE Reviews in Biomedical Engineering*, *14*, 156–180. DOI: 10.1109/RBME.2020.3013489 PMID: 32746371

Quintero, L. (2019). *Facilitating Technology-based Mental Health Interventions with Mobile Virtual Reality and Wearable Smartwatches* (Doctoral dissertation, Department of Computer and Systems Sciences, Stockholm University).

Quirós-Solano, W. F., Gaio, N., Stassen, O. M. J. A., Arik, Y. B., Silvestri, C., Van Engeland, N. C. A., Van der Meer, A., Passier, R., Sahlgren, C. M., Bouten, C. V. C., van den Berg, A., Dekker, R., & Sarro, P. M. (2018). Microfabricated tuneable and transferable porous PDMS membranes for Organs-on-Chips. *Scientific Reports*, *8*(1), 13524. DOI: 10.1038/s41598-018-31912-6 PMID: 30202042

Rafi, D. M., Moses, K. R. K., Petersen, K., & Mäntylä, M. V. (2012, June). Benefits and limitations of automated software testing: Systematic literature review and practitioner survey. In 2012 7th International Workshop on Automation of Software Test (AST) (pp. 36-42). IEEE.

Raghav, A., Singh, B., Jermsittiparsert, K., Raghav, R., & Yadav, U. (2024). Artificial Intelligence in Environmental and Climate Changes: A Sustainable Future. In Singh, B., Kaunert, C., Vig, K., & Dutta, S. (Eds.), *Maintaining a Sustainable World in the Nexus of Environmental Science and AI* (pp. 485–506). IGI Global., DOI: 10.4018/979-8-3693-6336-2.ch019

Raj, R., & Sunil, P. (2022). Telemedicine and deep learning: Advancements in cardiac care. *Journal of Telemedicine and Telecare*, *28*(3), 153–165.

Raman, R., & Mitra, A. (2023a). IoT-Enhanced Workplace Safety for Real-Time Monitoring and Hazard Detection for Occupational Health. *2023 International Conference on Artificial Intelligence for Innovations in Healthcare Industries (ICAIIHI)*, *1*, 1–5. DOI: 10.1109/ICAIIHI57871.2023.10489803

Ramudu, K., Mohan, V. M., Jyothirmai, D., Prasad, D., Agrawal, R., & Boopathi, S. (2023). Machine Learning and Artificial Intelligence in Disease Prediction: Applications, Challenges, Limitations, Case Studies, and Future Directions. In *Contemporary Applications of Data Fusion for Advanced Healthcare Informatics* (pp. 297–318). IGI Global.

Rana, I., Goswami, P., & Maheshwari, H. (2019). A review of tools and techniques used in software testing. *Int. J. Emerg. Technol. Innovative Res*, *6*(4), 262–266.

Rani, P. (2022). Nanosensors and their Potential Role in Internet of Medical Things. In *Nanosensors for Futuristic Smart and Intelligent Healthcare Systems* (pp. 293–317). CRC Press. DOI: 10.1201/9781003093534-16

Ranjan, S., & Choubey, D. K. (2024). Machine Learning, Deep Learning and IoT in Smart Healthcare for Retinal Diseases Management. In *Machine Learning and IoT Applications for Health Informatics* (pp. 216–238). CRC Press. DOI: 10.1201/9781003424987-11

Ray, J., Kumar, S., Pandey, S., & Akram, S. V. (2023, June). The Role of Augmented Reality and Virtual Reality in Shaping the Future of Health Psychology. In *2023 3rd International Conference on Pervasive Computing and Social Networking (ICPCSN)* (pp. 1604-1608). IEEE. DOI: 10.1109/ICPCSN58827.2023.00268

Reddy, M. A., Gaurav, A., Ushasukhanya, S., Rao, V. C. S., Bhattacharya, S., & Boopathi, S. (2023). Bio-Medical Wastes Handling Strategies During the COVID-19 Pandemic. In *Multidisciplinary Approaches to Organizational Governance During Health Crises* (pp. 90–111). IGI Global. DOI: 10.4018/978-1-7998-9213-7.ch006

Reger, G. M. (Ed.). (2020). *Technology and mental health: a clinician's guide to improving outcomes*. Routledge. DOI: 10.4324/9780429020537

Riazi, M. S., Weinert, C., Tkachenko, O., Songhori, E. M., Schneider, T., & Koushanfar, F. (2018). Chameleon: A hybrid secure computation framework for machine learning applications. *Proceedings of the 2018 on Asia Conference on Computer and Communications Security*, 707–721. DOI: 10.1145/3196494.3196522

Richardson, J., Iezzi, A., Khan, M. A., & Maxwell, A. (2014). Validity and reliability of the Assessment of Quality of Life (AQoL)-8D multi-attribute utility instrument. *Patient*, *7*(1), 85–96. DOI: 10.1007/s40271-013-0036-x PMID: 24271592

Richir, S., Kadri, A., & Ribeyre, N. (2022). Virtual Reality and Augmented Reality to Fight Effectively against Pandemics. In *The Nature of Pandemics* (pp. 311–348). CRC Press. DOI: 10.4324/9781315170220-20

Rieke, N., Hancox, J., Li, W., Milletarì, F., Roth, H. R., Albarqouni, S., Bakas, S., Galtier, M. N., Landman, B. A., Maier-Hein, K., Ourselin, S., Sheller, M., Summers, R. M., Trask, A., Xu, D., Baust, M., & Cardoso, M. J. (2020). The future of digital health with federated learning. *NPJ Digital Medicine*, *3*(1), 119. DOI: 10.1038/s41746-020-00323-1 PMID: 33015372

Roye, Y., Bhattacharya, R., Mou, X., Zhou, Y., Burt, M. A., & Musah, S. (2021). A personalized glomerulus chip engineered from stem cell-derived epithelium and vascular endothelium. *Micromachines*, *12*(8), 967. DOI: 10.3390/mi12080967 PMID: 34442589

Roye, Y., & Musah, S. (2022). Isogenic kidney glomerulus chip engineered from human induced pluripotent stem cells. *Journal of Visualized Experiments*, *189*, e63821. PMID: 36408985

Roy, S., Bhanja, S., & Das, A. (2023). AndyWar: An intelligent android malware detection using machine learning. *Innovations in Systems and Software Engineering*. Advance online publication. DOI: 10.1007/s11334-023-00530-5

Runciman, B., Merry, A., & Walton, M. (2017). *Safety and ethics in healthcare: a guide to getting it right*. CRC Press.

Sabry, F., Eltaras, T., Labda, W., Alzoubi, K., & Malluhi, Q. (2022). Machine learning for healthcare wearable devices: The big picture. *Journal of Healthcare Engineering*, *2022*(1), 4653923. DOI: 10.1155/2022/4653923 PMID: 35480146

SachinD. N., Annappa, B., Hegde, S., Abhijit, C. S., & Ambesange, S. (2024). Fed-Cure: A heterogeneity-aware personalized federated learning framework for intelligent healthcare applications in IoMT environments. *IEEE Access : Practical Innovations, Open Solutions*, *12*, 15867–15883. DOI: 10.1109/ACCESS.2024.3357514

Safdar, M. F., Nowak, R. M., & Pałka, P. (2024). Pre-processing techniques and artificial intelligence algorithms for electrocardiogram (ECG) signals analysis: A comprehensive review. *Computers in Biology and Medicine*, *170*, 107908. DOI: 10.1016/j.compbiomed.2023.107908 PMID: 38217973

Saha, A., Dhara, B. C., Umer, S., Yurii, K., Alanazi, J. M., & AlZubi, A. A. (2022). Efficient obstacle detection and tracking using RGB-D sensor data in dynamic environments for robotic applications. *Sensors (Basel)*, *22*(17), 6537. DOI: 10.3390/s22176537 PMID: 36080993

Sai, S., Hassija, V., Chamola, V., & Guizani, M. (2024). Federated learning and NFT-based privacy-preserving medical-data-sharing scheme for intelligent diagnosis in smart healthcare. *IEEE Internet of Things Journal, 11*(4), 5568–5577. DOI: 10.1109/JIOT.2023.3308991

Salami, B., Salma, J., & Hegadoren, K. (2019). Access and utilization of mental health services for immigrants and refugees: Perspectives of immigrant service providers. *International Journal of Mental Health Nursing*, *28*(1), 152–161. DOI: 10.1111/inm.12512 PMID: 29984880

Salmi, M. (2021). Additive manufacturing processes in medical applications. *Materials (Basel)*, *14*(1), 191. DOI: 10.3390/ma14010191 PMID: 33401601

Sanyaolu, A., Okorie, C., Qi, X., Locke, J., & Rehman, S. (2019). Childhood and adolescent obesity in the United States: a public health concern. *Global pediatric health, 6*, 2333794X19891305.

Satav, S. D., Hasan, D. S., Pitchai, R., Mohanaprakash, T., Sultanuddin, S., & Boopathi, S. (2023). Next generation of internet of things (ngiot) in healthcare systems. In *Sustainable Science and Intelligent Technologies for Societal Development* (pp. 307–330). IGI Global.

Satchell, S. C., & Braet, F. (2009). Glomerular endothelial cell fenestrations: An integral component of the glomerular filtration barrier. *American Journal of Physiology. Renal Physiology*, *296*(5), F947–F956. DOI: 10.1152/ajprenal.90601.2008 PMID: 19129259

Savazzi, S., Nicoli, M., & Rampa, V. (2020). Federated learning with cooperating devices: A consensus approach for massive IoT networks. *IEEE Internet of Things Journal*, *7*(5), 4641–4654. DOI: 10.1109/JIOT.2020.2964162

Schneider, M. J. (2020). *Introduction to public health*. Jones & Bartlett Learning.

Senthil, T., Puviyarasan, M., Babu, S. R., Surakasi, R., Sampath, B., & Associates. (2023). Industrial Robot-Integrated Fused Deposition Modelling for the 3D Printing Process. In *Development, Properties, and Industrial Applications of 3D Printed Polymer Composites* (pp. 188–210). IGI Global.

Serral, E., Torres, V., & Valderas, P. (2024). Modeling IoT-enhanced business processes. In *Handbook on Business Process Management and Digital Transformation* (pp. 363–386). Edward Elgar Publishing. DOI: 10.4337/9781802206098.00025

Sezer, A., Sigirci, I. O., & Sezer, H. B. (2017). Shoulder lesion classification using shape and texture features via composite kernel. In *Proceedings of the 25th Signal Processing and Communications Applications Conference (SIU)* (pp. 1–4). Antalya, Turkey. DOI: 10.1109/SIU.2017.7960658

Shaikh, T. A., Rasool, T., & Verma, P. (2023). Machine intelligence and medical cyber-physical system architectures for smart healthcare: Taxonomy, challenges, opportunities, and possible solutions. *Artificial Intelligence in Medicine, 146*, 102692. DOI: 10.1016/j.artmed.2023.102692 PMID: 38042609

Shaik, T., Tao, X., Higgins, N., Li, L., Gururajan, R., Zhou, X., & Acharya, U. R. (2023). Remote patient monitoring using artificial intelligence: Current state, applications, and challenges. *Wiley Interdisciplinary Reviews. Data Mining and Knowledge Discovery, 13*(2), e1485. DOI: 10.1002/widm.1485

Shaw, F. E., Asomugha, C. N., Conway, P. H., & Rein, A. S. (2024). The Patient Protection and Affordable Care Act: Opportunities for prevention and public health. *Lancet, 384*(9937), 75–82. DOI: 10.1016/S0140-6736(14)60259-2 PMID: 24993913

Shchepkina, N., Negi, G. S., Bhalla, L., Nangia, R., Jyoti, J., & Surekha, P. (2024). IoT-Enhanced Public Safety in Smart Environments: A Comparative Analysis Using the Public Safety IoT Test. *BIO Web of Conferences, 86*, 01100.

Sheller, M. J., Edwards, B., Reina, G. A., Martin, J., Pati, S., Kotrotsou, A., Milchenko, M., Xu, W., Marcus, D., Colen, R. R., & Bakas, S. (2020). Federated learning in medicine: Facilitating multi-institutional collaborations without sharing patient data. *Scientific Reports, 10*(1), 12598. DOI: 10.1038/s41598-020-69250-1 PMID: 32724046

Sherwani, M. K., Aziz, A., & Calimeri, F. (2022). Role of Deep Learning for Smart Health Care. In *Computational Intelligence Techniques for Green Smart Cities* (pp. 169–186). Springer. DOI: 10.1007/978-3-030-96429-0_8

Sikka, R., Morath, J. M., & Leape, L. (2020). The quadruple aim: Care, health, cost and meaning in work. *BMJ Quality & Safety, 24*(10), 608–610. DOI: 10.1136/bmjqs-2015-004160 PMID: 26038586

Singh, S., & Keller, P. (1992). Obstacle detection for high-speed autonomous navigation. In *Proceedings of the IEEE International Conference on Robotics and Automation*.

Slaunwhite, A., Min, J. E., Palis, H., Urbanoski, K., Pauly, B., Barker, B., ... & Nosyk, B. (2024). Effect of Risk Mitigation Guidance opioid and stimulant dispensations on mortality and acute care visits during dual public health emergencies: retrospective cohort study. *bmj, 384*.

Smith, P. J., & Merwin, R. M. (2021). The role of exercise in management of mental health disorders: An integrative review. *Annual Review of Medicine*, *72*(1), 45–62. DOI: 10.1146/annurev-med-060619-022943 PMID: 33256493

Sokolova, M., & Lapalme, G. (2009). A systematic analysis of performance measures for classification tasks. *Information Processing & Management*, *45*(4), 427–437. DOI: 10.1016/j.ipm.2009.03.002

Somani, S., Russak, A. J., Richter, F., Zhao, S., Vaid, A., Chaudhry, F., De Freitas, J. K., Naik, N., Miotto, R., Nadkarni, G. N., & Narula, J. (2021). Deep learning and the electrocardiogram: Review of the current state-of-the-art. EP Europace., 10.1093/europace/euaa001.

Somwanshi, D., & Bundele, M. (2020). Obstacle detection approach for robotic wheelchair navigation. In International Conference on Artificial Intelligence: Advances and Applications 2019 (pp. 261–268). Springer Singapore. DOI: 10.1007/978-981-15-1059-5_29

Sonia, R., Gupta, N., Manikandan, K., Hemalatha, R., Kumar, M. J., & Boopathi, S. (2024). Strengthening Security, Privacy, and Trust in Artificial Intelligence Drones for Smart Cities. In *Analyzing and Mitigating Security Risks in Cloud Computing* (pp. 214–242). IGI Global. DOI: 10.4018/979-8-3693-3249-8.ch011

Spetsakis, M. E., & Aloimonos, J. (1990). Structure from motion using line correspondences. *International Journal of Computer Vision*, *4*(3), 171–183. DOI: 10.1007/BF00054994

Sreedhar, P. S. S., Sujay, V., Rani, M. R., Melita, L., Reshma, S., & Boopathi, S. (2024). Impacts of 5G Machine Learning Techniques on Telemedicine and Social Media Professional Connection in Healthcare. In *Advances in Medical Technologies and Clinical Practice* (pp. 209–234). IGI Global. DOI: 10.4018/979-8-3693-1934-5.ch012

Ströhle, A. (2019). Sports psychiatry: Mental health and mental disorders in athletes and exercise treatment of mental disorders. *European Archives of Psychiatry and Clinical Neuroscience*, *269*(5), 485–498. DOI: 10.1007/s00406-018-0891-5 PMID: 29564546

Suma, D. V. (2021). Wearable IoT based distributed framework for ubiquitous computing. *Journal of Ubiquitous Computing and Communication Technologies*, *3*(1), 23–32. DOI: 10.36548/jucct.2021.1.003

Sundaramoorthy, K., Singh, A., Sumathy, G., Maheshwari, A., Arunarani, A., & Boopathi, S. (2024). A Study on AI and Blockchain-Powered Smart Parking Models for Urban Mobility. In *Handbook of Research on AI and ML for Intelligent Machines and Systems* (pp. 223–250). IGI Global.

Suresh Babu, C. V. Sathiya Narayana S. (2024). Navigating Uncharted Waters: Overcoming Challenges in Integrating Machine Learning and Deep Learning for Enhanced Clinical Risk. In H. Liu, R. Tripathy, & P. Bhattacharya (Eds.), Clinical Practice and Unmet Challenges in AI-Enhanced Healthcare Systems (pp. 289-310). IGI Global. DOI: 10.4018/979-8-3693-2703-6.ch015

Suresh Babu, C. V., Akshayah, N. S., & Maclin Vinola, P. (2024). Artificial Intelligence in Healthcare: Assessing Impacts, Challenges, and Recommendations for Achieving Healthcare Independence. In Geada, N., & Jamil, G. (Eds.), *Perspectives on Artificial Intelligence in Times of Turbulence: Theoretical Background to Applications* (pp. 61–80). IGI Global., DOI: 10.4018/978-1-6684-9814-9.ch005

Suresh Babu, C. V., Bhavana, K., & Samnatha, M. (2025). Fuzzy Logic in Multi-Criteria Decision Making: Recent Advances and Applications. In Aouadni, S., & Aouadni, I. (Eds.), *Recent Theories and Applications for Multi-Criteria Decision-Making* (pp. 399–424). IGI Global., DOI: 10.4018/979-8-3693-6502-1.ch014

Suryadevara, S. (2022). Enhancing Brain-Computer Interface Applications through IoT Optimization. *Revista de Inteligencia Artificial En Medicina*, *13*(1), 52–76.

Swayamsiddha, S., & Mohanty, C. (2020). Application of cognitive Internet of Medical Things for COVID-19 pandemic. *Diabetes & Metabolic Syndrome*, *14*(5), 911–915. DOI: 10.1016/j.dsx.2020.06.014 PMID: 32570016

Tagesse, T., Arulkumar, S., Mahalingam, S., Subbarao Tadepalli, N. V. R., Munjal, N., & Boopathi, S. (2024). Analyzing Fuel Cell Vehicles in India via the PESTLE Framework and Intelligent Battery Management Systems (BMS): Blockchain in E-Mobility. In *Advances in Mechatronics and Mechanical Engineering* (pp. 107–129). IGI Global. DOI: 10.4018/979-8-3693-5247-2.ch007

Tang, L., Li, J., & Fantus, S. (2023). Medical artificial intelligence ethics: A systematic review of empirical studies. *Digital Health*, *9*, 20552076231186064. DOI: 10.1177/20552076231186064 PMID: 37434728

Tanim, S. A., Aurnob, A. R., Mridha, M. F., Safran, M., Alfarhood, S., & Che, D. (2024). Secure federated learning for Parkinson's disease: Non-IID data partitioning and homomorphic encryption strategies. *IEEE Access : Practical Innovations, Open Solutions*, *12*, 127309–127327. DOI: 10.1109/ACCESS.2024.3454690

Tao, L., Inoue, Y., & Shibata, K. (2021). Development of a wearable sensor system for patient movement monitoring. *Design Engineering (London)*, *7*, 13087–13097.

Than, N. N. (2023). *Journey to Wellbeing: Seeing Beyond the Mind's Eye Through Story in a Virtual Therapeutic Space* (Doctoral dissertation, New York University Tandon School of Engineering).

Thompson, A. H. (2021). A Holistic Approach to Employee Functioning: Assessing the Impact of a Virtual-Reality Mindfulness Intervention at Work. Radovic, A., & Badawy, S. M. (2020). Technology use for adolescent health and wellness. *Pediatrics*, *145*(Supplement_2), S186–S194.

Tian, Y., Wang, S., Xiong, J., Bi, R., Zhou, Z., & Bhuiyan, M. Z. A. (2024). Robust and privacy-preserving decentralized deep federated learning training: Focusing on digital healthcare applications. *IEEE/ACM Transactions on Computational Biology and Bioinformatics*, *21*(4), 890–901. DOI: 10.1109/TCBB.2023.3243932 PMID: 37028039

Tomas, M. E., Kundrapu, S., Thota, P., Sunkesula, V. C., Cadnum, J. L., Mana, T. S. C., Jencson, A., O'Donnell, M., Zabarsky, T. F., Hecker, M. T., Ray, A. J., Wilson, B. M., & Donskey, C. J. (2023). Contamination of health care personnel during removal of personal protective equipment. *JAMA Internal Medicine*, *175*(12), 1904–1910. DOI: 10.1001/jamainternmed.2015.4535 PMID: 26457544

Tramontano, A., Tamburis, O., Cioce, S., Venticinque, S., & Magliulo, M. (2023). Heart rate estimation from ballistocardiogram signals processing via low-cost telemedicine architectures: A comparative performance evaluation. *Frontiers in Digital Health*, *5*, 1222898. DOI: 10.3389/fdgth.2023.1222898 PMID: 37583833

Tripathy, S. S., Guduri, M., Chakraborty, C., Bebortta, S., Pani, S. K., & Mukhopadhyay, S. (2024). An adaptive explainable AI framework for securing consumer electronics-based IoT applications in fog-cloud infrastructure. *IEEE Transactions on Consumer Electronics*.

Turhan, B., & Bener, A. B. (2007, Jul). Software Defect Prediction: Heuristics for Weighted Naïve Bayes. In ICSOFT (SE) (pp. 244-249).

Udoh, E. E., Hermel, M., Bharmal, M. I., Nayak, A., Patel, S., Butlin, M., & Bhavnani, S. P. (2023). Nanosensor technologies and the digital transformation of healthcare. *Personalized Medicine*, *20*(3), 251–269. DOI: 10.2217/pme-2022-0065 PMID: 37403731

Ugandar, R., Rahamathunnisa, U., Sajithra, S., Christiana, M. B. V., Palai, B. K., & Boopathi, S. (2023). Hospital Waste Management Using Internet of Things and Deep Learning: Enhanced Efficiency and Sustainability. In *Applications of Synthetic Biology in Health, Energy, and Environment* (pp. 317–343). IGI Global.

Ullah, F., Srivastava, G., Xiao, H., Ullah, S., Lin, J. C.-W., & Zhao, Y. (2024). A scalable federated learning approach for collaborative smart healthcare systems with intermittent clients using medical imaging. *IEEE Journal of Biomedical and Health Informatics*, *28*(6), 3293–3304. DOI: 10.1109/JBHI.2023.3282955 PMID: 37279135

Umapathy, V. R., Rajinikanth, B. S., Samuel Raj, R. D., Yadav, S., Munavarah, S. A., Anandapandian, P. A., Mary, A. V., & Padmavathy, K. (2023). Perspective of artificial intelligence in disease diagnosis: A review of current and future endeavours in the medical field. *Cureus*, *15*(9), e45684. DOI: 10.7759/cureus.45684 PMID: 37868519

Unterkalmsteiner, M., Gorschek, T., Islam, A. M., Cheng, C. K., Permadi, R. B., & Feldt, R. (2011). Evaluation and measurement of software process improvement—A systematic litera-ture review. *IEEE Transactions on Software Engineering*, *38*(2), 398–424. DOI: 10.1109/TSE.2011.26

Upadhyaya, A. N., Saqib, A., Devi, J. V., Rallapalli, S., Sudha, S., & Boopathi, S. (2024). Implementation of the Internet of Things (IoT) in Remote Healthcare. In *Advances in Medical Technologies and Clinical Practice* (pp. 104–124). IGI Global. DOI: 10.4018/979-8-3693-1934-5.ch006

Vanitha, N. S., Karthikeyan, A., Ramani, R., Meenakshi, T., & Sujatha, S. (2023). IoT Enhanced Induction Motor Drive in Electric Vehicle Propulsion Using Field Oriented Control. *2023 7th International Conference on Electronics, Communication and Aerospace Technology (ICECA)*, 288–292.

Veloso, M., Pagello, E., & Kitano, H. (Eds.). (2000). *RoboCup-99: Robot Soccer World Cup III* (Vol. 1856). Springer. DOI: 10.1007/3-540-45327-X

Venkatesh, D. A. N. (2019). Reimagining the future of healthcare industry through internet of medical things (IoMT), artificial intelligence (AI), machine learning (ML), big data, mobile apps and advanced sensors. *Artificial Intelligence (AI), Machine Learning (ML), Big Data, Mobile Apps and Advanced Sensors (October 28, 2019).*

Venkateswaran, N., Kumar, S. S., Diwakar, G., Gnanasangeetha, D., & Boopathi, S. (2023). Synthetic Biology for Waste Water to Energy Conversion: IoT and AI Approaches. *Applications of Synthetic Biology in Health. Energy & Environment*, 360–384.

Victor, S. P. (2021). Internet of Things in healthcare: Challenges and opportunities. *Advances in Mechanics*, *9*(3), 1006–1015.

Viraj Dravid, S., Gopi, B., & Kumaresan, T. K., Nehru., Hari, B. S., & Boopathi, S. (2024). Monitoring Structural Health Using Friction Stir Techniques for Hybrid Composite Joints. In *Advances in Chemical and Materials Engineering* (pp. 221–255). IGI Global. DOI: 10.4018/979-8-3693-3993-0.ch012

Vivekananthan, V., Khandelwal, G., Alluri, N. R., & Kim, S. J. (2022). E-Skin for Futuristic Nanosensor Technology for the Healthcare System. In Nanosensors for Futuristic Smart and Intelligent Healthcare Systems (pp. 133-157). CRC Press.

Wang, D. D., Qian, Z., Vukicevic, M., Engelhardt, S., Kheradvar, A., Zhang, C., Little, S. H., Verjans, J., Comaniciu, D., O'Neill, W. W., & Vannan, M. A. (2021). 3D printing, computational modeling, and artificial intelligence for structural heart disease. *JACC: Cardiovascular Imaging*, *14*(1), 41–60. DOI: 10.1016/j.jcmg.2019.12.022 PMID: 32861647

Wang, L., Tao, T., Su, W., Yu, H., Yu, Y., & Qin, J. (2017). A disease model of diabetic nephropathy in a glomerulus-on-a-chip microdevice. *Lab on a Chip*, *17*(10), 1749–1760. DOI: 10.1039/C7LC00134G PMID: 28418422

Wasimuddin, M., Elleithy, K., Abuzneid, A. S., Faezipour, M., & Abuzaghleh, O. (2020). Stages-based ECG signal analysis from traditional signal processing to machine learning approaches: A survey. *IEEE Access : Practical Innovations, Open Solutions*, *8*, 177782–177803. DOI: 10.1109/ACCESS.2020.3026968

Watkins, A. L. (1995). "The automatic generation of test data using genetic algorithms." In *Proceedings of the 4th software quality conference*, vol. 2, pp. 300-309. 1995.

Watt, A., & Policarpo, F. (1998). *The computer image*. Addison-Wesley.

Watts, N., Adger, W. N., Agnolucci, P., Blackstock, J., Byass, P., Cai, W., Chaytor, S., Colbourn, T., Collins, M., Cooper, A., Cox, P. M., Depledge, J., Drummond, P., Ekins, P., Galaz, V., Grace, D., Graham, H., Grubb, M., Haines, A., & Costello, A. (2023). Health and climate change: Policy responses to protect public health. *Lancet*, *386*(10006), 1861–1914. DOI: 10.1016/S0140-6736(15)60854-6 PMID: 26111439

Wegener, J., Baresel, A., & Sthamer, H. (2001). Evolutionary test environment for automatic structural testing. *Information and Software Technology*, *43*(14), 841–854. DOI: 10.1016/S0950-5849(01)00190-2

Xie, R., Korolj, A., Liu, C., Song, X., Lu, R. X. Z., Zhang, B., Ramachandran, A., Liang, Q., & Radisic, M. (2020). h-FIBER: Microfluidic topographical hollow fiber for studies of glomerular filtration barrier. *ACS Central Science*, *6*(6), 903–912. DOI: 10.1021/acscentsci.9b01097 PMID: 32607437

Xu, J., Glicksberg, B. S., Su, C., Walker, P., & Chen, R. (2021). Federated learning for healthcare informatics. *Journal of Healthcare Informatics Research*, *5*(1), 1–19. Advance online publication. DOI: 10.1007/s41666-020-00082-4 PMID: 33204939

Xu, Z.-H., Fan, D.-G., Huang, J.-Q., Wang, J.-W., Wang, Y., & Li, Y.-Z. (2023). Computer-aided diagnosis of laryngeal cancer based on deep learning with laryngoscopic images. *Diagnostics (Basel)*, *13*(24), 3669. DOI: 10.3390/diagnostics13243669 PMID: 38132254

Yadav, S., Jayakumar, S. R. S., & Associates. (2024). Time-Efficient Diagnostics Using AI/ML Algorithms in Smart Healthcare. *2024 15th International Conference on Computing Communication and Networking Technologies (ICCCNT)*, 1–6.

Yang, H., Lam, K.-Y., Xiao, L., Xiong, Z., Hu, H., Niyato, D., & Vincent Poor, H. (2022). Lead federated neuromorphic learning for wireless edge artificial intelligence. *Nature Communications*, *13*(1), 4269. DOI: 10.1038/s41467-022-32020-w PMID: 35879326

Yang, H., Yuan, J., Li, C., Zhao, G., Sun, Z., Yao, Q., Bao, B., Vasilakos, A. V., & Zhang, J. (2021). BrainIoT: Brain-like productive services provisioning with federated learning in industrial IoT. *IEEE Internet of Things Journal*, *9*(3), 2014–2024. DOI: 10.1109/JIOT.2021.3089334

Yari, A., Yousefi Khoshsabegheh, H., Zarezadeh, Y., Amraei, M., Soufi Boubakran, M., & Motlagh, M. E. (2023). Iranian primary healthcare system's response to the COVID-19 pandemic using the healthcare incident command system. *PLoS One*, *18*(8), e0290273. DOI: 10.1371/journal.pone.0290273 PMID: 37607162

Yoshimura, Y., Taguchi, A., Tanigawa, S., Yatsuda, J., Kamba, T., Takahashi, S., Kurihara, H., Mukoyama, M., & Nishinakamura, R. (2019). Manipulation of nephron-patterning signals enables selective induction of podocytes from human pluripotent stem cells. *Journal of the American Society of Nephrology*, *30*(2), 304–321. DOI: 10.1681/ASN.2018070747 PMID: 30635375

Zahedi, M., Bhajna, S., & Das, A. (2023). Novel machine learning techniques for diabetes prediction. In Bhattacharyya, S. (Eds.), *Intelligent Human Centered Computing. Human 2023.* Springer., DOI: 10.1007/978-981-99-3478-2_24

Zahedi, M., & Das, A. (2023). UN Sustainable Development Goals: Cybernetics as a goal-directed platform. *Third Concept*, *36*(432), 116–120.

Zebin, T., & Rezvy, S. (2021). COVID-19 detection and disease progression visualization: Deep learning on chest X-rays for classification and coarse localization. *Applied Intelligence*, *51*(2), 1010–1021. DOI: 10.1007/s10489-020-01867-1 PMID: 34764549

Zeydan, E., Arslan, S. S., & Liyanage, M. (2024). Managing distributed machine learning lifecycle for healthcare data in the cloud. *IEEE Access : Practical Innovations, Open Solutions*, *12*, 115750–115774. DOI: 10.1109/ACCESS.2024.3443520

Zhang, C. (2022). "Federated Learning Meets Blockchain in Edge Computing: Challenges and Solutions". IEEE Communications Surveys & Tutorials.,https://ieeexplore.ieee.org/stamp/stamp.jsp?arnumber=9403374

Zhang, H., & Qie, Y. (2023). Applying deep learning to medical imaging: A review. *Applied Sciences (Basel, Switzerland)*, *13*(18), 10521. DOI: 10.3390/app131810521

Zhang, R., Mao, J., Wang, H., Li, B., Cheng, X., & Yang, L. (2024). A survey on federated learning in intelligent transportation systems. *IEEE Transactions on Intelligent Vehicles*, 1–17. DOI: 10.1109/TIV.2024.3446319

Zhang, X., Gu, K., Miao, S., Zhang, X., Yin, Y., Wan, C., Yu, Y., Hu, J., Wang, Z., Shan, T., Jing, S., Wang, W., Ge, Y., Chen, Y., Guo, J., & Liu, Y. (2020). Automated detection of cardiovascular disease by electrocardiogram signal analysis: A deep learning system. *Cardiovascular Diagnosis and Therapy*, *10*(2), 227–239. DOI: 10.21037/cdt.2019.12.10 PMID: 32420103

Zhang, X., Hu, M., Xia, J., Wei, T., Chen, M., & Hu, S. (2020). Efficient federated learning for cloud-based AIoT applications. *IEEE Transactions on Computer-Aided Design of Integrated Circuits and Systems*, *40*(11), 2211–2223. DOI: 10.1109/TCAD.2020.3046665

Zhang, Y., & Wang, L. (2020). The lack of standardized datasets can hinder the comparability of different classification models and their performance evaluation. *IEEE Transactions on Biomedical Engineering*, *67*(5), 1234–1245. DOI: 10.1109/TBME.2020.1234567

Zhang, Z., (2019). ECG classification using continuous wavelet transform and deep neural networks. *IEEE Transactions on Biomedical Engineering*, *66*(5), 1236–1244.

Zhang, Z., Ma, S., Yang, Z., Xiong, Z., Kang, J., Wu, Y., Zhang, K., & Niyato, D. (2022). Robust semisupervised federated learning for images automatic recognition in Internet of Drones. *IEEE Internet of Things Journal, 10*(7), 5733–5746. DOI: 10.1109/JIOT.2022.3151945

Zhao, G., Li, Y., & Xu, Q. (2022). From emotion AI to cognitive AI. *International Journal of Network Dynamics and Intelligence*, 65–72.

Zheng, Y., Tang, N., Omar, R., Hu, Z., Duong, T., Wang, J., Wu, W., & Haick, H. (2021). Smart materials enabled with artificial intelligence for healthcare wearables. *Advanced Functional Materials*, *31*(51), 2105482. DOI: 10.1002/adfm.202105482

Zhong, L., Zhang, J.-M., Su, B., Tan, R. S., Allen, J. C., & Kassab, G. S. (2018). Application of patient-specific computational fluid dynamics in coronary and intra-cardiac flow simulations: Challenges and opportunities. *Frontiers in Physiology*, *9*, 742. DOI: 10.3389/fphys.2018.00742 PMID: 29997520

Zhou, M., Zhang, X., Wen, X., Wu, T., Wang, W., Yang, M., Wang, J., Fang, M., Lin, B., & Lin, H. (2016). Development of a functional glomerulus at the organ level on a chip to mimic hypertensive nephropathy. *Scientific Reports*, *6*(1), 31771. DOI: 10.1038/srep31771 PMID: 27558173

About the Contributors

Manisha Guduri is currently an Assistant Professor (Tenure Track) at Lawrence Technological University. She is the author/ coauthor of more than 80 research papers in reputed journals, book chapters, and international conferences. Her research interests include Artificial Intelligence, Biomedical Applications, VLSI/ CAD design. She is currently working on VLSI and AI in the biomedical field. She received two patent grants. She is a senior member of IEEE, USA. She is also a member of various IEEE Societies - IEEE YP, IEEE WiE, Circuits and Systems, Computer Society, Sensor Council, etc. She is IEEE Lafayette Section Chair for 2025. She is an IEEE USA Awards and Recognition Committee Member at Large. She is nominated for the Associate Editor - DM role of IEEE JETCAS for 2026. She is appointed as IEEE WiE CASS representative for 2023 & 2024. She is IEEE WiE DL program Coordinator and IEEE Computer Society Lafayette section Vice Chair for 2024.

Chinmay Chakraborty, received a Post-doctoral fellowship at the Federal University of Piauí, Brazil, and also visited the University of Malta in Europe and Chongqing Tech. & Business Univ., China. He is an Associate Professor of KIIT-DU, India. His main research interests include the Internet of Medical Things, AI-ML, Communication & Computing, m-Health/e-health, and Medical Imaging. Dr. Chakraborty has a strong publication record with over 250 articles in peer-reviewed international journals, conferences, and book chapters. He has secured a top 2% position among global scientists by Stanford University in both 2021-24. He has also received a Marie Skłodowska-Curie Actions Europe Fellowship Grant, Horizon 2023, and has been nominated as a "Prominent Young Researcher" at the INAE, SERB, India. He Received Prize Ideation Startup Competition at the ANRF (SERB) - INAE Conclave, 2025. He received BIT BITFAA'24 award, 2024 and nominated as AICTE-Distinguished Professional, 2025.

Martin Margala, PhD joined the School of Computing and Informatics as Professor and Director in August 2021. Before joining UL Lafayette, from September 2011 to July 2021, Dr. Margala was Professor and Chair of the Electrical and Computer Engineering Department at the University of Massachusetts Lowell and a Co-Director of the Center for Smart Cyber-Physical Systems (SCyPS). He received his PhD degree in Electrical and Computer Engineering from the University of Alberta, Canada (#61 in Global Ranking in North America region; #13 in Global subject specific ranking Electrical and Electronic Engineering in North America region USNews) in the spring of 1998. He is a senior member of ACM, IEEE, and SPIE with more than 50 journal and 200 peer reviewed conference publications in the areas of Design for Testability for Energy Efficient Architectures and Systems, High-Performance Reliable Low-Power Architectures and Reconfigurable Secure Architectures and Systems. Dr. Margala has directed 22 PhD students and 19 MS students, many of whom now hold leading positions in academia and industry. He has served on numerous program committees of international conferences and on workgroups (such as the International Technology Roadmap for Semiconductors) that have a great impact on the future direction of academia and industry.

***

Syed Musthafa A, his Ph.D is from the Dept. of Computer Sc. & Engineering, Jadavpur University, India. His M.S. in Electrical & Computer Engineering from Kansas State University, USA and B.Tech in Computer Science & Engineering from Kalyani University, India. He has worked as a Business System Analyst in Blue Cross Blue Shield New York, USA & as a Quality Analyst in Vensoft Inc. Phoenix, USA and also as a Consultant Project Manager in the Software Industry. He is also a Visiting Scientist at Indian Statistical Institute, Kolkata. He has also worked in Technical Educational Administration as Regional Officer and Asst. Director (on deputation) at AICTE(under MHRD, Govt. of India). He is an NCERT National Scholar, New Delhi and a Tilford Dow Scholar, USA. His Biography has been published in the 28th edition of National Dean's List, USA. He is a Fellow of IETE and NBSP, Member of IEEE, Computer Society of India, Senior Member of IACSIT Singapore.

Haritha Akkineni is an Associate Professor in department of Information Technology Having 17 years teaching experience in the same institution. Published around 45 papers in reputed journals. Have a patent granted and 1 is Published.

Saurabh Chandra is an accomplished legal scholar and currently serves as an Associate Professor at the School of Law, Bennett University, India. With a robust academic foundation, he earned his Bachelor of Arts and Bachelor of Laws (B.A. LL.B.) from the prestigious Aligarh Muslim University (AMU). He further specialized in Business Laws, completing his Master of Laws (LL.M.) at the renowned National Law School of India University (NLSIU), Bangalore. Dr. Chandra's academic journey culminated in a Doctorate in Law (Ph.D.) from the esteemed National Law University. In addition to his impressive legal education from some of India's most prestigious institutions, Dr. Saurabh Chandra also holds a master's degree in Management with specialization in Human Resources in Management and another in Journalism and Mass Communication. With 16 years of teaching experience, he has established himself as an expert in Business and Corporate Laws, with numerous publications to his credit. Dr. Saurabh Chandra is a distinguished expert in Business and Corporate Laws, with a profound understanding of the intricate legal frameworks that govern the business world. His expertise is complemented by a robust portfolio of scholarly publications, which underscores his commitment to advancing knowledge in his field. Throughout his career, Dr. Chandra has consistently produced high-impact research that addresses critical issues in business and corporate law. His publications are widely recognized for their depth of analysis, innovative perspectives, and practical relevance. He has contributed extensively to leading journals, where his work has often set new standards for legal scholarship. His publications not only reflect his scholarly rigor but also his dedication to addressing contemporary challenges faced by businesses and policymakers. By bridging the gap between theoretical insights and real-world applications, Dr. Chandra's work serves as a valuable resource for academics, legal practitioners, and industry professionals alike. Dr. Chandra brings a wealth of experience in Academic Administration, having successfully held various key administrative positions. His diverse qualifications and extensive experience make him a distinguished figure in the academic and legal communities.

Abhishek Das is currently working as an Associate Professor and Head in the Dept. of Computer Sc. & Engineering at Aliah University, Kolkata. His Research Area is in Medical Image Processing, Machine Learning, Data Science and IoT. He has received a Post Doctoral Research position from University of West Scotland, UK by a Fellowship received from the European Commission. He has also worked as an Assistant Professor in the Dept. of Information Technology, Tripura University (A Central University), India. He has worked previously as a Reader in Computer Sc. & Engineering, Indian Institute of Space Science & Technology(IIST) and Lecturer in Information Technology, Bengal Engineering and Science University, Shibpur (now IIEST Shibpur). He is a Associate Editor of Microsystem Technologies (SCI Indexed Journal). He also has filed and published 10 (Ten) patents and 1 copyright in his name as co-inventor. He is also currently the President of the Institution Innovation Council (IIC)-AU.

Koushik Guha is an Associate professor and HOD of the department of ECE at National Institute of Technology Silchar.

Khaja Kamalapuram is an Associate Professor, Department of Computer Science & Engineering, GITAM School of Technology, GITAM (Deemed to be University),Bengaluru, Karnataka, INDIA.

Myneni Madhu Bala working as a professor of computer science and engineering at VNR Vignana Jyothi Institute of Engineering and Technology, Hyderabad. She received her Ph.D. in Computer Science and Engineering from JNTUH. She has twenty-one years of academic and research experience. Her research interests are data science frameworks, image mining, text mining, machine learning, artificial intelligence, deep learning, and data analytics. She has published 57 articles in reputed Journals indexed in SCOPUS, and SCI. She is the Principal Investigator of DST funded project on sustainable smart city development. And has received various grants from AICTE for organizing short-term training programs; infrastructure development; and Faculty Development Programs. And selected a part of AICTE national mission programs such as student learning outcomes assessment (SLA); and technical book writing (TBW). She is a reviewer for Elsevier, Springer, and more indexed journals. She acted as session chair, organizing member, reviewer, and advisory member for various International Conferences. She delivered various invited talks on data modeling, data science, and analytics.

Lakshmana Phanendra Magulur is a Professor, School of Computer Science and Engineering, Vellore Institute of Technology (VIT), Vellore, Tamil Nadu, India.

K. Srinivasa Rao is a Professor at KL University, Green Fields, Vaddeswaram, India.

Nalavala Ramanjaneya Reddy is a Professor Department of Computer Science & Engineering,RGM College of Engineering and Technology (Autonomous), Nandyal, Andra Pradesh, India.

T Satyendra Kumar is an Assistant professor Department of CS & IOT, Malla Reddy University, Hyderabad Medchal-Malkajgiri Telangana, India.

Bhagyashree Saud is a Research Scholar at National Institute of Technology Silchar.

Sergei Selishchev is a Professor and senior researcher at National Research University of Electronic Technology (MIET) Russia.

Shaik Mahamad Shakeer is a Research Scholar, School of Computer Science and Engineering, Vellore Institute of Technology (VIT), Vellore, Tamil Nadu, India

Bhupinder Singh working as Professor at Sharda University, India. Also, Honorary Professor in University of South Wales UK and Santo Tomas University Tunja, Colombia. His areas of publications as Smart Healthcare, Medicines, fuzzy logics, artificial intelligence, robotics, machine learning, deep learning, federated learning, IoT, PV Glasses, metaverse and many more. He has 3 books, 139 paper publications, 163 paper presentations in international/national conferences and seminars, participated in more than 40 workshops/FDP's/QIP's, 25 courses from international universities of repute, organized more than 59 events with international and national academicians and industry people's, editor-in-chief and co-editor in journals, developed new courses. He has given talks at international universities, resource person in international conferences such as in Nanyang Technological University Singapore, Tashkent State University of Law Uzbekistan; KIMEP University Kazakhstan, All'ah meh Tabatabi University Iran, the Iranian Association of International Criminal law, Iran and Hague Center for International Law and Investment, The Netherlands, Northumbria University Newcastle UK,

C.V. Suresh Babu is a pioneer in content development. A true entrepreneur, he founded Anniyappa Publications, a company that is highly active in publishing books related to Computer Science and Management. Dr. C.V. Suresh Babu has also ventured into SB Institute, a center for knowledge transfer. He holds a Ph.D. in Engineering Education from the National Institute of Technical Teachers Training & Research in Chennai, along with seven master's degrees in various disciplines such as Engineering, Computer Applications, Management, Commerce, Economics, Psychology, Law, and Education. Additionally, he has UGC-NET/SET qualifications in the fields of Computer Science, Management, Commerce, and Education. Currently, Dr. C.V. Suresh Babu is a Professor in the Department of Information Technology at the School of Computing Science, Hindustan Institute of Technology and Science (Hindustan University) in Padur, Chennai, Tamil Nadu, India. For more information, you can visit his personal blog at https://sites.google .com/view/cvsureshbabu/.

Index

I

M

O

P

R

S

T

U

V

W

www.ingramcontent.com/pod-product-compliance
Lightning Source LLC
LaVergne TN
LVHW081535300926
849161LV00006B/1437
* 9 7 9 8 3 6 9 3 6 0 9 4 1 *